The
Cardiorenal
Syndrome

The
Cardiorenal Syndrome

A Clinician's Guide to Pathophysiology and Management

editors

J. Thomas Heywood MD

Director, Heart Failure Recovery & Research Program,
Scripps Clinic, La Jolla, California; Clinical Professor of Medicine,
Loma Linda University Medical Center, Loma Linda, California

John C. Burnett Jr. MD

Marriott Family Professor of Cardiovascular Research,
Mayo Clinic College of Medicine;
Mayo Heart and Lung Research Center Director,
Mayo Clinic, Rochester, Minnesota

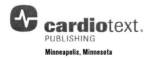

cardiotext.
PUBLISHING
Minneapolis, Minnesota

Cardiotext Publishing, LLC
3405 W. 44th Street
Minneapolis, Minnesota 55410
USA
www.cardiotextpublishing.com

Any updates to this book may be found at:
www.cardiotextpublishing.com/titles/detail/9780979016479

Comments, inquiries, and requests for bulk sales can be directed to the publisher at:
info@cardiotextpublishing.com.

Cover art: Heart, Alfred Pasieka / Photo Researchers, Inc.
           Kidney, SPL/Photo Researchers, Inc.

Unless otherwise stated, all figures and tables in this book are used courtesy of the authors.

Cover design by Beth Wright, Trio Bookworks
Book design by Ann Delgehausen, Trio Bookworks

Library of Congress Control Number: 2011940468

ISBN: 978-0-9790164-7-9

Printed in the U.S.A.

16   15   14   13   12   11   1   2   3   4   5   6   7   8   9   10

This book would not have happened
without the myriad of individual patients
who teach me about medicine and life every single day.
Daily I learn, and my heart is touched by their complexity
and courage. In the final accounting, though,
it is not where you go in the morning that is most important
but those who welcome you at the end of the day.
Therefore, this book is dedicated to my dear wife, Stephanie,
and my wonderful daughters, Kazia, Magda, and Jana.

—J. Thomas Heywood

Contents

Contributors

editors

J. Thomas Heywood MD
Director, Heart Failure Recovery & Research Program, Scripps Clinic, La Jolla, California; Clinical Professor of Medicine, Loma Linda University Medical Center, Loma Linda, California

John C. Burnett Jr. MD
Marriott Family Professor of Cardiovascular Research, Mayo Clinic College of Medicine; Mayo Heart and Lung Research Center Director, Mayo Clinic, Rochester, Minnesota

contributors

Piergiuseppe Agostoni MD, PhD
Associated Professor of Cardiology, Centro Cardiologico Monzino, IRCCS, Department of Cardiovascular Sciences, University of Milan, Milan, Italy; Department of Critical Care and Respiratory Medicine, University of Washington, Seattle, Washington

Luis R. Alvarez-Contreras MD
Interventional Cardiology Fellow, Instituto Clinic del Tórax, Hospital Clínic de Barcelona, Universidad de Barcelona, Barcelona, Spain

Shweta Bansal MD
Assistant Professor, Department of Medicine, Division of Nephrology, University of Texas Health Sciences Center, San Antonio, Texas

Kalkidan G. Bishu MD
Cardiovascular Fellow, Cardiorenal Research Laboratory, Mayo Clinic, Rochester, Minnesota

John Blair MD
Assistant Professor, Uniformed Services University for Health Sciences, Wilford Hall
Medical Center, Department of Cardiology, Lackland Air Force Base, Texas

Jeremy S. Bock MD
Fellow in Cardiovascular Disease, Division of Cardiology, Department of Medicine,
University of Maryland School of Medicine, Baltimore, Maryland

Maria Rosa Costanzo MD, FACC, FAHA
Medical Director, Midwest Heart Specialists Heart Failure and Pulmonary Arterial
Hypertension Programs; Medical Director, Edward Hospital Center for Advanced Heart
Failure, Naperville, Illinois

Uri Elkayam MD, FACC
Professor of Medicine, Division of Cardiology, Department of Medicine,
University of Southern California, Keck School of Medicine, Los Angeles County,
University of Southern California Medical Center, Los Angeles, California

Gary S. Francis MD
Professor of Medicine, Cardiovascular Division, University of Minnesota,
Minneapolis, Minnesota

Mihai Gheorghiade MD
Professor of Medicine and Surgery, Director of Experimental Therapeutics,
Center for Cardiovascular Innovation, Northwestern University Feinberg School
of Medicine, Chicago, Illinois

Stephen S. Gottlieb MD
Professor of Medicine; Director, Cardiomyopathy and Pulmonary Hypertension;
Director, Clinical Research Program in Cardiology, Department of Medicine,
Division of Cardiology, University of Maryland, Baltimore, Maryland

Gretchen Hageman BSBME
Biomedical Engineer, Innovative BioTherapies, Inc., Ann Arbor, Michigan

H. David Humes MD
Professor of Internal Medicine (Nephrology), University of Michigan,
Ann Arbor, Michigan

Brian E. Jaski MD, FACC
Medical Director, Advanced Heart Failure and Cardiac Transplant Program,
Sharp Memorial Hospital, San Diego Cardiac Center, San Diego, California

Mariell Jessup MD
Professor of Medicine, University of Pennsylvania School of Medicine, Philadelphia, Pennsylvania; Associate Chief–Clinical Affairs, Division of Cardiovascular Medicine, Medical Director, Heart and Vascular Center, Penn Medicine, Philadelphia, Pennsylvania

Mrunalini A. Joshi MS
Division of Heart Valve Therapy, Edwards Lifesciences, Irvine, California

Richard E. Katholi MD
Clinical Professor of Pharmacology and Medicine, Southern Illinois University School of Medicine, Springfield, Illnois

Tariq A. Khan MD
Clinical Assistant Professor, Department of Medicine, Eastern Kansas VA Health Care System affiliated with University of Kansas, Leavenworth, Kansas

Nudrat Khatri MBBS
Research Associate, Division of Cardiovascular Medicine, Keck School of Medicine, University of Southern California, Los Angeles, California

Andrew J. King MD
Head, Division of Nephrology, Scripps Clinic and Green Hospital, San Diego, California; Clinical Professor of Medicine, UCSD School of Medicine, La Jolla, California

Henry Krum MBBS, PhD, FRACP, FESC
Director, CCRE Therapeutics, Monash University, Melbourne, Australia

Tong Liu MD
Department of Cardiology, Capital Medical University Affiliated Beijing Anzhen Hospital, Beijing Institute of Heart, Lung and Blood Vessel Disease, Beijing, China

Giancarlo Marenzi MD, FESC
Centro Cardiologico Monzino, IRCCS, Department of Cardiovascular Sciences, University of Milan, Milan, Italy

Fernando L. Martin MD
Department of Cardiovascular Diseases, Division of Internal Medicine, Mayo Clinic, Rochester, Minnesota

Paul M. McKie MD
Cardiorenal Research Laboratory, Division of Cardiology, Mayo Clinic, Rochester, Minnesota

Tien M. H. Ng PharmD, FCCP, BCPS
Associate Professor of Clinical Pharmacy, University of Southern California,
School of Pharmacy, Los Angeles, California

Peter S. Pang MD, FACEP, FAAEM
Associate Chief, Associate Professor of Emergency Medicine, Associate Director
of Experimental Therapeutics/Center for Cardiovascular Innovation, Associate Professor
of Medicine, Northwestern University Feinberg School of Medicine, Chicago, Illinois

Jigar Patel DO
Division of Cardiovascular Diseases, Scripps Clinic and Scripps Green Hospital,
La Jolla, California

Margaret M. Redfield MD
Professor of Medicine, Division of Cardiovascular Diseases, Department of Internal
Medicine, Mayo Clinic, Rochester, Minnesota

Claudio Ronco MD
Head of Department of Nephrology, Dialysis and Renal Transplant, Director of
International Renal Research Institute of Vicenza (IRRIV), San Bortolo Hospital,
Vicenza, Italy

Markus P. Schlaich MD
Associate Professor of Medicine; Head, Neurovascular Hypertension & Kidney Disease,
Baker IDI Heart & Diabetes Institute, Melbourne, Australia

Robert W. Schrier MD, MACP
Professor of Medicine, Department of Medicine, Division of Renal Diseases and
Hypertension, University of Colorado School of Medicine, Aurora, Colorado

Domenic A. Sica MD
Professor of Medicine and Pharmacology; Chairman, Section of Clinical Pharmacology
and Hypertension, Division of Nephrology, Virginia Commonwealth University Health
System, Richmond, Virginia

Paul A. Sobotka MD, FACP, FACC
Professor of Medicine, Division of Cardiology, Clinical, The Ohio State University,
Columbus, Ohio; Medical Advisor, Medtronic Inc.

W. H. Wilson Tang MD, FACC, FAHA
Associate Professor of Medicine, Cleveland Clinic Lerner College of Medicine
at Case Western Reserve University, Cleveland, Ohio

Abbreviations

ACE	angiotensin-converting enzyme	CI	confidence interval
ACEI	ACE inhibitor	CKD	chronic kidney disease
ACTH	adrenocorticotropic hormone	CNP	C-type natriuretic peptide
ADHF	acute decompensated heart failure	CNS	central nervous system
		CO	cardiac output
ADP	antidiuretic hormone	CrCl	creatinine clearance
AGE	advanced glycation end-product	CRP	C-reactive protein
AKI	acute kidney injury	CVD	cardiovascular disease
AMI	acute myocardial infarction	CVP	central venous pressure
ANP	atrial natriuretic peptide	DNP	*Dendroaspis* natriuretic peptide
AR	adenosine receptor	DRI	direct renin inhibitor
ARB	angiotensin receptor blocker	ECFV	extracellular fluid volume
ATP	adenosine triphosphate	EDPVR	end-diastolic pressure-volume relationship
AUC	area under the curve		
AVP	arginine vasopressin	EF	ejection fraction
BMI	body mass index	ERPF	effective renal plasma flow
BNP	brain natriuretic peptide	ESRD	end-stage renal disease
BUN	blood urea nitrogen	FDA	Food and Drug Administration
CABG	coronary artery bypass grafting	GC	guanylyl cyclase
cAMP	cyclic adenosine monophosphate	GFR	glomerular filtration rate
cGMP	cyclic guanosine monophosphate	HR	hazard ratio
		JVD	jugular venous distention
CHF	congestive heart failure	LOH	loop of Henle

LV	left ventricular	PRA	plasma renin activity
LVAD	left ventricular assist device	PRR	plasma refill rate
LVEF	left ventricular ejection fraction	PTCA	percutaneous transluminal
LVOT	left ventricular outflow tract		coronary angioplasty
MAP	mean arterial pressure	RAAS	renin-angiotensin-aldosterone
MI	myocardial infarction		system
MOF	multiorgan failure	RAD	renal assist device
MSNA	muscle sympathetic	RAP	right arterial pressure
	nerve activity	RBF	renal blood flow
NGAL	neutrophil gelatinase–regulated	RI	renal insufficiency
	lipocalin	RPF	renal plasma flow
NO	nitric oxide	RV	right ventricular
NP	natriuretic peptide	RVG	radionuclide ventriculography
NYHA	New York Heart Association	SNS	sympathetic nervous system
OR	odds ratio	TGF	tubuloglomerular feedback
PCI	percutaneous coronary	TNF-α	tumor necrosis factor–alpha
	intervention	TVI	time velocity integral
PCWP	pulmonary capillary wedge	vWF	von Willebrand factor
	pressure	WRF	worsening renal function

Foreword

Inder Anand MD

Professor of Medicine at the University of Minnesota
Director of the Heart Failure Program at the Minneapolis VA Medical Center

During the last two decades, remarkable advances in the management of heart failure have resulted in considerable improvement in the mortality of patients with this very common disease. Nevertheless, clinical trial and registry data demonstrate that renal dysfunction is becoming increasingly common. The development of renal impairment, particularly in the setting of acute decompensated heart failure, is associated with poor outcomes. The term *cardiorenal syndrome* is often used to describe the renal insufficiency in heart failure, although previously the syndrome has not been well defined and it has been even less well understood. It is not surprising that renal dysfunction is an integral part of heart failure, given that the kidney plays such an important role in salt

The Cardiorenal Syndrome: A Clinician's Guide to Pathophysiology and Management, 1st ed. © 2012
J. Thomas Heywood and John C. Burnett Jr., eds.
Cardiotext Publishing, ISBN: 978-0-9790164-7-9.

and water regulation. The neurohormonal compensatory mechanisms activated in heart failure affect not just the heart but also the kidney in a complex interaction where the function of one organ influences that of the other.

The management of patients with cardiorenal syndrome remains unclear. On the one hand, until recently the focus has been largely on the heart despite the fact that drugs that "improve" cardiac function acutely often come at the cost of reduced survival. On the other, the therapy that is most obviously nephrocentric, namely diuretics, remains to this day the only means by which symptoms are improved most rapidly and effectively. When employed poorly, however, diuretics can worsen renal function and impair the very organ whose function is critical to symptom relief.

It is therefore important that physicians involved in the care of patients with heart failure better understand the definition, epidemiology, pathogenesis, clinical features, and mechanisms underlying various evolving novel therapies for this increasingly common and serious condition: the cardiorenal syndrome. It is equally important that investigators, whether basic or clinical scientists, also understand the relationship between abnormalities at the molecular, cellular, organ, and clinical level.

The publication of *The Cardiorenal Syndrome: A Clinicians' Guide to Pathophysiology and Management* is most timely in fulfilling the need and lacuna in the field. Indeed, it is greatly welcomed. Drs. Heywood and Burnett, both distinguished and highly respected experts in this area, have assembled comprehensive chapters by eminent investigators and clinicians covering all aspects of this perplexing syndrome. Areas of certainty, of controversy, and of future research are addressed. Each chapter is complete in its own right and includes an invaluable up-to-date reference list. Pathophysiology and epidemiology are well covered, providing an excellent basis for the later chapters that describe the essential aspects of the disease from drug and mechanical therapies to transplant of either or both organs. Here, clinicians will readily find what has been learned about the cardiac and renal interactions in heart failure. Dr. Heywood's own chapter provides the clinicians a very useful and practical approach to heart failure patients who present with worsening renal function. Perhaps the most useful lesson from the book is that there are many diverse varieties of this disorder with radically different therapies. For example, worsening renal function can be the result of either too little or too much diuretic. The skill lies in the ability to assess the difference in a particular patient. The authors endeavor to give the reader knowledge for making this key distinction. Left ventricular assist devices can definitively cure renal failure in carefully chosen patients, but they can expensively fail to do so when deployed in the wrong patient.

This book stands as a landmark in the study of the cardiorenal syndrome. It will no doubt be extremely useful to the cardiovascular specialist and internist caring for the growing number of these patients. And it will be just as useful to the scientists and the trainees interested in this condition. The authors are to be congratulated for their success in putting together, with such dexterity and finesse, so much relevant and crucial information on the subject in one volume.

Preface

The last several decades have seen important successes in the effort to treat those suffering from congestive heart failure. Ironically, because heart failure is both so deadly and yet so common, it is particularly well suited for the discovery of new therapies by means of randomized controlled trials. Dating back to the early 1980s, a few key treatments have been identified and vindicated while considerably more procedures and medications have been studied and abandoned. Stable heart failure patients enrolled in clinical trials and benefiting from evidence-based therapy and devices currently have yearly mortalities of 5% or less.[1]

This steady progress can in no way allay the sad reality that heart failure remains a frequent cause for hospital admission and

is the direct cause of 50,000 deaths per year in the United States alone. In the past decade appreciation of the role of worsening renal function both as a risk factor and also as a cause of poor outcomes in congestive heart failure have been increasing. The term *cardiorenal syndrome* has been applied to the concurrence of significant renal and cardiac dysfunction, which portends a marked increase in mortality. In the Acute Decompensated Heart Failure National Registry (ADHERE) study, an elevated BUN (blood urea nitrogen) and creatinine were 2 of the 3 most significant predictors of in-hospital mortality.[2] Of course, it is not surprising that renal dysfunction is an integral part of the syndrome of congestive heart failure given the key role that the kidney plays in fluid and electrolyte balance in mammalian physiology. However, the same clinical trials that so importantly crafted modern therapy for heart failure via neurohormonal blockade and later device implantation at the same

The Cardiorenal Syndrome: A Clinician's Guide to Pathophysiology and Management, 1st ed. © 2012 J. Thomas Heywood and John C. Burnett Jr., eds. Cardiotext Publishing, ISBN: 978-0-9790164-7-9.

time obscured the role of renal dysfunction in the progression of heart failure for the simple reason that patients with significant kidney dysfunction were routinely excluded from these trials.

Recognition of the role of renal dysfunction in the progression of heart failure is a critical advance, but it is only a first step; many questions remain. How to define cardiorenal syndrome: is it a cardiovascular problem (low blood pressure, low cardiac output) or one renal pathophysiology? Is blockade of the renin–angiotensin–aldosterone system useful or detrimental in this syndrome? Is cardiorenal syndrome a medical emergency requiring organ transplantation, or a should hospice be utilized instead? Cardiac function can currently be largely supported by implantation of a left ventricular assist device. In these cases clinicians must make critical decisions about the potential reversibility of renal dysfunction before inserting these costly devices.

Of course there are no single answers to these questions. But that does not mean they are the wrong questions or should not be asked. The first line of Tolstoy's *Anna Karenina* is: "Happy families are all alike, every unhappy family is unhappy in their own way." In the same way each patient with cardiorenal syndrome is unique and often requires very different treatment than the patient who appears tomorrow with the same BUN, creatinine, and ejection fraction.

From this realization, *The Cardiorenal Syndrome: A Clinician's Guide to Pathophysiology and Management* took its genesis. In an era when information technology is changing rapidly,

it still seemed that a book was the best way to collect key information about what is known and not known about this complex and deadly syndrome, that is, What is cardiorenal syndrome clinically, and how should it be defined and recognized? Are there therapies to counteract it and when, and more importantly, for whom should they be applied? The book contains very clinically oriented chapters on the risks and benefits of organ transplantation and assist device implantation in high-risk individuals; there are also intriguing suggestions that new therapies may be added to our armamentarium in the form of designer peptides and stem cell technologies.

At the core of *The Cardiorenal Syndrome: A Clinician's Guide to Pathophysiology and Management* is the realization that for practicing clinicians, an understanding of the syndrome is not an academic exercise. The well-being and at times the lives of people depend on it. Our hope and belief is that wrestling this most dangerous foe and winning a bit more often will reduce suffering and save lives.

References

1. Moss AJ, Hall WJ, Cannom DS, et al. Cardiac-resynchronization therapy for the prevention heart-failure events. *New Eng J Med.* 2009;361:1329–1338.
2. Fonarow GC, Adams KF Jr, Abraham WT, et al. Risk stratification for in-hospital mortality in acutely decompensated heart failure: classification and regression tree analysis. *JAMA.* 2005; 293:572–580.

The Role of the Kidney in Heart Failure

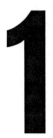

ROBERT W. SCHRIER

SHWETA BANSAL

The Normal Relationship of the Heart and Kidney

Because the kidneys receive 20% of cardiac output, heart and kidney function are interdependent. Changes in volume and pressure in the cardiac atria initiate reflexes that alter renal function. Gauer and colleagues were the first to demonstrate that an increase in left atrial pressure was associated with a water diuresis; this effect was shown to be associated with a suppression of the antidiuretic hormone, arginine vasopressin (AVP). This so-called Henry-Gauer reflex is mediated via the vagus nerve to the central source of AVP synthesis and release in the hypothalamo-neurohypophyseal system. Thus, vagatomy

The Cardiorenal Syndrome: A Clinician's Guide to Pathophysiology and Management, 1st ed. © 2012 J. Thomas Heywood and John C. Burnett Jr., eds. Cardiotext Publishing, ISBN: 978-0-9790164-7-9.

abolishes this atrial-renal reflex.[1] The water diuresis, which has been associated with paroxysmal atrial tachycardia, is probably related to this same reflex.[2] There is also evidence that atrial transmural pressure exerts an effect on renal sympathetic tone. Specifically, an increase in atrial pressure is associated with a decrease in renal sympathetic activity, thereby attenuating any neurally mediated vasoconstriction of the kidney.[3] This atrial-renal reflex would also be expected to dampen any effect of beta-adrenergic stimulation to increase renin release.[4]

Granules had been observed in cardiac atria, but their function was not known. De Bold[5] wondered whether these granules might contain hormones and proceeded to test this hypothesis. He discovered that rats injected with these granules demonstrated a profound increase in urinary sodium and water excretion. This substance was thus named atrial natriuretic peptide (ANP). In addition to the natriuretic effect, ANP was found to exert other properties, including suppression of both the renin-angiotensin-aldosterone system (RAAS) and sympathetic neural activity, as well as being a potent renal and systemic vasodilator. The cardiac ventricles have been found to be the source of another natriuretic peptide termed brain natriuretic peptide (BNP; or B-type natriutretic peptide), since it was first found in the brain. BNP and ANP have similar properties.

The role of BNP to attenuate renal sodium retention secondary to a decrease in systemic arterial pressure was demonstrated by Clavell et al.[6] Mean arterial pressure was lowered to the same level by either decreasing cardiac function or constricting the thoracic vena cava. Atrial pressure rose with the cardiac, but not the caval, maneuver. Thus, plasma BNP increased with hypotension secondary to decreased cardiac function, but not with caval constriction. Renal sodium retention was significantly greater with the caval constriction despite comparable hypotension. To test whether this was due to the difference in plasma BNP concentrations, the caval animals were administered exogenous BNP to mimic the plasma level observed in the cardiac-mediated hypotension. The sodium excretion typically produced by BNP was blunted in these animals while the hypotensive effect persisted.

The Effect of Central Venous Pressure

Increased right-sided cardiac volume and pressure also can exert effects on the kidney. With the atrial-renal reflexes discussed, the kidney responses tend to lower cardiac-filling pressure by increasing sodium and water excretion. However, a rise in central, and thus renal, venous pressure during increased cardiac preload may actually enhance renal sodium and water retention. Experimental studies have shown that an increase in renal

venous pressure is associated with a rise in interstitial pressure, activation of the RAAS, and a fall in glomerular filtration rate (GFR) and renal sodium retention.[7,8]

The Effect of Decreased Cardiac Output

In addition to the atrial-renal reflexes and the effects on renal venous pressure, the heart can also affect the kidney by activating high-pressure arterial baroreceptors.[9-11] Arterial stretch baroreceptors are found in the carotid sinus, aortic arch, and afferent arteriole of the glomerulus. Normally, the vagus and glossopharyngeal afferent pathways from these high-pressure receptors inhibit sympathetic outflow from the central nervous system (CNS). With a decrease in stroke volume or a decline in arterial pressure, this CNS inhibition is removed and an increase in sympathetic efferent outflow as well as nonosmotic AVP release occurs. The increase in sympathetic tone stimulates the RAAS via the renal beta-adrenergic pathway.[4] This neurohumoral stimulation, which results from diminished cardiac function, exerts multiple effects on the kidney. Adrenergic and angiotensin receptors on the proximal tubule epithelium, when stimulated, enhance proximal tubule sodium reabsorption. In addition to these direct effects on sodium balance, the resultant decreased fluid and sodium delivery to the distal nephron also has an effect on urinary sodium excretion. The sodium-retaining effect of aldosterone is only temporary because of the "escape phenomenon." Normally, the expansion of extracellular fluid volume (ECFV) secondary to aldosterone increases GFR, decreases proximal tubule reabsorption, and enhances sodium delivery to the distal nephron, the site of aldosterone activity. This effect, along with the rise in plasma ANP, which occurs with ECFV expansion, overrides the effect of aldosterone to enhance tubular sodium reabsorption and accounts for aldosterone escape. In contrast, the diminished distal sodium delivery that occurs with neurohumoral activation abolishes the normal aldosterone escape, leading to continued aldosterone-mediated renal sodium retention. Micropuncture studies have also shown that a decrease in renal arterial perfusion pressure, as may occur with a decrease in cardiac output, causes enhanced proximal tubule sodium reabsorption.[8]

As with aldosterone, the site of action of natriuretic peptides is also in the distal nephron—namely the collecting duct. Thus, the natriuretic response of these peptides is also dependent on distal sodium delivery, and the resistance to the natriuretic response of ANP and BNP in cardiac failure appears to be secondary to the neurohumoral-mediated diminished sodium delivery to the collecting duct site of their action.

There are numerous pathways, therefore, whereby the heart can affect the function of the normal kidney. In fact, when this occurs, either acutely or chronically, the term *cardiorenal syndrome* has been used in clinical medicine.[11] This is different than when acute or chronic renal parenchymal disease is associated with increased cardiovascular complications, which can most appropriately be termed renocardiac syndrome. The experimental information described here can be used to understand the effects on kidney function that occur with cardiovascular disease. We now focus on how abnormal cardiac function can affect kidney function in human disease.

Kidney Function with Congestive Heart Failure

In patients with asymptomatic or symptomatic congestive heart failure (CHF), a mild or moderate decrease in kidney function correlates with a highly significant increase in morbidity and mortality.[12,13] Reduced kidney function after an acute myocardial infarction is also associated with increased mortality.[13] Minimal increases in serum creatinine (> 0.5 mg/dL) within 48 hours after cardiothoracic surgery in patients with baseline serum creatinine < 1.3 mg/dL was associated with an 10-fold increase in 30-day mortality independent of other variables.[14] There has been considerable discussion as to whether the worsening of renal function in CHF patients is merely a marker for poor outcomes or actually a pathogenetic factor in causing the progression of functional cardiac dysfunction.

The Role of Neurohumoral Axis in Congestive Heart Failure

The seeming paradox of increased blood volume with renal sodium and water retention in cardiac failure has been explained by the body fluid volume regulation hypothesis.[9,10,15] This hypothesis proposes that the kidney does not respond to changes in total blood volume but rather responds to what has been termed *effective arterial blood volume*. In general terms, approximately 85% of circulating blood volume is in the low-pressure venous side of the circulation, whereas only 15% is in the high-pressure arterial circulation. The integrity of the arterial circulation depends on cardiac output and systemic vascular resistance and is modulated by arterial stretch baroreceptors in the carotid sinus, aortic arch, and afferent arteriole of the glomerulus. Thus, despite an increase in total blood volume, arterial underfilling may develop secondary to a decrease in cardiac output in heart failure or decreased systemic vascular resistance in high-output heart failure. With arterial underfilling secondary to either condition, arterial baroreceptor-mediated activation of the neurohumoral axis occurs. The resultant increase in RAAS leads to sodium retention, and the increase in the nonosmotic release of AVP is associated with water retention and hyponatremia in advanced left ventricular failure.

Considerable evidence shows that renal activation of the RAAS, which occurs with diminished cardiac function, contributes to increased morbidity and mortality. Angiotensin II activates the sympathetic nervous system (SNS), and mortality in heart failure correlates both with increased plasma renin activity[16] and with norepinephrine concentrations.[17] Angiotensin II also is known to cause cardiac remodeling, a known pathogenetic factor in CHF.[18] Even though chymases, rather than angiotensin-converting enzyme (ACE), are known primarily to convert angiotensin I to the bioactive angiotensin II in the heart, ACE inhibition has been shown in prospective randomized studies to improve left ventricular function, attenuate left ventricular remodeling, and increase survival in patients with CHF.[19] Some of these beneficial effects with ACE inhibition may be due to increased bradykinin, because bradykinin degradation is decreased with ACE inhibition.[20,21] Blockade of angiotensin-induced AT1 receptor activation inhibits synthesis of tumor necrosis factor-alpha, inducible nitric oxide, free radical formation, and transforming growth factor-beta, all of which are stimulated by angiotensin II and are deleterious to the heart.[22] Similarly, beta-adrenergic blockade in randomized studies with controlled-release metoprolol[23] and carvedilol[24] has been shown to improve survival in patients with CHF.

Angiotensin II and the SNS, which are activated by a decrease in cardiac stroke volume, increase systemic vascular resistance and maintain arterial pressure. However, the trade-offs of this response are not only the effects on the kidney relating to sodium and water retention, failure to escape from the sodium-retaining effect of aldosterone, and resistance to the natriuretic effect of ANP and BNP but also the increase in cardiac afterload. An increase in cardiac afterload in an already ischemic heart in CHF patients can further impair cardiac function.

The Specific Role of Aldosterone in Congestive Heart Failure

The renal activation of the renin–angiotensin system secondary to impaired cardiac function is associated with increased plasma aldosterone concentration, which is also related to increased mortality in CHF patients.[16] The Randomized Aldactone (spironolactone) Evaluation Study (RALES) used doses (25–50 mg/24 h) of the aldosterone antagonist, spironolactone, which did not alter urinary sodium excretion.[25,26] The results demonstrated improved survival in CHF patients, indicating a protective effect of aldosterone, which has an antifibrotic effect on the heart and blood vessels. There are, however, results that also suggest that secondary hyperaldosteronism is an important renal sodium-retaining mechanism in patients with CHF.[27,28] A lowering of plasma aldosterone with ACE inhibition in CHF, however, may not cause a natriuresis for at least 2 reasons. First, a decrease in angiotensin II with ACE inhibitor diminishes mean arterial pressure, and thus lowers renal perfusion pressure, which may obscure the expected natriuresis normally associated with decreased plasma aldosterone. Second, in 30% to 40% of patients receiving an ACE inhibitor, plasma aldosterone will initially decrease but later the plasma aldosterone level will increase to baseline. This phenomenon, termed aldosterone "breakthrough," can have important clinical consequences given aldosterone's profibrotic actions on diverse organ systems, including the heart and kidney, as well as the hormone's sodium-retaining effect.[29]

Aldosterone antagonists, such as spironolactone or eplerenone, compete with endogenous aldosterone for the mineralocorticoid receptors, and adding them to conventional heart and kidney failure regimens can improve clinical outcomes. However, doses used in RALES were not natriuretic. Secondary hyperaldosteronism is known to be involved in the resistance to loop diuretics (Figure 1.1). In patients with advanced CHF larger doses (100–400 mg/24 h) of spironolactone have been shown to reverse the resistance to loop diuretics and result in significant natriuresis.[27,30,31] While these studies document the role of secondary hyperaldosteronism in advanced heart failure, natriuretic doses of mineralocorticoid antagonists are generally not used in CHF patients. This is the case, even though hospitalized patients with acute decompensated heart failure are frequently loop diuretic resistant and nearly 50% of these patients are discharged without a significant loss of body weight, a circumstance predictive of early readmission.[32] The potential of hyperkalemia with the use

of mineralocorticoid antagonists in CHF patients receiving ACE inhibitors and/or beta-blockers must be considered. Van Vliet et al[27] demonstrated in diuretic–resistant CHF patients receiving low–dose ACE inhibitors that the addition of 100 mg spironolactone/24 h caused a natriuresis with very little change in plasma potassium concentration. Reversal of loop diuretic resistance, including increased urinary potassium loss and a low-potassium diet, may attenuate any rise in serum potassium in CHF patients with spironolactone or eplerenone. An epidemiological study reported a correlation between the time of the RALES results with the onset of more potassium–related hospitalizations and mortality.[33] This observational study, however, has several caveats that question the relationship of increased plasma potassium concentration with the use of spironolactone at the 25- to 50-mg dose. Because tubular potassium secretion is passive and relates to increased tubular sodium reabsorption, the absence of a natriuresis in RALES with the spironolactone doses used calls into question

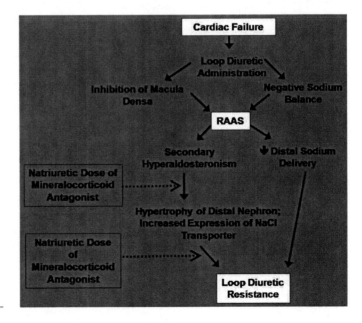

Figure 1.1 Mechanisms of diuretic resistance; role of secondary hyperaldosteronism in the resistance and potential benefit of mineralocorticoid antagonism. Dotted line indicates inhibition.

an effect to decrease potassium secretion and raise serum potassium concentration. The median plasma potassium concentration in RALES increased by only 0.3 mmol/L.

Attenuation of Atrial-Renal Reflexes in CHF

The rise in atrial pressures in CHF patients might be expected to activate the aforementioned atrial-renal reflexes, which increase urinary sodium and water excretion. In spite of elevated atrial pressures, however, patients with CHF retain sodium and water; this indicates either a blunting of these atrial reflexes during heart failure, which has been shown experimentally,[34] and/or an overriding of the low-pressure atrial reflexes by arterial baroreceptor–mediated events. These high-pressure arterial reflexes not only increase RAAS and sympathetic activations but also stimulate the nonosmotic AVP release. In hyponatremic CHF patients, the low plasma osmolality does not suppress AVP release; rather, the baroreceptor-mediated nonosmotic release of AVP occurs and leads to water retention.[35]

Heart Failure with Normal Left Ventricular Ejection Fraction

While much attention has been paid to the consequences relating to decreased cardiac output activating arterial baroreceptor reflexes, including RAAS, SNS, and AVP, in heart failure patients, it must be acknowledged that many of these patients exhibit normal ejection fraction. These patients are, however, seen only at a snapshot in time and not at the time of initiation of heart failure. Studies in experimental heart failure have

shown that an early decrease in cardiac output activates the RAAS, and the resultant renal sodium retention returns the cardiac output and RAAS activity back to normal; this occurs, however, at the expense of an increase in cardiac preload (Figure 1.2).[36] The increased preload has several consequences. The resultant cardiac dilatation is associated with cardiac remodeling, functional mitral insufficiency, and increased ventricular wall stress, which can lead to ventricular wall hypertrophy. Hypertrophied cardiac muscle is known to have a relative decrease in capillarity, and thus to be more predisposed to ischemic insults. The relationship between an increase in central venous pressure, diminished renal function, and mortality has been reported.[37,38] In addition to the effects of increased preload on the heart, there is an associated increase in renal venous pressure. Renal perfusion pressure equals renal arterial pressure minus renal venous pressure, thus an increase in central, and thus renal, venous pressure can decrease renal perfusion. Moreover, a rise in renal venous pressure increases interstitial and tubular pressure, which results in a decrease in GFR and activation of the RAAS.

Less is known about how right-sided failure secondary to pulmonary arterial hypertension affects the kidney.[39] The effect of increased central venous pressure associated with pulmonary hypertension on renal function and the RAAS certainly would be expected with isolated right ventricular failure. Another effect could be explained by interventricular asynchrony and/or pericardium-mediated right ventricle–left ventricle interaction. The mechanism behind this asynchrony is that right ventricular pressure overload leads to prolonged contraction of right ventricular free wall. At the time that the left ventricle has entered its early diastolic phase, right ventricle pressure exceeds left ventricular pressure, leading to para-

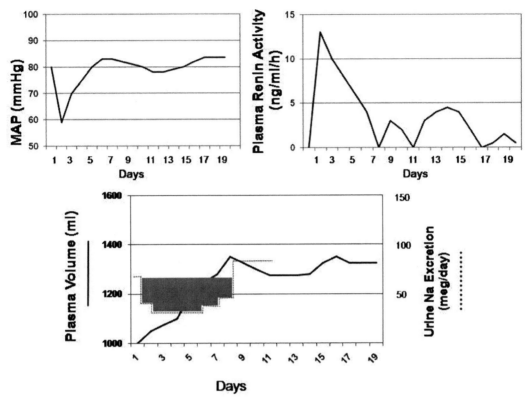

Figure 1.2. Initial decrease in cardiac output associated with a decline in mean arterial pressure (MAP) (upper left panel), which was associated with activation of the RAAS (upper right panel), which in turn led to a positive sodium balance (lower panel). The resultant increase in plasma volume (lower panel) was associated with a return of MAP and the RAAS to baseline. The positive sodium balance is shown by the shaded area (lower panel). Compiled from experimental heart failure data from Damman K, van Deursen VM, Navis G, Voors AA, van Veldhuisen DJ, Hillege HL. Increased central venous pressure is associated with impaired renal function and mortality in a broad spectrum of patients with cardiovascular disease. *J Am Coll Cardiol.* 2009;53:582–588.

doxic septum movement. The consequence of this leftward septal bowing is not only ineffective right ventricular end-systolic contraction but also impaired left ventricular early diastolic filling. A decreased left ventricular end-diastolic volume directly impairs left ventricular output according to the Frank–Starling mechanism and leads to arterial underfilling. The potential effect of right ventricular failure to activate the RAAS, sympathetic activation, and nonosmotic release of AVP are shown in Figure 1.3. However, this pathophysiological pathway,

whereby right ventricular failure alters renal function, is in need of further study.

High-Output Cardiac Failure

Another potential dilemma whereby the heart affects the kidney in clinical medicine is high-output cardiac failure, as occurs with beriberi or thyrotoxicosis. The pathophysiology of low- and high-output cardiac failure appears to be quite similar.[10] The arterial

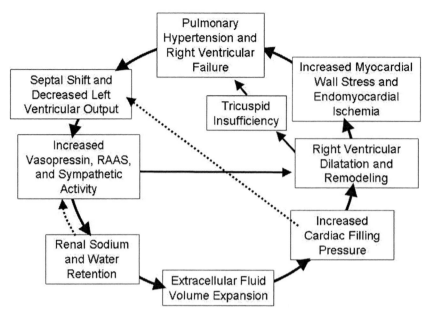

Figure 1.3. Feedback mechanisms for normalizing neurohormones and cardiac index with myocardial injury. The dashed lines indicate the compensatory responses that could return cardiac index and RAAS to within normal range. Klein L, Massie BM, Leimberger JD, O'Connor CM, Piña IL, Adams KF Jr, Califf RM, Gheorghiade M; OPTIME-CHF Investigators. Admission or changes in renal function during hospitalization for worsening heart failure predict postdischarge survival: Results from the outcomes of a prospective trial of intravenous milrinone for exacerbations of chronic heart failure (OPTIME-CHF). *Circ Heart Fail.* 2008;1:25–33. With permission.

stretch baroreceptors sense either a decrease in cardiac output or systemic arterial vasodilation as arterial underfilling with resultant activation of the neurohumoral axis (Figure 1.4). In patients with high-output cardiac failure, the arterial underfilling results from systemic arterial vasodilatation.

The Beneficial Role of Fluid Removal

The Frank-Starling curve has not been found to have a descending limb, therefore fluid removal by a diuretic or ultrafiltration would be expected to either maintain cardiac output (flat part of the curve) or decrease it (ascending limb of curve). In the latter circumstance, the decrease in cardiac output is associated with a decrease in kidney function and a rise in blood urea nitrogen (BUN) and serum creatinine. Because of the effect of AVP to increase the urea transporter and slow tubular flow in the collecting duct during CHF, urea reabsorption is enhanced. Thus, BUN may rise faster than the serum creatinine concentration in patients with CHF. In fact, in a recent analysis of results from a randomized study, cardiac failure, the admission BUN, and BUN change during hospitalization for cardiac failure were more sensitive than serum creatinine or estimated GFR in predicting 60–day mortality.[40,41]

In patients with cardiac failure and increased BUN and serum creatinine, there is hesitation to remove fluid or treat with ACE inhibitor in spite of substantial fluid over-

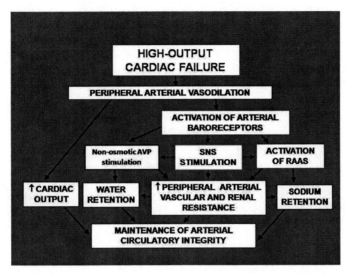

Figure 1.4. Neurohumoral activation in response to arterial underfilling secondary to systemic arterial vasodilatation from high-output cardiac failure. Adapted from Swedberg K, Eneroth P, Kjekshus J, Wilhelmsen L. Hormones regulating cardiovascular function in patients with severe congestive heart failure and their relation to mortality. CONSENSUS Trial Study Group. *Circulation*. 1990;82:1730–1736. With permission.

load. Of note, however, some heart failure patients may respond to fluid removal by improving cardiac output and kidney function; this may be due to decreased cardiac preload, less cardiac dilatation, and reversal of functional mitral insufficiency as well as diminished ventricular wall stress (Figure 1.5). In addition to the expected improved renal arterial perfusion as cardiac output rises, the decrease in renal venous pressure with fluid removal may also contribute to the observed improvement in renal function in CHF patients.

The purported more-beneficial effect of ultrafiltration over loop diuretic–induced fluid removal in CHF patients is in need of confirmation. However, 2 important differences exist between ultrafiltration and loop diuretic–induced fluid removal. Diuretic-induced urinary losses are generally hypotonic, whereas ultrafiltration fluid removal is isotonic. Thus, for the same volume of fluid removed, more sodium, the major determinant of ECFV, is removed with ultrafiltration. Secondly, loop diuretics block the macular densa and therefore always stimulate the RAAS independent of fluid removal.[42] Moreover, loop diuretics are more likely to cause electrolyte abnormalities secondary to urinary potassium, calcium, and magnesium losses. Studies in CHF suggest that movement of interstitial fluid into the vascular compartment can average 14 to 15 mL/min. Thus, ultrafiltration fluid removal that does not exceed this rate may not stimulate the RAAS, and in fact if cardiac output increases and renal venous pressure decreases, there can actually be a decline in RAAS activity.

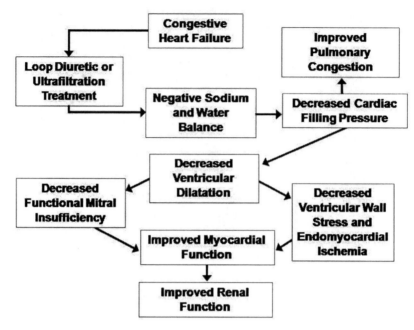

Figure 1.5. Mechanisms in CHF whereby negative sodium and water balance by loop diuretics or ultrafiltration therapy may improve myocardial function. Schrier RW. Role of diminished renal function in cardiovascular mortality: marker or pathogenetic factor? *J Am Coll Cardiol.* 2006;47:1–8. With permission.

Conclusion

CHF is a complex and diverse pathophysiologic state manifested by concomitant heart and kidney failure. An appreciation of the interaction between the heart and kidney during dysfunction of each or both organ has practical clinical implications for patients as well as healthcare costs. Because there are 6 million Americans with CHF and 600,000 annual admissions secondary to heart failure, the depth of knowledge and complexity of care necessary to offer best therapy to these patients demands a multidisciplinary approach, combining the expertise of cardiology, nephrology, and critical care.

References

1. Henry JP, Gauer OH, Reeves JL. Evidence of the atrial location of receptors influencing urine flow. *Circ Res.* 1956;4:85–90.

2. Wood P. Polyuria in paroxysmal tachycardia and paroxysmal atrial flutter and fibrillation. *Br Heart J.* 1963;25:689–690.

3. Linden RJ, Kappagoda CT, eds. *Atrial Receptors.* London: Cambridge University Press; 1982.

4. Henrich WL, Anderson RJ, Berns AS, et al. The role of renal nerves and prostaglandins in control of renal hemodynamics and plasma renin

activity during hypotensive hemorrhage in the dog. *J Clin Invest.* 1978;61:744-750.

5. de Bold AJ. Atrial natriuretic factor: a hormone produced by the heart. *Science.* 1985;230:767-770.

6. Clavell AL, Stingo AJ, Aarhus LL, Burnett JC Jr. Biological actions of brain natriuretic peptide in thoracic inferior vena caval constriction. *Am J Physiol.* 1993;265:R1416-R1422.

7. Firth JD, Raine AE, Ledingham JG. Raised venous pressure: a direct cause of renal sodium retention in oedema? *Lancet.* 1988;1:1033-1035.

8. Schrier RW, De Wardener HE. Tubular reabsorption of sodium ion: influence of factors other than aldosterone and glomerular filtration rate. 2. *N Engl J Med.* 1971;285:1292-1303.

9. Schrier RW, Abraham WT. Hormones and hemodynamics in heart failure. *N Engl J Med.* 1999;341:577-585.

10. Schrier RW. Pathogenesis of sodium and water retention in high-output and low-output cardiac failure, nephrotic syndrome, cirrhosis, and pregnancy (2). *N Engl J Med.* 1988;319:1127-1134.

11. Schrier RW. Role of diminished renal function in cardiovascular mortality: marker or pathogenetic factor? *J Am Coll Cardiol.* 2006;47:1-8.

12. Wong ND, Wilson PW, Kannel WB. Serum cholesterol as a prognostic factor after myocardial infarction: the Framingham Study. *Ann Intern Med.* 1991;115:687-693.

13. Pfeffer MA, McMurray JJ, Velazquez EJ, et al; Valsartan in Acute Myocardial Infarction Trial Investigators. Valsartan, captopril, or both in myocardial infarction complicated by heart failure, left ventricular dysfunction, or both. *N Engl J Med.* 2003;349:1893-1906.

14. Lassnigg A, Schmidlin D, Mouhieddine M, et al. Minimal changes of serum creatinine predict prognosis in patients after cardiothoracic surgery: a prospective cohort study. *J Am Soc Nephrol.* 2004;15:1597-1605.

15. Schrier RW. Body fluid volume regulation in health and disease: a unifying hypothesis. *Ann Intern Med.* 1990;113:155-159.

16. Swedberg K, Eneroth P, Kjekshus J, Wilhelmsen L. Hormones regulating cardiovascular function in patients with severe congestive heart failure and their relation to mortality. CONSENSUS Trial Study Group. *Circulation.* 1990;82: 1730-1736.

17. Cohn JN, Levine TB, Olivari MT, et al. Plasma norepinephrine as a guide to prognosis in patients with chronic congestive heart failure. *N Engl J Med.* 1984;311:819-823.

18. Hirsch AT, Pinto YM, Schunkert H, Dzau VJ. Potential role of the tissue renin-angiotensin system in the pathophysiology of congestive heart failure. *Am J Cardiol.* 1990;66:22D-30D; discussion 30D-32D.

19. Mielniczuk L, Stevenson LW. Angiotensin-converting enzyme inhibitors and angiotensin II type I receptor blockers in the management of congestive heart failure patients: what have we learned from recent clinical trials? *Curr Opin Cardiol.* 2005;20:250-255.

20. Baumgarten CR, Linz W, Kunkel G, Scholkens BA, Wiemer G. Ramiprilat increases bradykinin outflow from isolated hearts of rat. *Br J Pharmacol.* 1993;108:293-295.

21. Liu YH, Yang XP, Shesely EG, Sankey SS, Carretero OA. Role of angiotensin II type 2 receptors and kinins in the cardioprotective effect of angiotensin II type 1 receptor antagonists in rats with heart failure. *J Am Coll Cardiol.* 2004;43: 1473-1480.

22. Schulz R, Heusch G. Angiotensin II in the failing heart. Short communication. *Kidney Blood Press Res.* 2005;28:349-352.

23. Hjalmarson A, Goldstein S, Fagerberg B, et al. Effects of controlled-release metoprolol on total mortality, hospitalizations, and well-being in patients with heart failure: the Metoprolol CR/XL Randomized Intervention Trial in congestive heart failure (MERIT-HF). MERIT-HF Study Group. *JAMA.* 2000;283:1295-1302.

24. Packer M, Bristow MR, Cohn JN, et al. The effect of carvedilol on morbidity and mortality in patients with chronic heart failure. US Carvedilol Heart Failure Study Group. *N Engl J Med.* 1996;334:1349-1355.

25. Effectiveness of spironolactone added to an angiotensin-converting enzyme inhibitor and a loop diuretic for severe chronic congestive heart failure (the Randomized Aldactone Evaluation Study [RALES]). *Am J Cardiol.* 1996;78: 902-907.

26. Pitt B, Zannad F, Remme WJ, et al. The effect of spironolactone on morbidity and mortality in patients with severe heart failure. Randomized Aldactone Evaluation Study Investigators. *N Engl J Med.* 1999;341:709-717.

27. van Vliet AA, Donker AJ, Nauta JJ, Verheugt FW. Spironolactone in congestive heart failure refractory to high-dose loop diuretic and low-dose angiotensin-converting enzyme inhibitor. *Am J Cardiol.* 1993;71:21A-28A.

28. Abdallah JG, Schrier RW, Edelstein C, Jennings SD, Wyse B, Ellison DH. Loop diuretic infusion increases thiazide-sensitive Na(+)/Cl(-)-cotransporter abundance: role of aldosterone. *J Am Soc Nephrol.* 2001;12:1335-1341.

29. Bomback AS, Klemmer PJ. The incidence and implications of aldosterone breakthrough. *Nat Clin Pract Nephrol.* 2007;3:486-492.

30. Hensen J, Abraham WT, Durr JA, Schrier RW. Aldosterone in congestive heart failure: analysis of determinants and role in sodium retention. *Am J Nephrol.* 1991;11:441-446.

31. Braunwald E, Plauth WH Jr, Morrow AG. A method for the detection and quantification of impaired sodium excretion. Results of an oral sodium tolerance test in normal subjects and in patients with heart disease. *Circulation.* 1965;32:223-231.

32. Adams KF Jr, Fonarow GC, Emerman CL, et al; ADHERE Scientific Advisory Committee and Investigators. Characteristics and outcomes of patients hospitalized for heart failure in the United States: rationale, design, and preliminary observations from the first 100,000 cases in the Acute Decompensated Heart Failure National Registry (ADHERE). *Am Heart J.* 2005; 149:209-216.

33. Juurlink DN, Mamdani MM, Lee DS, et al. Rates of hyperkalemia after publication of the Randomized Aldactone Evaluation Study. *N Engl J Med.* 2004;351:543-551.

34. Zucker IH, Gorman AJ, Cornish KG, Lang M. Impaired atrial receptor modulation or renal nerve activity in dogs with chronic volume overload. *Cardiovasc Res.* 1985;19:411-418.

35. Schrier RW, Gross P, Gheorghiade M, et al; SALT Investigators. Tolvaptan, a selective oral vasopressin V2-receptor antagonist, for hyponatremia. *N Engl J Med.* 2006;355:2099-2112.

36. Watkins L Jr, Burton JA, Haber E, Cant JR, Smith FW, Barger AC. The renin-angiotensin-aldosterone system in congestive failure in conscious dogs. *J Clin Invest.* 1976;57:1606-1617.

37. Damman K, van Deursen VM, Navis G, Voors AA, van Veldhuisen DJ, Hillege HL. Increased central venous pressure is associated with impaired renal function and mortality in a broad spectrum of patients with cardiovascular disease. *J Am Coll Cardiol.* 2009;53:582–588.

38. Mullens W, Abrahams Z, Francis GS, et al. Importance of venous congestion for worsening of renal function in advanced decompensated heart failure. *J Am Coll Cardiol.* 2009;53:589–596.

39. Schrier RW, Bansal S. Pulmonary hypertension, right ventricular failure, and kidney: different from left ventricular failure? *Clin J Am Soc Nephrol.* 2008;3:1232–1237.

40. Klein L, Massie BM, Leimberger JD, et al; OPTIME-CHF Investigators. Admission or changes in renal function during hospitalization for worsening heart failure predict postdischarge survival: results from the outcomes of a prospective trial of intravenous milrinone for exacerbations of chronic heart failure (OPTIME-CHF). *Circ Heart Fail.* 2008;1:25–33.

41. Schrier RW. Blood urea nitrogen and serum creatinine. Not married in heart failure. *Circ Heart Fail.* 2008;1:2–5.

42. He XR, Greenberg SG, Briggs JP, Schnermann J. Effects of furosemide and verapamil on the NaCl dependency of macula densa–mediated renin secretion. *Hypertension.* 1995;26:137–142.

The Role of Renal Nerves in Cardiorenal Syndrome in Heart Failure

2

RICHARD E. KATHOLI

PAUL A. SOBOTKA

HENRY KRUM

MARKUS P. SCHLAICH

The kidney and heart are connected in terms of hemodynamic and regulatory functions. The kidney has an important role in electrolyte balance, volume, and blood pressure regulation. Communication between the kidney and the heart occurs at multiple levels, including the sympathetic nervous system (SNS), the renin–angiotensin–aldosterone system (RAAS), antidiuretic hormone, nitric oxide, endothelin, and the natriuretic peptides. This chapter will elucidate the role of renal sympathetic efferent and afferent sensory nerves in modulating renal and cardiac function. Stimulation of the renal sympathetic efferent nerves cause renin release, sodium retention, and reduced renal blood flow,[1] all hallmarks of the renal manifestations of heart failure and cardiorenal syndrome.[2-4] Elevated afferent renal sensory nerve signaling increases sympathetic drive via central integration in the hypothalamic region,[5-7] thereby mediating an increase in sympathetic outflow directed to various regions, including the skeletal muscle vasculature, the kidneys, and the heart, which contributes substantially to elevated peripheral vascular resistance, vascular remodeling, and left ventricular hypertrophy,[8,9] as well as accelerating the decline of left ventricular function.[2-4]

Efferent Renal Nerves in the Pathogenesis of Congestive Heart Failure

In congestive heart failure (CHF), the SNS is activated earlier than the RAAS.[10] The increased sympathetic activity affects all vascular beds, with greater activity noted in the

The Cardiorenal Syndrome: A Clinician's Guide to Pathophysiology and Management, 1st ed. © 2012 J. Thomas Heywood and John C. Burnett Jr., eds. Cardiotext Publishing, ISBN: 978-0-9790164-7-9.

heart and kidney as demonstrated by an exaggerated increase in norepinephrine overflow from the heart and kidney to plasma in this patient group.[11] Mammalian kidneys are richly innervated with postganglionic sympathetic fibers to the afferent and efferent renal arterioles, juxtaglomerular apparatus, proximal renal tubule, loop of Henle, and distal renal tubule. Accordingly, the efferent renal sympathetic nerves can affect control of renal vascular resistance and increase renin release; and they have been shown to regulate sodium and water excretion both by producing arteriolar vasoconstriction, resulting in a change in intrarenal hemodynamics, and by a direct effect on renal proximal tubular sodium reabsorption and ascending portion of the cortical loop of Henle sodium and chloride reabsorption (Figure 2.1).[5,12,13]

There are many inputs to the control of efferent renal nerve activity. Investigators have demonstrated the important role played by the aortic and carotid baroreflexes in the modulation of central sympathetic outflow and, thus, efferent renal nerve activity.[14,15] Findings indicate that tonic arterial chemoreceptor activation may be involved in sympathetic activation associated with renal impairment. Deactivation of arterial chemoreceptors via inhalation of 100% oxygen has been demonstrated to substantially decrease muscle sympathetic nerve activity in patients with chronic renal disease, whereas muscle sympathetic nerve activity was unchanged during 100% oxygen inhalation in healthy control subjects.[14] Importantly, peripheral chemoreceptor hypersensitivity has been shown to determine cardiovascular prognosis in CHF.[15]

In addition, cardiac stretch receptors with vagal afferents that modulate efferent renal sympathetic nerve activity have been identified.[16] More recently, renorenal reflexes that alter the level of efferent nerve activity in the contralateral kidney have been described.[1,17]

Fine-tuning of sympathetic activity is achieved through regionalization and preferential activation of sympathetic outflow to specific organs. Some vascular beds such as the renal vasculature often receive greater sympathetic activation than others, particularly so in the presence of heart failure.[5,18] A disproportionate increase in renal sympathetic activity results in increased renal vascular resistance compared to the general circulation, causing increased plasma renin activity and facilitating sodium and water retention.[19] These observations suggest that increased SNS activity with disproportionately greater stimulation to the kidney may be an important mechanism by which the SNS could initiate CHF or allow CHF to be sustained by preventing compensatory natriuresis from occurring, and reducing GFR.[20,21] This dynamic SNS connection defines the functional renal component of cardiorenal syndrome.

Examination of the relationship between renal efferent sympathetic activity and CHF in rats identified that increased renal sympathetic activity is associated with resistance to the natriuretic action of atrial natriuretic peptide (ANP).[22] Subsequent work documented the salutary effects of bilateral renal denervation in rats with heart failure following left anterior descending artery ligation.[23] The investigation revealed that sodium retention was attributable in part to renal sympathetic efferent nerve activity, which was abolished by renal denervation. Similar conclusions were derived from work on renal denervated dogs with an arteriovenous fistula and the syndrome of compensated high-output heart failure.[24] The renal denervation protected against expression of postprandial natriuretic resistance and the development of congestion or rises in ventricular filling pressures. The therapeutic

Renal Sympathetic Efferent Nerves

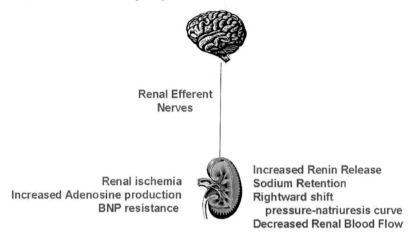

Renal Efferent
Nerves

Renal ischemia
Increased Adenosine production
BNP resistance

Increased Renin Release
Sodium Retention
Rightward shift
    pressure-natriuresis curve
Decreased Renal Blood Flow

Renal Somatic-Sympathetic Afferent Effects

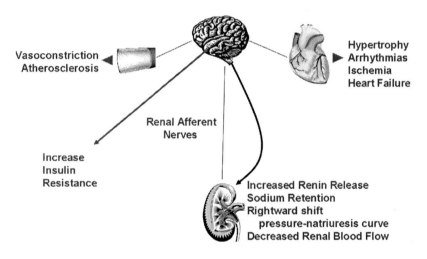

Vasoconstriction
Atherosclerosis

Hypertrophy
Arrhythmias
Ischemia
Heart Failure

Renal Afferent
Nerves

Increase
Insulin
Resistance

Increased Renin Release
Sodium Retention
Rightward shift
    pressure-natriuresis curve
Decreased Renal Blood Flow

Figure 2.1. Stimulation of the renal sympathetic efferent nerves causes renin release, sodium retention, and reduced renal blood flow, all hallmarks of the renal manifestations of cardiorenal syndrome in heart failure (upper panel). Elevated afferent renal sensory nerve signals are centrally integrated in the hypothalamic region and result in increased sympathetic outflow directed to various regions, including the kidneys, the skeletal muscle vasculature, and the heart, which contributes substantially to elevated peripheral vascular resistance, vascular remodeling and left ventricular hypertrophy, as well as accelerating the decline of left ventricular function (lower panel).

value of renal denervation in heart failure was evaluated in 2 similar experimental models of coronary ligation–induced myocardial infarction in rats.[25,26] These studies, in which renal denervation was performed before the onset of myocardial infarction, demonstrated reduced ventricular filling pressure and improved ventricular function compared to nondenervated controls. In these studies in experimental animals, renal denervation has been used to gain physiologic insights into a pathological condition. At the same time, however, these studies reveal a potential and attractive therapeutic target, namely, the renal efferent sympathetic and afferent sensory nerves and their modulation. The report of reduction of renal noradrenaline spillover of 47% ($P <$ 0.023) in patients undergoing percutaneous renal sympathetic denervation for resistant hypertension confirms that an intervention may become available to address this therapeutic target.[27]

Although there are obvious limitations in studying the role of the SNS and of the efferent renal sympathetic nerves in patients with CHF, much indirect evidence suggests that the efferent renal sympathetic nerves function similarly in humans, as has been defined by direct techniques in experimental models of CHF. Activation of cardiorenal sympathetic nerve activity is pronounced in heart failure as demonstrated by an exaggerated increase of norepinephrine overflow from the heart and kidney to plasma in these patients.[11] In support of a role for increased renal sympathetic nerve activity in the sodium and water retention in humans with CHF is the observation that intrarenal adrenergic blockade results in a natriuresis.[28] Further, treatment with centrally acting alpha-2-adrenoceptor agonist clonidine, at modest doses, significantly attenuates cardiac and renal sympathetic activity in patients with CHF.[29] In addition to the beneficial ef-

fects of antiadrenergic therapy on the heart, the renal sympatholytic effects counteract the salt and water retention that is a hallmark of the condition. Consistent with this thought is the demonstration of a strong negative predictive value of renal sympathetic activation on all-cause mortality in patients with CHF, which is independent of overall sympathetic activity, glomerular filtration rate (GFR), and left ventricular ejection fraction.[20] These findings clearly suggest that treatment regimens that further reduce renal sympathetic activity have the potential to improve survival in patients with CHF.

The reduction of renal blood flow and GFR as a result of renal sympathetic efferent activity may play a role in the functional loss of renal function in cardiorenal syndrome, that is, renal dysfunction as a progressive complication of chronic CHF, with a clinical course that typically fluctuates with the patient's clinical status and treatment. Increased renal sympathetic efferent activity also stimulates renin secretion and renin mRNA expression through beta-adrenoreceptors and consequently through cAMP.[30,31] Thus, angiotensin–converting enzyme (ACE) inhibitors and beta-blockers without intrinsic sympathomimetic activities are potent therapies in patients with CHF.[32] ACE inhibitors and certain beta-blockers (carvedilol, metoprolol succinate, and bisoprolol) lower total mortality and heart failure hospitalizations by 25% to 40% across all ages, functional capacities, degrees of left ventricular dysfunction, and causes.[32,33]

While ACE inhibitors and beta-blockers are important therapies in patients with CHF, there are putative reasons why beta-blockers may lead to greater survival and improved quality of life.[32,33] Evidence suggests that there is less "escape" and greater suppression of angiotensin II by ACE inhibitors when the renal sympathetic efferent stimulus for renin release is also blocked by beta-blockers.[34] Cardiorenal complications of heart failure may be avoided because rises in serum creatinine with ACE inhibitors may be decreased by pretreatment with a beta-blocker. Beta-blockers may have a greater impact on ventricular remodeling than ACE inhibitors.[35] In contrast to ACE inhibitors, beta-blockers also appear to have a greater impact on the lowering of sudden death risk, which accounts for one-half to two-thirds of total mortality in patients with CHF.

What other pharmacological approaches can be used to attenuate sympathetic-neural effects beyond beta-blockers' decreasing renin release? Initial beta-blocker (cardioselective or nonselective) therapy in patients with CHF causes increased renal vascular resistance due to unopposed alpha-1-mediated vasoconstriction.[33] In contrast, renal vascular resistance is maintained or decreased during initiation of therapy with carvedilol, which blocks alpha-1 receptors as well as beta-1 and beta-2 receptors.[35,36] This gives insight to the contribution of renal sympathetic efferent nerve activity to heart failure but likely does not explain the possible carvedilol mortality benefits compared to metoprolol tartrate.[37] Increased alpha-1 activity causes peripheral and renal vasoconstriction and myocardial hypertrophy. However, it is unlikely that carvedilol's alpha-1 adrenergic blocking property is important for the long-term treatment of CHF. Pure alpha-1 antagonists have not been associated with favorable effects on either the incidence of heart failure or its outcome.[33] There are also important data comparing the effects of metoprolol versus carvedilol on systemic and cardiac spillover demonstrating that carvedilol but not metoprolol decreased both measures without changes in MSNA, indicating that the effect may be due to blocking peripheral prejunctional beta-adrenergic receptors.[38] In addition, there are data showing the development of

tolerance to the peripheral and renal hemodynamic alpha-1-mediated effects of carvedilol in patients with CHF.[36] However, carvedilol appears to have renoprotective properties in patients with chronic systolic CHF, as evidenced by increases in GFR.[37] The improvement in GFR with carvedilol is independent of the improvement in left ventricular ejection fraction. Proposed renoprotective mechanisms of carvedilol include antagonizing prejunctional beta-adrenergic receptors, which facilitate renal neural norepinephrine release.[35,36,37] Carvedilol has also been shown to reduce urinary albumin excretion and expression of profibrotic factors such as renal tissue growth factor-beta, likely due to its antioxidant properties.[39]

Clinical trial data indicate that spironolactone has an additive beneficial effect on mortality in patients with moderate or severe CHF who are receiving ACE inhibitor and beta-blocker therapy.[40] Aldosterone blockade reduces sudden death and death from progressive heart failure. Although the mechanisms are incompletely understood, increases in potassium and magnesium may play an important role as well as attenuation of myocardial hypertrophy and fibrosis. Aldosterone blockade also improves baroreceptor function in patients with CHF,[41] thus increasing parasympathetic activity and decreasing central sympathetic outflow, resulting in less renal efferent sympathetic activity. Similar increases in spontaneous baroreflex sensitivity of MSNA were observed following selective renal denervation in humans with resistant hypertension.[42,43]

Exercise training improves survival in patients with CHF. Aerobic exercise training also preferentially reduces resting renal but not cardiac sympathetic efferent activity in humans.[44] After 1 month of endurance exercise training, renal norepinephrine spillover to plasma fell by an average of 41% and renal vascular conductance increased by 10%. The reduction in resting sympathetic activity with exercise training is largely confined to the kidney. Thus, regular aerobic exercise is a nonpharmacological mechanism by which to decrease renal sympathetic efferent activity. Weight loss in overweight and obese subjects has also been associated with a reduction in sympathetic activity, which may also be beneficial in the scenario of heart failure.[45]

While carvedilol, spironolactone, and aerobic exercise attenuate renal sympathetic efferent activity in the treatment of cardiorenal syndrome in patients with CHF, selective renal denervation would likely prevent much of the decline in renal function that is associated with chronic CHF, while preserving or improving baroreceptor function.

Renal Sensory Afferent Nerve Activity in Congestive Heart Failure

Chronic elevation in SNS activity is associated with the development and progression of chronic CHF. The mechanisms involved in sympathetic dysfunction in this disorder appear to be complex and multifactorial, including alterations in multiple autonomic reflex pathways, central integratory sites, and chemical mediators that control sympathetic outflow.[16,46] It is well known that restraint of central sympathetic outflow by arterial and cardiopulmonary baroreflexes is depressed in patients with CHF.[46] Moreover, maladaptive changes also occur in the central nervous system (CNS) at integrative sites for autonomic control in heart failure. It has also been demonstrated that sympathoexcitatory cardiac, somatic, and central/peripheral chemoreceptor reflexes are enhanced, contributing to increased SNS activity in patients with CHF.[16,46] Thus, while increased SNS activity may start as a compensatory response in the development of CHF,[20] it becomes part of a pathological positive feedback cycle as cardiac deterioration continues.

In recent years, studies suggest that, in addition to depressed baroreflex sensitivity, an increase in the activity of sympathoexcitatory chemoreflexes also contributes the sympathetic activation in CHF.[16,46] Activation of and/or enhancement in the sensitivity of these chemoreflexes is due to changes in the interstitial milieu in which the afferents reside. Increases in the local production of substances such as bradykinin, nitric oxide, prostaglandins, and adenosine have been implicated as excitatory substances for cardiac and peripheral chemoreceptor afferents in CHF.

Although increased activity of renal sensory afferent nerves being centrally integrated with resulting increased central sympathetic outflow has been studied in experimental animals, their respective role in humans with CHF warrants further study. However, the kidney as another source of afferent activity contributing to increased SNS activity in patients with CHF needs important consideration. These renal afferent signals in CHF are likely due to chemoreceptor activation because mechanoreceptors typically reset. The kidneys communicate with integral structures in the CNS via unmyelinated renal sensory afferent nerves. Thus, renal sensory afferent nerve activity directly influences central sympathetic outflow directed toward the kidneys, thereby inducing renin secretion, sodium retention, and vasoconstriction, but is also directed toward other organs that have a dense sympathetic innervation, such as the heart and the peripheral vasculature, resulting in the described adverse effects of sympathetic activation.[1,5,13] Thus, a pathological positive feedback cycle at the level of the kidney may contribute to cardiorenal syndrome in patients with CHF. The importance of heightened renal sympathetic nerve activity for alteration of left ventricular structure and function[8] is probably most evident in patients with end-stage renal disease who have high levels of sympathetic activity and ~80% of whom develop heart failure within the first 36 months of renal replacement therapy.[9] Increasing evidence indicates that the kidney is a sensory organ.[1,5,13] Mechanoreceptors and chemoreceptors have been demonstrated in the kidney; mechanoreceptors are located both in the renal cortex and in the renal pelvis, while chemoreceptive nerve endings may be found primarily in the submucosal layers of the renal pelvis. Studies have shown that the renal nerves contain multiple afferent fibers that carry impulses centrally from renal receptors of different varieties and specificities. There is strong evidence that the afferent renal nerves are involved not only in renorenal regulation but also in cardiovascular regulation. Numerous studies have provided functional evidence for projections of afferent renal nerves to central structures known to be involved in cardiovascular regulation. Indeed, reductions in MSNA have been reported in a patient with resistant hypertension who underwent therapeutic renal denervation,[42] which suggests either a direct renal-to-CNS communication or that the reduction of renal angiotensin II levels following efferent sympathetic nerve ablation reduced central sympathetic gain. Either possibility confirms a renal contribution to central sympathetic drive and provides partial explanation of cardiorenal syndrome.

If one hypothesizes that afferent renal nerve signals from a hemodynamically stressed kidney enhance SNS activity in patients with CHF, what could be a stimulus? Because the signals would probably be continuously sent from the afferent renal nerves to play a long-term role in CHF, the receptor likely is a chemoreceptor. Adenosine, which is readily released by renal proximal tubular cells directly into the tubular fluid during increased metabolic activity,[47] is a possible agent to stimulate chemoreceptive nerve endings in patients with CHF. Intrarenal adenosine has been found to be elevated in patients with CHF.[48,49] Studies in experimental animals have demonstrated that adenosine-sensitive nerve endings located within or near the renal pelvis, when stimulated, activate central SNS activity via the afferent renal nerves.[6,7] Theophylline, a competitive antagonist of purinergic adenosine receptors, does not alter the sympathetic response to intrarenal adenosine, suggesting that this excitatory action of adenosine is on a different type of receptor.[6] Consistent with this possibility is the observation that theophylline does not significantly alter the excitatory action of adenosine on cat carotid chemoreceptors.[50] The contribution of intrarenal adenosine-induced SNS activation in the pathogenesis of CHF merits further study.

Conclusion

Much evidence suggests roles for both renal efferent sympathetic activity and renal sensory afferent nerve activity in patients with CHF and cardiorenal syndrome. To study the role of the renal nerves in patients with CHF more definitely will require minimally invasive percutaneous renal denervation as a therapeutic strategy. The physiology of patients with CHF suggests that (1) denervation of efferent sympathetic nerves will reduce inappropriate renin release, salt retention, and improve renal blood flow and that (2) denervation of afferent sensory nerves will attenuate the kidney's contribution to centrally mediated SNS activity. A reduction of central sympathetic outflow to heart, vasculature, and kidney in combination with evidence-based medicines like ACE inhibitors, carvedilol, and spironolactone may attenuate cardiorenal syndrome. Direct and significant interference with the cardiac-renal-neuro axis will require renal sympathetic nerve ablation; fortunately, studies of this approach are to be eagerly anticipated.

References

1. DiBona GF. Neural control of the kidney: past, present, and future. *Hypertension.* 2003;41(3 Pt 2):621–624.

2. Boerrigter G, Burnett JC Jr. Cardiorenal syndrome in decompensated heart failure: prognostic and therapeutic implications. *Curr Heart Fail Rep.* 2004;1:113–120.

3. Heywood JT, Fonarow GC, Costanzo MR, Mathur VS, Wigneswaran JR, Wynne J. High prevalence of renal dysfunction and its impact on outcome in 118,465 patients hospitalized with acute decompensated heart failure: a report from the ADHERE database. *J Card Fail.* 2007;13:422–430.

4. Wencker D. Acute cardio-renal syndrome: progression from congestive heart failure to congestive kidney failure. *Curr Heart Fail Rep.* 2007;4:134–138.

5. Katholi RE. Renal nerves in the pathogenesis of hypertension in experimental animals and humans. *Am J Physiol.* 1983;245:F1–F14.

6. Katholi RE, Hageman GR, Whitlow PL, Woods WT. Hemodynamic and afferent renal nerve responses to intrarenal adenosine in the dog. *Hypertension.* 1983;s5(2 Pt 2):I149–I154.

7. Katholi RE, Whitlow PL, Hageman GR, Woods WT. Intrarenal adenosine produces hypertension by activating the sympathetic nervous system via the renal nerves in the dog. *J Hypertens.* 1984;2:349–359.

8. Schlaich MP, Kaye DM, Lambert E, Sommerville M, Socratous F, Esler MD. Relation between cardiac sympathetic activity and hypertensive left ventricular hypertrophy. *Circulation.* 2003;108:560–565.

9. Schlaich MP, Socratous F, Hennebry S, et al. Sympathetic activation in chronic renal failure. *J Am Soc Nephrol.* 2009;20:933–939.

10. Francis GS, Benedict C, Johnstone DE, et al. Comparison of neuroendocrine activation in patients with left ventricular dysfunction with and without congestive heart failure. A substudy of the Studies of Left Ventricular Dysfunction (SOLVD). *Circulation.* 1990;82:1724–1729.

11. Hasking GJ, Esler MD, Jennings GL, Burton D, Johns JA, Korner PI. Norepinephrine spillover to plasma in patients with congestive heart failure: evidence of increased overall and cardiorenal sympathetic nervous activity. *Circulation.* 1986;73:615–621.

12. Bello-Reuss E, Trevino DL, Gottschalk CW. Effect of renal sympathetic nerve stimulation on proximal water and sodium reabsorption. *J Clin Invest.* 1976;57:1104–1107.

13. Katholi RE. Renal nerves and hypertension: an update. *Fed Proc.* 1985;44:2846–2850.

14. Hering D, Zdrojewski Z, Król E, et al. Tonic chemoreflex activation contributes to the elevated muscle sympathetic nerve activity in patients with chronic renal failure. *J Hypertens.* 2007;25:157–161.

15. Ponikowski P, Chua TP, Anker SD, et al. Peripheral chemoreceptor hypersensitivity: an ominous sign in patients with chronic heart failure. *Circulation.* 2001;104:544–549.

16. Zucker IH. Novel mechanisms of sympathetic regulation in chronic heart failure. *Hypertension*. 2006;48:1005-1011.

17. Kopp UC, Cicha MZ, Smith LA, Mulder J, Hokfelt T. Renal sympathetic nerve activity modulates afferent renal nerve activity by PGE2-dependent activation of alpha1- and alpha2-adrenoceptors on renal sensory nerve fibers. *Am J Physiol Regul Integr Comp Physiol*. 2007;293:R1561-R1572.

18. Kon V. Neural control of renal circulation. *Miner Electrolyte Metab*. 1989;15:33-43.

19. Kirchheim H, Ehmke H, Persson P. Sympathetic modulation of renal hemodynamics, renin release and sodium excretion. *Klin Wochenschr*. 1989;67:858-864.

20. Petersson M, Friberg P, Eisenhofer G, Lambert G, Rundqvist B. Long-term outcome in relation to renal sympathetic activity in patients with chronic heart failure. *Eur Heart J*. 2005;26:906-913.

21. Shlipak MG, Massie BM. The clinical challenge of cardiorenal syndrome. *Circulation*. 2004;110:1514-1517.

22. Pettersson A, Hedner J, Hedner T. Renal interaction between sympathetic activity and ANP in rats with chronic ischaemic heart failure. *Acta Physiol Scand*. 1989;135:487-492.

23. DiBona GF, Sawin LL. Role of renal nerves in sodium retention of cirrhosis and congestive heart failure. *Am J Physiol*. 1991;260(2 Pt 2):R298-R305.

24. Villarreal D, Freeman RH, Johnson RA, Simmons JC. Effects of renal denervation on postprandial sodium excretion in experimental heart failure. *Am J Physiol*. 1994;266(5 Pt 2):R1599-R1604.

25. Nozawa T, Igawa A, Fujii N, et al. Effects of long-term renal sympathetic denervation on heart failure after myocardial infarction in rats. *Heart Vessels*. 2002;16:51-56.

26. Souza DR, Mill JG, Cabral AM. Chronic experimental myocardial infarction produces antinatriuresis by a renal nerve-dependent mechanism. *Braz J Med Biol Res*. 2004;37:285-293.

27. Krum H, Schlaich M, Whitbourn R, et al. Catheter-based renal sympathetic denervation for resistant hypertension: a multicentre safety and proof-of-principle cohort study. *Lancet*. 2009;373:1275-1281.

28. Schrier RW. Pathogenesis of sodium and water retention in high-output and low-output cardiac failure, nephrotic syndrome, cirrhosis, and pregnancy (1). *N Engl J Med*. 1988;319:1065-1072.

29. Aggarwal A, Esler MD, Morris MJ, Lambert G, Kaye DM. Regional sympathetic effects of low-dose clonidine in heart failure. *Hypertension*. 2003;41:553-557.

30. Holmer S, Rinne B, Eckardt KU, et al. Role of renal nerves for the expression of renin in adult rat kidney. *Am J Physiol*. 1994;266(5 Pt 2):F738-F745.

31. Zanchetti AS. Neural regulation of renin release: experimental evidence and clinical implications in arterial hypertension. *Circulation*. 1977;56: 691-698.

32. Fang JC. Angiotensin-converting enzyme inhibitors or beta-blockers in heart failure: does it matter who goes first? *Circulation*. 2005;112:2380-2382.

33. Metra M, Dei Cas L, Cleland JG. Pharmacokinetic and pharmacodynamic characteristics of beta-blockers: when differences may matter. *J Card Fail*. 2006;12:177-181.

34. Knight EL, Glynn RJ, McIntyre KM, Mogun H, Avorn J. Predictors of decreased renal function in patients

with heart failure during angiotensin-converting enzyme inhibitor therapy: results from the studies of left ventricular dysfunction (SOLVD). *Am Heart J.* 1999;138(5 Pt 1):849–855.

35. Remme WJ, Riegger G, Hildebrandt P, et al. The benefits of early combination treatment of carvedilol and an ACE-inhibitor in mild heart failure and left ventricular systolic dysfunction. The carvedilol and ACE-inhibitor remodelling mild heart failure evaluation trial (CARMEN). *Cardiovasc Drugs Ther.* 2004;18:57–66.

36. Abraham WT, Tsvetkova T, Lowes BD, Ferguson DA, Gilbert EM, Bristow MR. Carvedilol improves renal hemodynamics in patients with chronic heart failure (abstract). *J Card Fail.* 1998;4(suppl 1):3 abstract 005.

37. Di Lenarda A, Charlesworth A, Cleland JG, et al. Prognostic significance and the evolution of renal insufficiency in COMET trial. Heart Society of America (HFSA) 8th Annual Scientific Meeting. Toronto, Canada. September 12-15, 2004;Abstract #221.

38. Azevedo ER, Kubo T, Mak S, et al. Nonselective versus selective beta-adrenergic receptor blockade in congestive heart failure: differential effects on sympathetic activity. *Circulation.* 2001;104:2194-2199.

39. Bakris GL, Fonseca V, Katholi RE, et al. Differential effects of beta-blockers on albuminuria in patients with type 2 diabetes. *Hypertension.* 2005;46:1309–1315.

40. Pitt B, Zannad F, Remme WJ, et al. The effect of spironolactone on morbidity and mortality in patients with severe heart failure. Randomized Aldactone Evaluation Study Investigators. *N Engl J Med.* 1999;341:709-717.

41. MacFadyen RJ, Barr CS, Struthers AD. Aldosterone blockade reduces vascular collagen turnover, improves heart rate variability and reduces early morning rise in heart rate in heart failure patients. *Cardiovasc Res.* 1997;35:30-34.

42. Esler M, Schlaich M, Sobotka P, et al. Catheter-based renal denervation reduces total body and renal noradrenaline spillover and blood pressure in resistant hypertension. *J Hypertens.* 2009;27(suppl 4):s167.

43. Schlaich MP, Sobotka PA, Krum H, Lambert E, Esler MD. Renal sympathetic nerve ablation for the treatment of uncontrolled hypertension. *New Engl J Med.* 2009: 36; 9, 932-934

44. Meredith IT, Friberg P, Jennings GL, et al. Exercise training lowers resting renal but not cardiac sympathetic activity in humans. *Hypertension.* 1991; 18:575-582.

45. Straznicky NE, Lambert EA, Lambert GW, Masuo K, Esler MD, Nestel PJ. Effects of dietary weight loss on sympathetic activity and cardiac risk factors associated with the metabolic syndrome. *J Clin Endocrinol Metab.* 2005;90:5998-6005.

46. Schultz HD, Li YL, Ding Y. Arterial chemoreceptors and sympathetic nerve activity: implications for hypertension and heart failure. *Hypertension.* 2007;50: 6-13.

47. Katholi RE, Taylor GJ, McCann WP, et al. Nephrotoxicity from contrast media: attenuation with theophylline. *Radiology.* 1995;195:17-22.

48. Funaya H, Kitakaze M, Node K, Minamino T, Komamura K, Hori M. Plasma adenosine levels increase in patients with chronic heart failure. *Circulation.* 1997;95:1363-1365.

49. Rajaram V, Joseph J. Role of adenosine antagonism in the cardio-renal syndrome: pathophysiology and therapeutic potential. *Curr Heart Fail Rep.* 2007;4:153–157.

50. McQueen DS, Ribeiro JA. Effect of adenosine on carotid chemoreceptor activity in the cat. *Br J Pharmacol.* 1981;74:129–136.

Diagnosis and Prognosis of Cardiorenal Syndrome

3

Maria Rosa Costanzo
Claudio Ronco

The term *cardiorenal syndrome* often refers to a condition in which renal impairment occurs as a result of cardiac dysfunction.[1] This view is supported by the observation that a previously impaired renal function improves after a cardiac assist device is implanted in a patient with end-stage heart failure (HF).[2] The expression "cardiorenal syndrome" has also been used to describe the negative effects of renal disorders on heart structure and function.[3] Thus, although the term *cardiorenal syndrome* is loosely applied to many pathological interactions between the heart and the kidney, until recently a comprehensive definition was lacking. To be inclusive of the damage/dysfunction produced in either the heart or the kidney by an acute or chronic disease of the other organ, car-

diorenal syndrome should be classified according to whether the impairment of each organ is primary or secondary, or whether abnormal heart and kidney functions occur simultaneously as a result of a systemic disease.[4] For example, acute HF decompensation can cause both acute renal injury and chronic kidney disease (CKD): a decreased cardiac output is associated with renal arterial underfilling and increased venous pressure, which, in turn, result in a reduced glomerular filtration rate (GFR).[5] Activation of the renin–angiotensin–aldosterone system (RAAS), initially aimed at restoring GFR, eventually leads to increased renal expression of endothelin 1 (ET-1), a potent proinflammatory and profibrotic vasoconstrictor peptide known to mediate acute and chronic kidney injury.[4]

In chronic HF, increased sympathetic nervous system and RAAS activity augment oxidative stress to the kidneys and impair action of nitric oxide on the vascular endo-

The Cardiorenal Syndrome: A Clinician's Guide to Pathophysiology and Management, 1st ed. © 2012 J. Thomas Heywood and John C. Burnett Jr., eds. Cardiotext Publishing, ISBN: 978-0-9790164-7-9.

thelium.[5] Activation of the RAAS, which increases production of angiotensin II and aldosterone within the kidney, is a key factor in the development of end-organ damage in the heart, vasculature, and kidneys.[6] Chronic HF is often complicated by anemia, known to independently worsen hemodynamic and clinical outcomes, and by the release of inflammatory cytokines including tumor necrosis factor-alpha (TNF-α), interleukin 1 (IL-1), and interleukin 6 (IL-6). This inflammation leads to gradual toxic injury to renal cells and eventually to chronic kidney damage and functional loss.[4]

Conversely, acute kidney injury (AKI) can provoke cardiac failure. Models of postischemic renal injury have demonstrated the intrarenal accumulation of neutrophils, macrophages/monocytes, and lymphocytes and increased circulating levels of inflammatory cytokines, which can impair cardiac contractility and trigger myocytes apoptosis.[4]

CKD independently increases the risk of cardiovascular disease by promoting myocardial hypertrophy, coronary atherosclerosis, and fluid overload. Anemia, advanced glycation end-products (AGEs), abnormal calcium–phosphate metabolism, nutritional factors, extracellular fluid accumulation, inflammation, insulin resistance, hyperhomocysteinemia, oxidative stress, and dyslipidemia have all been implicated in the amplification of cardiovascular morbidity by CKD.[5] In addition, by inhibiting Na–K-ATPase, uremic toxins may increase contractile force and impair relaxation of cardiac myocytes, thus contributing to the diastolic dysfunction commonly encountered in patients with CKD.[4]

Finally, highly prevalent conditions, such as diabetes and hypertension, and less common ones, including autoimmune diseases, amyloidosis, pulmonary arterial hypertension, and sepsis, can simultaneously damage the heart and kidneys.[4,5]

This chapter will examine the methods currently used to diagnose the presence of renal dysfunction in patients with cardiovascular disease (CVD), describe a newly proposed classification of cardiorenal syndrome, summarize the evidence for the impact of renal disease on cardiovascular outcomes, and describe the data showing that renal dysfunction worsens the outcomes of HF patients.

Diagnosis by Primary Organ Dysfunction and Acuity of Events

Although generally defined as a condition characterized by the initiation and/or progression of renal insufficiency secondary to HF, the term *cardiorenal syndrome* is also used to describe the negative effects of reduced renal function on the cardiovascular system.[4] The direct and indirect effects of each dysfunctional organ can initiate and perpetuate the combined disorder of the 2 organs through complex neurohormonal feedback mechanisms. Consequently the subdivision of cardiorenal syndrome into 5 different subtypes may facilitate care of individual patients (Table 3.1).

Type 1 cardiorenal syndrome (acute cardiorenal syndrome) defines a rapid deterioration in cardiac function, which produces AKI. Regardless of whether acute HF presents as hypertensive pulmonary edema with preserved left ventricular (LV) systolic function, exacerbation of chronic HF, cardiogenic shock, or predominantly right ventricular (RV) failure, premorbid CKD is common and increases the risk of AKI.[7,8] Severity of AKI is greater in patients with impaired than in those with preserved LV systolic function, and it occurs in more than 70% of patients with cardiogenic shock.[7] As discussed later

Table 3.1: Cardiorenal Syndrome

Type 1: acute cardiorenal syndrome

Abrupt worsening of cardiac function
(eg, acute cardiogenic shock, or ADHF)
leading to acute kidney injury

Type 2: chronic cardiorenal syndrome

Chronic abnormalities in cardiac function
(eg, chronic HF) causing progressive
and potentially permanent chronic kidney
disease

Type 3: acute renocardiac syndrome

Abrupt worsening of renal function
(eg, acute kidney ischemia or
glomerulonephritis) causing acute cardiac
disorders (eg, HF, arrhythmia, ischemia)

Type 4: chronic renocardiac syndrome

Chronic kidney disease (eg, chronic
glomerular or interstitial disease)
contributing to decreased cardiac
function, cardiac hypertrophy, and/or
increased risk of adverse cardiovascular
events

Type 5: secondary cardiorenal syndrome

Systemic conditions (eg, diabetes mellitus,
sepsis) causing both cardiac and renal
dysfunction

Adapted from Ronco C, Haapio M, House AA:
Cardiorenal syndrome. *J Am Coll Cardiol*. 2008;
52:1527–1539. With permission from Elsevier.

in this chapter, renal dysfunction consistently and independently predicts 1–year mortality in patients with acute decompensated heart failure (ADHF), possibly because an acute decline in renal function accelerates progression of CVD through activation of inflammatory pathways.[5] Key concerns regarding AKI are whether it represents inadequate renal perfusion due to either a low cardiac output (CO) and/or marked increase in central venous pressure (CVP), decreased diuretic responsiveness, or intravascular volume depletion from overzealous diuresis.[3] Accurate diagnosis and appropriate treatment of type 1 cardiorenal syndrome may require measurement of CO and CVP.[4] In addition, renal function and potassium levels should be closely monitored to minimize avoidance of lifesaving medications such as angiotensin–converting enzyme inhibitors (ACEIs), angiotensin receptor blockers (ARBs), and aldosterone blockers.[4] However, initiation of beta–blockers, particularly atenolol and sotalol, which undergo renal excretion, should be deferred until hemodynamic stability is achieved.[4] Kidney function should be closely monitored also in patients with acute myocardial infarction (AMI), and in those undergoing cardiac surgery, percutaneous coronary intervention (PCI), or radiocontrast cardiac imaging, because in these settings an increase in serum creatinine signals the onset of AKI, which, in turn, may accelerate cardiovascular injury through activation of neurohormonal, immunological, and inflammatory pathways.[3-5] As discussed later in this chapter, even a modest increase in serum creatinine (> 0.3 mg/dL) is an independent predictor of unfavorable cardiovascular outcomes. Attempts to attenuate renal damage are largely futile because renal function markers such as serum creatinine rise only after AKI has occurred.[4] However, the discovery of novel AKI biomarkers may permit an earlier diagnosis of cardiorenal syndrome (Table 3.2). The use of a complementary deoxyribonucleic acid (DNA) microarray has identified a subset of genes whose expression is up–regulated within the first few hours after the onset of AKI.[9] Urine and serum neutrophil gelatinase–associated lipocalin (NGAL) levels are early predictors of AKI after use of radiocontrast and cardiac surgery. In critically ill patients elevation of

Table 3.2 Protein Biomarkers
for the Early Detection of Acute Kidney Injury

Biomarker	Associated Injury
Cystatin C	Proximal tubule injury
KIM-1	Ischemia and nephrotoxins
NGAL (lipocalin)	Ischemia and nephrotoxins
NHE3	Ischemia, pre-renal, post-renal AKI
Cytokines (IL-6, IL-8, IL-18)	Toxic, delayed graft function
Actin-actin depolymerizing F	Ischemia and delayed graft function
α-GST	Proximal tubule injury, acute rejection
Π-GST	Distal tubule injury, acute rejection
L-FABP	Ischemia and nephrotoxins
Netrin-1	Ischemia and nephrotoxins, sepsis
Keratin-derived chemokine	Ischemia and delayed graft function

GST = glutathione S-transferase; IL = interleukin; KIM = kidney injury molecule; L-FABP = L-type fatty acid binding protein; NGAL = neutrophil gelatinase-associated lipocalin; NHE = sodium-hydrogen exchanger. Ronco C, Haapio M, House AA. Cardiorenal syndrome. *J Am Coll Cardiol.* 2008;52:1527–1539. With permission from Elsevier.

NGAL levels precedes that of serum creatinine by 48 to 72 hours.[10] Cystatin C also predicts AKI and the requirement for renal replacement therapy earlier than serum creatinine elevation[11] (Figure 3.1). After cardiac surgery both cystatin C and NGAL predicted renal damage at 12 hours, but NGAL was superior to cystatin C at earlier time points.[4] Kidney injury molecule 1, a protein detectable in the urine after proximal tubular cells injury, may be highly specific for ischemic AKI. Biomarkers such as N-acetyl-β-(D)glucosaminidase, IL-18, and others have been evaluated for their ability to detect AKI and CKD progression. Use of a "panel" of biomarkers that includes several serum and urinary molecules may ultimately permit detection of AKI before irreversible renal damage has occurred.[4]

Type 2 cardiorenal syndrome (chronic cardiorenal syndrome) refers to progressive CKD occurring in approximately 25% of HF patients.[12] Its presence and worsening renal function (WRF) in HF patients are consistently associated with adverse outcomes, as discussed in detail later in this chapter. Chronic HF may be associated with longstanding renal hypoperfusion often aggravated by co-existing micro- and macrovascular disease.[4] Other causes of the onset and progression of renal dysfunction in chronic HF include neurohormonal activation; resistance to natriuretic peptides; iatrogenic hypovolemia and hypotension and down-regulation of

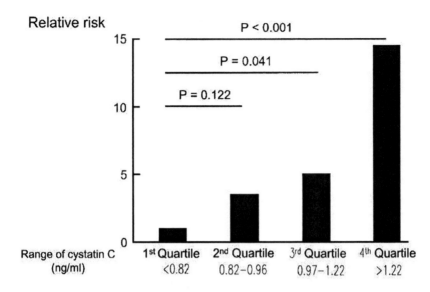

Figure 3.1. Quartile analysis of serum cystatin C levels and all-cause cardiac events in HF patients. The relative risk of all-cause cardiac events was significantly elevated in the fourth quartile (cystatin C > 1.22 ng/mL). Arimoto T, Takeishi Y, Niizeki T, et al. Cystatin C, a novel measure of renal function is an independent predictor of cardiac events in patients with heart failure. *J Cardiac Fail.* 2005:11:595–601. With permission from Elsevier.

the cardiac erythropoietin receptor, a mediator of decreased apoptosis, fibrosis, and inflammation.[3–5] Preliminary data show that erythropoiesis–stimulating agents in patients with chronic HF, CKD, and anemia lead to improved cardiac function and reduction in LV size and B–type natriuretic peptide (BNP) levels.[15]

Type 3 cardiorenal syndrome (acute renocardiac syndrome) consists of a rapid worsening of kidney function due to AKI, ischemia, or glomerulonephritis, which leads to acute cardiac abnormalities including ischemia, arrhythmia, and HF. According to the Risk, Injury, and Failure; Loss; and End–stage kidney disease (RIFLE) consensus definition, AKI can be identified in approximately 9% of ADHF patients and in more than 35% of those requiring care in an intensive care unit.[14] In patients with acute renocardiac syndrome, fluid overload can result in pulmonary edema, and hyperkalemia can cause arrhythmias and even cardiac

arrest. Untreated uremia results in the accumulation of myocardial depressant factors and pericarditis.[15] Deleterious effects of acidemia include pulmonary vasoconstriction, which increases the risk of right–sided HF, and negative inotropic effects, which may be proarrhythmic, especially if associated with electrolyte abnormalities.[4,15] In addition renal ischemia itself may enhance cardiac inflammation and apoptosis.[5] Patients with bilateral renal artery stenosis (or unilateral stenosis in a solitary kidney) are prone to decompensated diastolic HF due to neurohormonally mediated arterial hypertension, sodium and water retention from renal dysfunction, and acute myocardial ischemia caused by an increased myocardial oxygen demand resulting from intense peripheral vasoconstriction.[4,5] In these patients GFR is highly dependent upon angiotensin II, and its blockade causes rapid deterioration of renal function. Biomarkers of myocardial ischemia (troponin), or of myocyte stress (BNP), may permit earlier diagnosis and treatment of type 3 cardiorenal syndrome.[16] The detection early in cardiorenal syndrome of markers of oxidative stress (myeloperoxidase) or of inflammation (TNF-α, IL-1, and IL-6) suggests that these processes may contribute to both cardiac and renal injury.[17]

Detection of AKI can trigger reduction or even discontinuation of both diuretics and ACEIs, which exposes patients to a greater risk of ADHF and kidney injury due to hyperfiltration.[4] If AKI is severe enough to require renal replacement therapy, continuous techniques are safer than conventional dialysis because the avoidance of rapid fluid and electrolyte shifts minimizes the risk of hypotension, arrhythmias, and myocardial ischemia.[16]

Type 4 cardiorenal syndrome (chronic renocardiac syndrome) develops when primary CKD contributes to the aggravation of systolic and diastolic LV dysfunction, LV hypertrophy, and risk of adverse cardiovascular events, as detailed later in this chapter.[4] In type 4 cardiorenal syndrome increased BNP levels are associated with faster progression of nondiabetic CKD to end-stage kidney disease.[17] Increased levels of other biomarkers including troponins, asymmetric dimethylarginine, plasminogen-activator inhibitor type 1, homocysteine, natriuretic peptides, C-reactive protein, serum amyloid A protein, hemoglobin, and ischemia-modified albumin have also been correlated to unfavorable cardiovascular outcomes in CKD patients.[4] These findings suggest a possible link between chronic inflammation, subclinical infections, accelerated atherosclerosis, and adverse cardiorenal outcomes. Unfortunately, because of concerns about WRF, less than 50% of CKD patients are treated with therapies aimed at minimizing cardiovascular risk factors, including aspirin, beta-blockers, ACEIs, and statins.[18] In a cohort of more than 140,000 individuals,

the 1025 patients with proven CKD were less likely to receive these medications after an AMI than patients without CKD. Yet when receiving these drugs CKD patients had 30-day mortality risk reductions similar to those achieved in individuals with normal renal function. Notably, cardiovascular medications can be safely given to CKD patients if therapy is carefully adjusted and monitored.[18]

Type 5 cardiorenal syndrome (secondary cardiorenal syndrome) is characterized by concomitant cardiac and renal dysfunction due to acute or chronic systemic disorders such as sepsis, hypertension, diabetes, amyloidosis, and autoimmune diseases.

Severe sepsis can produce AKI and myocardial depression through the up-regulation of TNF-α and other proinflammatory mediators.[19] While decreased CO can further impair renal function, AKI can negatively affect cardiac performance. Hypotension-induced renal ischemia can further worsen myocardial injury in a vicious cycle harmful to both organs.[4,5] Therefore, early detection and interruption of this cycle is crucially important to improve cardiorenal outcomes.

Impact of Renal Impairment on Heart Failure Prognosis

The data summarized previously show that renal impairment increases the risk of cardiovascular disease in disparate clinical settings, including ischemic heart disease, acute coronary syndromes, surgical and percutaneous coronary arteries revascularization, cerebrovascular disease, and HF. In HF patients, renal dysfunction has become increasingly recognized as an independent risk factor for morbidity and mortality.[20-25] Given the growing epidemics of HF and CKD, both extraordinarily costly and morbid conditions, it is important to understand the impact of cardiorenal syndrome on outcomes in these patient groups[25,26] (Table 3.3).

A meta-analysis evaluated 16 cohort studies and retrospective analyses of randomized controlled trials whose primary objective was to analyze the association between serially assessed renal function and mortality in patients with an unequivocal HF diagnosis who were followed for at least 6 months. Secondary outcomes that were analyzed included cardiovascular mortality (all cardiovascular and pump failure mortality), hospital costs, and functional decline[27] (Table 3.4). In 12 studies more than 50% of patients had any renal impairment and 29% had moderate to severe renal impairment.[21-24,28-33] Prevalence of renal dysfunction was higher in hospitalized ADHF patients than in outpatients. In 11 studies all-cause 1-year mortality was 26%, 45%, and 51%, respectively, in patients with normal renal function, any renal impairment, and moderate to severe renal dysfunction.[21-26,28,30,31,33-39] This translated into a combined unadjusted relative mortality risk of 1.48 (95% confidence interval [CI], 1.45–1.52; $P < 0.001$) in patients with any renal impairment and of 1.81 (95% CI, 1.76–1.86; $P < 0.001$) in those with moderate to severe kidney dysfunction. In 9 studies, any renal impairment remained associated with higher mortality risk (1.56; 95% CI, 1.53–1.60; $P < 0.001$) after adjustment for demographic and clinical variables.[21-24,28,31,33,40] In 5 studies adjusted mortality risk was more than doubled in patients with moderate to severe renal impairment (2.31; 95% CI, 2.18–2.44; $P < 0.001$). Assessment of renal function as a continuous variable showed a 33% and 7% increase in mortality risk, respectively, for each 1-mg/dL increase in serum creatinine level and for each 10-mL/min decrease in GFR.[24,30,32,41,42] In one study, however, an increased mortality risk occurred only when estimated GFR was below 50 mL/min.[43] In 3 studies of hospitalized patients WRF during

Table 3.3: Etiologies of Comorbid Renal Insufficiency in Patients with Heart Failure

Intrinsic renal disease
- Renal vascular disease
- Nephron loss (diabetes mellitus, hypertension)
- Diuretic resistance

Inadequate renal perfusion
- Hypovolemia (inadequate preload)
- Inadequate cardiac output (excessive vasoconstriction)
- Hypotension
  - With normal cardiac output (vasodilator shock)
  - With low cardiac output (severe pump failure, cardiogenic shock)
- Abnormally high central venous pressure
- Drug-induced (nonsteroidal anti-inflammatory drugs [NSAIDs], cyclosporine, tacrolimus, ACEI, ARBs, etc)

hospitalization was associated with a significantly increased mortality risk (1.47; 95% CI, 1.26–1.72).[24,26,43]

In general, renal impairment predicted an increased risk of pump failure but not of arrhythmic death.[29,43,44] In hospitalized patients WRF was associated with increased hospitalizations costs and rehospitalization rates.[24,44] In ambulatory patients baseline renal dysfunction predicted an increased risk of the combined outcome of death or hospitalization for HF, and patients with severe renal impairment also had greater 6-month functional deterioration (odds ratio [OR] = 1.95; 95% CI, 1.16–3.28).[22,23,28]

Renal impairment significantly increases mortality risk in both ischemic and nonischemic HF patients. One study found

Table 3.4 Impact of Worsening Renal Function on Patients Clinical Outcomes and Resource Consumption

Outcomes	Total	WRF Absent	WRF Present	Adjusted Estimates*
In-hospital Mortality	68 (4%)	36 (3%)	32 (7%)	2.72 (1.62–4.58)
30 Day Mortality	123 (7%)	76 (6%)	47 (10%)	1.87 (1.25–2.80)
30 Day Readmission, all-cause	296 (18%)	201 (17%)	95 (20%)	1.29 (0.98–1.71)
30 Day Readmission, heart failure related	118 (7%)	80 (7%)	38 (8%)	1.17 (0.77–1.77)
6 Month Mortality	354 (21%)	235 (19%)	119 (25%)	1.56 (1.19–2.05)
6 Month Readmission, all-cause	790 (47%)	555 (46%)	235 (50%)	1.16 (0.93–1.44)
6 Month readmission, heart failure related	380 (23%)	264 (22%)	116 (25%)	1.07 (0.82–1.39)
Length of Hospital Stay, mean (SD) (d)	7.55 (4.70)	6.93 (3.92)	9.14 (6.01)	2.28 (0.25)†
Hospital cost, mean (SD)	$6,823 ($5,175)	$6,327 ($4,874)	$8,085 ($5,665)	$1,758 ($287.2)†

*Estimates were odds ratios and 95% confidence intervals for mortality and readmission outcomes, and regression coefficients and their standard errors for length of hospital stay and hospital cost outcomes; estimates adjusted for sex, age, diabetes, hypertension, rales, pulse, baseline creatinine, systolic blood pressure, and left ventricular ejection fraction.

†p < 0.0001.

Krumholz HM, Chen YT, Vaccarino V, et al. Correlates and impact on outcomes of worsening renal function in patients ≥ 65 years of age with heart failure. *Am J Cardiol.* 2000;85:1110–1113. With permission from Elsevier.

significantly higher mortality risk in whites versus blacks (2.61; 95% CI, 2.44–2.80 vs 1.99; 95% CI, 1.62–2.45; $P < 0.001$).[45] Women with HF and severe renal impairment have a significantly greater mortality risk than their male counterparts (2.40; 95% CI, 1.60–3.62).[28] Severity of HF symptoms appears to modify the effect of renal impairment on outcomes. In New York Heart Association (NYHA) functional class I and II patients mortality risk increases only with moderate to severe renal impairment (1.41; 95% CI, 1.15–1.73), whereas in NYHA functional class III and IV patients mortality risk increases with any renal impairment (2.10; 95% CI, 1.76–2.50) and to an even greater extent with severe renal impairment (3.23; 95% CI, 2.42–4.31). The presence of any renal impairment increased the risk of early mortality (< 1 year) more than that of late mortality (≥ 1 year): 1.84; 95% CI, 1.62–2.09; $P < 0.001$[20,46,47] (Figure 3.2).

The majority of HF patients included in the meta-analysis had some degree of renal impairment and should be considered as a high-risk group, given the 50% increased relative mortality risk compared to HF patients with normal renal function. In addition almost 30% of patients had moderate to severe renal impairment, which is associated with more than 100% increased relative mortality risk and an absolute 5-year mortality rate as high as 51%. White and symptomatic HF patients with renal dysfunction appear to have particularly poor outcomes. Given the prevalence and association of renal impairment with excess mortality in all HF patients, it is imperative to incorporate measures of renal function into risk-stratification models and to identify HF therapies tailored to this high-risk population. Though risk-stratification models in HF have increasingly included renal function for the prediction of mortality risk, therapies specifically aimed at reducing mortality in HF patients with renal impairment remain elusive.

Typically, HF patients with serum creatinine levels > 2.5 have been excluded from clinical trials and thus the benefits of drugs such as ACEIs and beta-blockers in patients with concomitant cardiac and renal dysfunction remain controversial.[20,23–25,30,32,48–50] It is possible that underutilization of these drugs itself contributes to the excess mortality occurring in HF patients with impaired renal function.

Notably, in the studies discussed, renal impairment was consistently associated with an increased mortality risk regardless of the highly variable definitions and measurements of renal impairment. However, identification of the best measure of renal function and standardization of the definitions of renal impairment may help to further characterize the impact of renal dysfunction on the prognosis of HF patients. Another open question is whether mortality risk escalates with increasing renal dysfunction or whether there is a threshold of GFR below which death rates are increased. One study found that mortality risk increases only when GFR drops below 50 mL/min.[45] In contrast, other analyses have shown that even at its mildest degrees renal impairment is associated with an incremental mortality risk. Importantly, newer measures of renal function, such as cystatin C, may be superior to currently used variables to assess the impact of renal dysfunction on HF prognosis.[51] Furthermore renal impairment may be a marker for worsening HF. Alternatively, renal impairment itself may worsen HF through the neurohormonal and inflammatory mechanisms outlined elsewhere in this book. The finding in healthy community subjects that baseline renal impairment increases the risk of developing HF provides initial evidence of a causal relationship between renal dysfunction and the onset of HF.[52]

Estimates of the prevalence of any renal impairment, despite the heterogeneity of

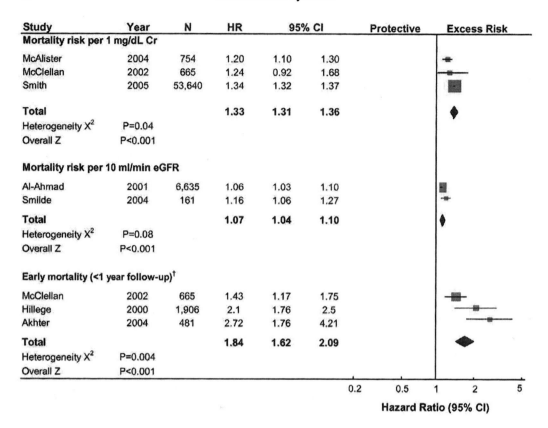

Study	Year	N	HR	95% CI		Protective	Excess Risk
Mortality risk per 1 mg/dL Cr							
McAlister	2004	754	1.20	1.10	1.30		
McClellan	2002	665	1.24	0.92	1.68		
Smith	2005	53,640	1.34	1.32	1.37		
Total			**1.33**	**1.31**	**1.36**		
Heterogeneity X^2	P=0.04						
Overall Z	P<0.001						
Mortality risk per 10 ml/min eGFR							
Al-Ahmad	2001	6,635	1.06	1.03	1.10		
Smilde	2004	161	1.16	1.06	1.27		
Total			**1.07**	**1.04**	**1.10**		
Heterogeneity X^2	P=0.08						
Overall Z	P<0.001						
Early mortality (<1 year follow-up)[†]							
McClellan	2002	665	1.43	1.17	1.75		
Hillege	2000	1,906	2.1	1.76	2.5		
Akhter	2004	481	2.72	1.76	4.21		
Total			**1.84**	**1.62**	**2.09**		
Heterogeneity X^2	P=0.004						
Overall Z	P<0.001						

0.2   0.5   1   2   5

Hazard Ratio (95% CI)

Figure 3.2. Incremental and early mortality risks. Smith GL, Lichtman JH, Bracken MB, et al. Renal impairment and outcomes in heart failure: systematic review and meta-analysis. *J Am Coll Cardiol.* 2006;47:1987–1996. With permission from Elsevier.

* Total HR = 1.20 (1.11, 1.30) when Smith et al[24] removed (disproportionately large sample size of hospitalized elderly) with heterogeneity X2, *P* = 0.84.

† Results not significantly different when using Smilde et al[45] for PRIME-I results instead of Hillege et al[21] or when Akhter et al[29] removed NYHA functional class IV only). When renal function was characterized continuously and linearly, renal impairment generally showed an incremental increase in mortality risk. A 33% increased mortality risk per 1 mg/dL creatinine (31%–36%, *P* < 0.001) (or 15% per every 0.5 mg/dL creatinine [14%–17%]) found in 3 studies[24,30,32] and a 7% increased mortality risk per 10 mL/min eGFR (4%–10%, *P* < 0.001) found in 2 studies[41,45] suggested a dose-response relationship.

CI = confidence interval; HR = hazard ratio.

definitions and populations, is surprisingly consistent in hospitalized and ambulatory patients, lending validity to the estimate that at least 50% of HF patients have renal impairment.

Renal impairment confers a clinically significant risk for excess mortality in patients with HF, and the magnitude of such risk is comparable to that imposed by traditional prognostic HF indicators, such as ejection fraction (Figure 3.3). Though more common in patients hospitalized for HF, at least some degree of renal impairment is still present in approximately 50% of stable HF patients. The prognostic importance of renal function in HF patients makes it imperative to identify the optimal methods for the detection and characterization of renal impairment in this patient population.

Renal Impairment and Prognosis in Acute Decompensated Heart Failure

An analysis from the Acute Decompensated Heart Failure National Registry (ADHERE), a large US database of patients hospitalized with a primary diagnosis of ADHF, showed that among 118,465 patients in whom admission GFR was estimated by the abbreviated Modification of Diet in Renal Disease (MDRD) formula, 10,660 patients (9.0%) had normal renal function (GFR ≥ 90), 32,423 (27.4%) had mild kidney dysfunction (GFR 60–89), 51,553 (43.5%) had moderate renal impairment (GFR 30–59), 15,553 (13.1%) had severe renal compromise (GFR 15–29), and 8276 (7.0%) had kidney failure (GFR < 15 or chronic dialysis). Notably, only 30% of the patients had been deemed to have renal impairment based upon admission serum creatinine level. Hospital mortality increased from 1.9% for patients with normal renal function to 7.6% and 6.5%, respectively, for patients with severe dysfunction and kidney failure, (P < 0.0001)[53] (Figure 3.4). These

findings draw attention to the fact that renal dysfunction is frequent in patients hospitalized for ADHF, is not adequately identified by serum creatinine level alone, and carries important prognostic implications.[53] A separate analysis of variables predicting mortality in patients from ADHERE showed that the best single predictor for mortality in this population was an admission BUN level (≥ 43 mg/dL) followed by low admission systolic blood pressure (< 115 mm Hg) and then by serum creatinine levels > 2.75 mg/dL. The risk tree analysis performed in this population identified patient groups with hospital mortality ranging from 2.1% (patients without the 3 risk factors) to 21.9% (patients with all 3 risk factors). The odds ratio for mortality between patients identified as high and low risk was 12.9 (95% CI, 10.4–15.9)[47] (Figure 3.5).

Interestingly, the finding that BUN is superior to serum creatinine in predicting the outcomes of hospitalized ADHF is consistent with the results of several other studies. A retrospective analysis of 949 patients from the Outcomes of a Prospective Trial of Intravenous Milrinone for Exacerbations of Chronic Heart Failure (OPTIME-CHF), investigating the relationship between admission values and changes in BUN and estimated GFR and death rates by 60 days after discharge, showed that both lower admission GFR and higher baseline BUN were associated with a greater 60-day mortality risk. However, when the prognostic value of these renal function variables was tested in a multivariable analysis, BUN emerged as a stronger predictor of 60-day mortality than GFR. Furthermore, independently of admission values, an increase of 10 mg/dL in BUN during hospitalization was associated with lower 60-day survival rates (hazard ratio [HR], 1.08; 95% CI, 1.01–1.16 per 5-mg/dL BUN increase).[54] The finding that admission BUN and change in BUN during hospitalization (independent of the admission value) was a

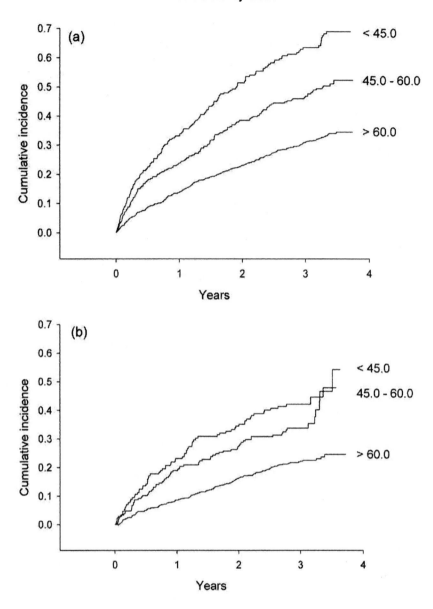

Figure 3.3. Kaplan-Meier plot of cumulative incidence of
cardiovascular death or unplanned admission to hospital
for the management of worsening HF stratified by < 45.0,
45.0 to 60.0, and > 60 mL/min per 1.73 m^2 eGFR in mL/
min per 1.73 m^2 in patients with (a) reduced LVEF (LVEF
≤ 40%) and (b) preserved LV systolic function (LVEF
> 40%). Hillege HL, Nitsch D, Pfeffer MA, et al. Renal
function as a predictor of outcome in a broad spectrum
of patients with heart failure. *Circulation.* 2006;113:671–
678. With permission.

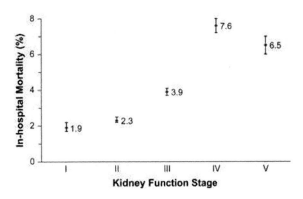

Figure 3.4. In-hospital mortality by kidney function stage for 118,465 hospitalizations for ADHF recorded in the Acute Decompensated Heart Failure National Registry (ADHERE). GFR was estimated using the abbreviated MDRD study formula. In-hospital mortality increased with severity of baseline renal dysfunction. Error bars depict the 95% CIs for the point estimates. Heywood JT, Fonarow GC, Costanzo MR et al. High prevalence of renal dysfunction and its impact on outcome in 118,465 patients hospitalized with acute decompensated heart failure: a report from the ADHERE database. *J Cardiac Fail.* 2007;13;422–430. With permission from Elsevier.

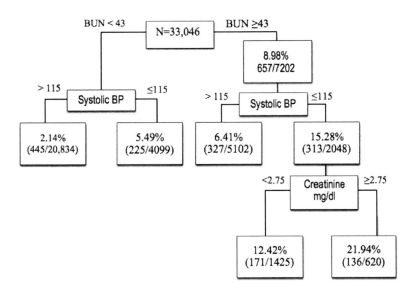

Figure 3.5. Predictors of in-hospital mortality developed and validated in the ADHERE heart failure registry. Using Classification and Regression Tree (CART) analysis multiple clinical and laboratory parameters were examined to determine their effect on mortality for patients admitted with decompensated heart failure. The most parsimonious model included only admission BUN, systolic blood pressure and serum creatinine. Multiple cut points for these parameters were evaluated. After the model was constructed with a derivation cohort (shown) it was validated in a second large cohort prospectively with very similar results. As can be seen renal parameters accounted for 2 of the three most important predictors of mortality, with a ten fold difference in mortality between the lowest and highest risk groups. Adapted from Fonarow GC, Adams KF Jr, Abraham WT, Yancy CW, Boscardin WJ. Risk stratification for in-hospital mortality in acutely decompensated heart failure classification and regression tree analysis. *JAMA.* 2005;293:572–580.

statistically superior predictor of outcomes than was GFR is at first surprising, because BUN is not as reliable as GFR in the assessment of renal function due to the influence on BUN levels of protein intake, catabolism, and tubular reabsorption of urea. The latter is flow dependent, so that more urea is reabsorbed at lower urine flow rates.[55] Most importantly, the reabsorption of urea in the collecting duct is mediated by the effect of arginine vasopressin (AVP) on the urea transporter in this portion of the nephron.[55] Thus the rise in BUN may serve as an index of the extent of neurohumoral activation over and above any fall in GFR. In fact, separation of patients in BUN quartiles revealed an increase in 60-day mortality with the rise in BUN quartile. Notably, the use of ACEIs decreased significantly as the admission BUN rose, despite the fact patients with the higher BUN values may have the greatest need for the antineurohormonal effects of ACEIs.[54] Another interesting observation in the OPTIME-CHF study is the significant rise in jugular venous pressure as quartile BUN values rose. The associated increase in renal venous pressure increases renal interstitial pressure and activates the RAAS.[55] Moreover, increases in cardiac preload and cardiac dilatation are known to be important risk factors for increased death rate in HF patients.[55] Notably, in 145 ADHF patients increased CVP, but not CO, was independently associated with renal dysfunction, WRF, and unfavorable outcomes[56] (Figure 3.6). The discordance between cardiac performance and renal function challenges the notion that, in HF, renal insufficiency solely represents hypoperfusion of the kidney as the result of poor forward flow or overzealous diuresis.[55] Instead, growing evidence shows that hyper-

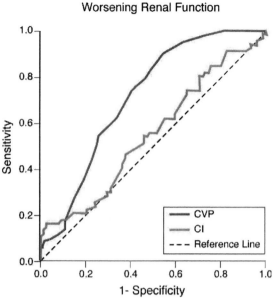

Worsening Renal Function

Figure 3.6. Receiver-operating characteristic (ROC) curves for central venous pressure (CVP) and cardiac index (CI) on admission for the development of WRF in 145 patients hospitalized for ADHF and treated with intensive medical therapy guided by pulmonary artery catheter. WRF was defined as an increase of serum creatinine ≥ 0.3 mg/dL during hospitalization. Fifty-eight patients (40%) developed WRF. Patients who developed WRF had a greater CVP on admission (18 ± 7 vs 12 ± 6 mm Hg, $P < 0.001$) and after intensive medical therapy (11 ± 8 vs 8 ± 5 mm Hg, $P = 0.04$). The development of WRF occurred less frequently in patients who achieved a CVP < 8 mm Hg ($P = 0.01$). Using ROC curve analysis, baseline CVP (0.734, $P < 0.0001$) but not baseline CI (0.552, $P = 0.6$) predicted the development of WRF (difference $P = 0.012$). Mullens W, Abrhams Z, Francis GS et al. Importance of venous congestion for worsening renal function in advanced decompensated heart failure. *J Am Coll Cardiol.* 2009;53: 589–596. With permission from Elsevier.

volemia by itself is independently associated with mortality.[57] Enhanced renal sodium and water reabsorption predominantly fills the compliant venous circulation, increasing CVP and atrial pressures. In the Evaluation Study of Congestive Heart Failure and Pulmonary Artery Catheterization Effectiveness (ESCAPE) trial, right atrial pressure emerged as the only hemodynamic variable correlated with baseline renal function, an independent predictor of mortality and HF hospitalization.[58] Indeed in this analysis from ESCAPE baseline renal insufficiency, defined as an estimated GFR < 60 mL/min but not WRF, defined as an increase in serum creatinine ≥ 0.3 mg/dL during treatment for ADHF, was associated with an increased risk of death and HF rehospitalization.[58]

Worsening Renal Function During Hospitalization and Prognosis

Several studies have documented that, during hospitalization for HF, > 70% of patients will experience some increase in serum creatinine, with approximately 20% to 30% having increments > 0.3 mg/dL. Deterioration in renal function occurs early in the course of the hospitalization and is independently associated with longer hospitalizations, greater costs, and higher short- and long-term mortality[34,35,43,44,59] (Figure 3.7). Nonetheless, it remains unclear whether WRF itself contributes to the increased mortality or whether it represents more advanced HF. Rates of WRF

during hospitalization are similar in patients with decreased or preserved LV ejection fraction, supporting the evidence that in HF forward flow is not the sole determinant of renal function.[27,35,59] On average, persons developing WRF are older and more often have prior HF, renal dysfunction, diabetes, and hypertension (Table 3.5). Cox regression analysis in 1004 heterogeneous HF patients permitted the development of a risk score for predicting which patients with ADHF are likely to develop WRF. With the allocation of 1 point each to HF history, diabetes, and systolic blood pressure > 160 mm Hg at admission, 2 points to creatinine level of 1.5 to 2.4 mg/dL, and 3 points to creatinine level ≥ 2.5 mg/dL, 35% of the patients had a score of ≥ 3 and a 43% likelihood of WRF.[34]

A prospective cohort study of 412 patients hospitalized for HF compared various definitions of WRF (absolute serum creatinine elevations ≥ 0.1–0.5 mg/dL and 25% relative elevation from baseline) to identify which index of WRF was most closely associated with 6-month mortality, rehospitalization, and functional decline. Serum creatinine elevation ≥ 0.1 mg/dL and ≥ 0.5

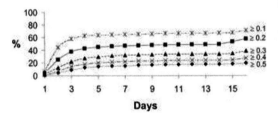

Figure 3.7. The time course of development of increasing serum creatinine of various extents. When the creatinine increased, it occurred soon after hospital admission. Of 1004 patients, 723 (72%) developed increased serum creatinine during the hospitalization, with 20% developing an increase of ≥ 0.5 mg/dL. Worsening renal function predicted both in-hospital mortality and length of stay > 10 days. Even an increased creatinine of 0.1 mg/dL was associated with worse outcome. Sensitivity for death decreased from 92% to 65% as the threshold for increased creatinine was raised from 0.1 to 0.5 mg/dL, with specificity increasing from 28% to 81%. At a threshold of a 0.3 mg/dL increase, sensitivity was 81% and specificity was 62% for death and 64% and 65% for length of stay > 10 days. Adding a requirement of final creatinine of ≥ 1.5 mg/dL improved specificity. Gottlieb SS, Abraham W, Butler J, et al. The prognostic importance of different definitions of worsening renal function in congestive heart failure. *J Card Fail.* 2002;8:136–141. With permission from Elsevier.

Table 3.5 Correlates of Worsening Renal Function

Characteristics	Adjusted OR*	95% CI	P value
Women	1.41	1.12–1.77	0.003
Systemic hypertension	1.64	1.12–2.40	0.003
Rales > basilar	1.28	1.02–1.61	0.03
Pulse > 100 beats/min	1.34	1.06–1.68	0.01
sCr ≥ 1.5 mg/dL	1.77	1.42–2.22	< 0.001
Systolic blood pressure > 200 mm Hg	1.63	1.13–2.35	0.009

Adjusted OR = odds ratio adjusted for other variables in the table;
CI= confidence interval; OR= odds ratio; sCr = serum creatinine

Krumholz HM, Chen YT, Vaccarino V, et al. Correlates and impact on outcomes of worsening renal function in patients > or = 65 years of age with heart failure. *Am J Cardiol*. 2000;85:1110–1113. With permission from Elsevier.

mg/dL occurred, respectively, in 75% and 24% of the patients. Risk of death increased with higher serum creatinine elevations (adjusted HR = 0.89, 1.19, 1.67, 1.91, and 2.90 for increases ≥ 0.1–0.5 mg/dL). In this study, although larger serum creatinine elevations predicted the highest risk of death, even minor renal function changes during hospitalization were associated with unfavorable outcomes.[44]

None of the studies summarized here, however, provide an answer to the question of whether WRF is more likely to occur in sicker patients who have poorer outcomes because of the severity of their underlying cardiac disease or whether WRF *itself* hastens HF progression and thus contributes to the occurrence of adverse outcomes.[27]

Worsening Renal Function and Diuretic Therapy

The use of high intravenous loop diuretic doses has been linked to the development of WRF in several studies.[60-63] In a nested case control study of 382 subjects hospitalized for HF, diuretic doses were higher in the 191 patients who developed WRF, defined as a rise in serum creatinine level > 0.3 mg/dL, than in those without WRF (199 ± 195 mg vs 143 ± 119 mg, $P < 0.05$), without differences in fluid intake/output or weight changes. Together with a history of diabetes mellitus or HF, systolic blood pressure > 160 mm Hg or serum creatinine levels > 2.5 mg/dL and use of calcium channel blockers, higher loop diuretic doses on the day preceding WRF independently predicted a higher risk for WRF.[38] The association between higher diuretic doses and development of WRF is not readily explainable. One possibility is that a subgroup of HF patients refractory to diuretics, and therefore requiring higher doses of these drugs during HF decompensation, are especially susceptible to the development of WRF. In fact, these patients had significantly higher admission serum creatinine levels and included a higher percentage of patients requiring thiazide—in addition to loop diuretics. Although higher diuretic doses may have increased the risk of WRF because of a greater diuresis, this possibility is unlikely

due to the observation that different diuretic doses produced similar fluid losses. Another plausible explanation is that patients with WRF required higher diuretic doses because of more advanced HF. However, indices of HF severity were similar in patients and control subjects. Therefore, the question of whether higher diuretic doses are responsible for WRF or are a marker of greater disease severity remains unanswered.[38] Among 395 ESCAPE patients treated with diuretics a strong correlation was identified between in-hospital diuretic dose and 6-month mortality ($P = 0.003$), especially at > 300 mg/day (Figure 3.8). Diuretic dose remained a significant predictor of mortality

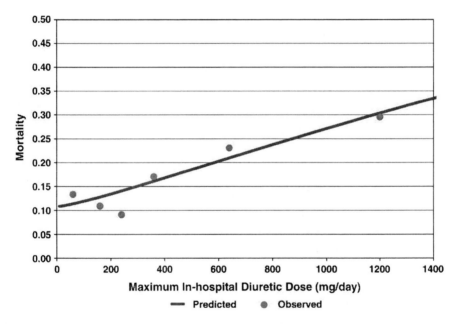

Figure 3.8. Mortality as a function of in-hospital diuretic dose in 395 patients from the ESCAPE trial who received diuretics during admission. Baseline weight, length of stay, and baseline BNP were significant predictors of weight loss. After adjusting for these factors, in-hospital diuretic dose was not a significant predictor of weight loss. A strong relation between dose and mortality was seen ($P = 0.003$), especially at > 300 mg/day. Dose remained a significant predictor of mortality after adjusting for baseline variables that significantly predicted mortality. Correlation between maximal dose and creatinine level change was not significant ($r = 0.043$; $P = 0.412$). Hasselblad V, Gattis Stough W, Shah M, et al. Relation between dose of loop diuretics and outcomes in a heart failure population: results of the ESCAPE trial. *Eur J Heart Fail*. 2007;9:1064–1069. By permission of Oxford University Press.

after adjusting for baseline variables that significantly predicted mortality, including age > 65 years and BUN and serum sodium levels. While this observational analysis cannot establish a cause-and-effect relation between high-dose diuretic and increased mortality, the results raise the concern that this relationship may exist.[58-65] In addition, in the analysis from ESCAPE diuretic dose was associated with increases in serum creatinine from baseline to discharge. As previously discussed, WRF has been shown to independently predict mortality in other studies.[44,47,52,53] These findings and the association between diuretic dose and mortality raise concerns regarding the additional observation from ESCAPE that higher diuretic doses are also associated with WRF.[61]

Other studies have examined the effects of high-dose loop diuretics. Twenty patients with decompensated HF were randomized to 1 of 3 groups: (1) low-dose dopamine and low-dose oral furosemide (40 mg orally twice daily); (2) low-dose dopamine and furosemide continuous infusion (5 mg/kg/day); and (3) high-dose furosemide continuous infusion (10 mg/kg/day). Despite similar improvement in congestive symptoms and weight loss the 2 groups treated with intravenous furosemide experienced significant decreases in mean arterial blood pressure and WRF.[62] A study comparing high-dose nitrates (3 mg bolus every 5 min) plus low-dose furosemide (40 mg bolus) with low-dose nitrates (1 mg/h, doubled every 10 min) plus high-dose furosemide (80 mg bolus every 15 min) showed that compared to the low-dose loop diuretic group, patients treated with higher furosemide doses included a greater percentage of patients requiring mechanical ventilation (40% vs 13%, $P = 0.0041$) and achieving the composite end point of death, mechanical ventilation, or myocardial infarction.[63] Data from the ADHERE database suggest that patients treated with intravenous diuretics had higher hospital mortality, longer hospitalization, and longer length of stay in the intensive care unit than patients not treated with intravenous diuretics, even after adjusting for other prognostic factors.[64]

Finally, in 318 ADHF patients, WRF (defined as the occurrence, at any time during the hospitalization, of both a ≥ 25% and a ≥ 0.3 mg/dL increase in serum creatinine from admission) was an independent predictor of death or HF rehospitalization (adjusted HR, 1.47; 95% CI, 1.13–1.81; $P = 0.024$). By multivariable logistic regression the independent predictors of WRF were history of CKD ($P = 0.002$), LVEF ($P = 0.012$), furosemide daily dose ($P = 0.03$), and NYHA class ($P = 0.05$) on admission.[65] The results of this study support the hypothesis that higher loop diuretic doses are associated with a worse prognosis because they aggravate renal impairment. However, the possibility that the administration of higher doses of furosemide is a consequence, rather than a cause, of more advanced HF and coexistent renal failure cannot be excluded, making high diuretic doses only a marker rather than a cause of poor outcomes. In this study the fact that signs of congestion were more frequent in patients with WRF, whereas weight loss was similar in patients with and without WRF, suggests that patients with WRF had diuretic resistance, not excessive fluid loss.

Conclusion

Renal impairment is common, occurring in 30% of ambulatory and > 50% of hospitalized HF patients, and remains frequently unrecognized. Even mild renal insufficiency worsens the outcomes of patients with CVD in general and of patients with HF in particular. Therapies such as ACEIs, ARBs, aldosterone antagonists, and beta-blockers have similar benefits in HF patients with and in those without renal impairment. Unfortunately HF patients with renal dysfunction are often deprived of these lifesaving medications, which instead should be used even more aggressively in individuals with cardiorenal syndrome due to their poorer prognosis. The unfavorable effects of renal insufficiency on outcomes are similar in patients with decreased and preserved LV systolic function. In addition, the prognostic impact of kidney dysfunction is independent of that of other variables affecting prognosis, including age, LV ejection fraction, serum sodium levels, and symptom status. In HF patients a rapid decline in GFR is associated with increased mortality independent of worsening HF and baseline renal function. It remains unclear whether the relationship between renal function and outcomes is graded or whether mortality increases sharply below a GFR threshold at which factors such as anemia, inflammation, and diuretic resistance are more likely to be present. In HF patients renal impairment and WRF not only decrease survival but also increase length of hospitalization, healthcare costs, and rehospitalization rates. In general WRF during hospitalization for ADHF appears to provide prognostic information independent of admission renal function values. To date a cause–and–effect relationship between high–dose loop diuretics and increased mortality has not been firmly established, but the results of several studies raise the concern that this relationship may exist. Cardiorenal syndrome has recently been classified according to whether the impairment of each organ is primary or secondary, or whether heart and kidney dysfunction occurs simultaneously as a result of a systemic disease. A consensus definition of each type of cardiorenal syndrome may help to design randomized controlled trials aimed at identifying pathophysiologically sound interventions targeting specific patient populations.

References

1. Sica DA. Sodium and water retention in heart failure and diuretic therapy: basic mechanisms. *Cleve Clin J Med.* 2006;73(suppl 2):S2–S7.

2. Farrar DJ, Hill JD. Recovery of major organ function in patients awaiting heart transplantation with Thoratec ventricular devices. Thoratec Ventricular Assist Device Principal Investigators. *J Heart Lung Transplant.* 1994;13:1125–1132.

3. Schrier RW. Role of diminished renal function in cardiovascular mortality: marker or pathogenic factor? *J Am Coll Cardiol.* 2006;47:1–8.

4. Ronco C, Haapio M, House AA. Cardiorenal syndrome. *J Am Coll Cardiol.* 2008;52: 1527–1539.

5. Bongartz LG, Cramer MJ, Doevendans PA, et al. The severe cardiorenal syndrome. "Guyton revisited." *Eur Heart J.* 2005;26:11–7.

6. Schrier RW, Abraham WT. Hormones and hemodynamics in heart failure. *N Engl J Med.* 1999;341:577–585.

7. Mebazaa A, Gheorghiade M, Pina IL, et al. Practical recommendations for prehospital and early in–hospital management of patients presenting with acute heart failure syndromes. *Crit Care Med.* 2008;36:S129–S139.

8. Fonarow GC, Stough WG, Abraham WT, et al. Characteristics, treatments, and outcomes of patients with preserved systolic function hospitalized for heart failure: a report from the OPTIMIZE-HF registry. *J Am Coll Cardiol.* 2007;50: 768–777

9. Nguyen MT, Ross GF, Dent CL, Devarajan P. Early prediction of acute renal injury using urinary proteomics. *Am J Nephrol.* 2005;25:318–326.

10. Mishra J, Dent C, Tarabishi R, et al. Neutrophil gelatinase–associated lipocalin (NGAL) as a biomarker for

acute renal injury after cardiac surgery. *Lancet*. 2005;365:1231–1238.

11. Dharnidharka VR, Kwon C, Stevens G. Serum cystatin C is superior to serum creatinine as a marker of kidney function: a meta-analysis *Am J Kidney Dis*. 2002;40:221–226.

12. Hillege HL, Nitsch D, Pfeffer MA, et al. Renal function as a predictor of outcome in a broad spectrum of patients with heart failure. *Circulation*. 2006;113:671–678.

13. Palazzuoli A, Silverberg DS, Iovine F, et al. Effects of beta-erythropoietin treatment on left ventricular remodeling, systolic function, and B-type natriuretic peptide levels in patients with the cardiorenal anemia syndrome. *Am Heart J*. 2007;154:645e9–15.

14. Bagshaw SM, George C, Dinu I, Bellomo R. A multi-centre evaluation of the RIFLE criteria for early acute kidney injury in critically ill patients. *Nephrol Dial Transplant*. 2008;23:1203–1210.

15. Meyer TW, Hostetter TH. Uremia. *N Engl J Med*. 2007;357:1316–1325.

16. Hirsch AT, Haskal ZJ, Hertzer NR, et al. ACC/AHA guidelines for the management of patients with peripheral arterial disease (lower extremity, renal, mesenteric, and abdominal aortic): a collaborative report from the American Association for Vascular Surgery/Society for Vascular Surgery, Society for Cardiovascular Angiography and Interventions, Society of Interventional Radiology, Society for Vascular Medicine and Biology, and the American College of Cardiology/American Heart Association Task Force on Practice Guidelines (Writing Committee to Develop Guidelines for the Management of Patients With Peripheral Arterial Disease). *J Am Coll Cardiol*. 2006;47:e1–e192.

17. Braunwald E. Biomarkers in heart failure. *N Engl J Med*. 2008;358:2148–2159.

18. Berger AK, Duval S, Krumholz HM. Aspirin, beta-blocker, and angiotensin-converting enzyme inhibitor therapy in patients with end-stage renal disease and an acute myocardial infarction. *J Am Coll Cardiol*. 2003;42:201–208.

19. Kumar A, Paladugu B, Mensing J, Kumar A, Parrillo JE. Nitric oxide–dependent and –independent mechanisms are involved in TNF-alpha–induced depression of cardiac myocyte contractility. *Am J Physiol Regul Integr Comp Physiol*. 2007;292:R1900–R1906.

20. Shlipak MG. Pharmacotherapy for heart failure in patients with renal insufficiency. *Ann Intern Med*. 2003;138:917–924.

21. Hillege HL, Girbes AR, de Kam PJ, et al. Renal function, neurohormonal activation, and survival in patients with chronic heart failure. *Circulation*. 2000;102:203–210.

22. Bibbins-Domingo K, Lin F, Vittinghoff E, Barrett-Connor E, Grady D, Shlipak MG. Renal insufficiency as an independent predictor of mortality among women with heart failure. *J Am Coll Cardiol*. 2004;44:1593–1600.

23. Shlipak MG, Smith GL, Rathore SS, Massie BM, Krumholz HM. Renal function, digoxin therapy, and heart failure outcomes: evidence from the digoxin intervention group trial. *J Am Soc Nephrol*. 2004;15:2195–2203.

24. Smith GL, Shlipak MG, Havranek EP, et al. Race and renal impairment in heart failure: mortality in blacks versus whites. *Circulation*. 2005;111:1270–1277.

25. Ezekowitz J, McAlister FA, Humphries KH, et al. The association among renal insufficiency, pharmacotherapy, and outcomes in 6,427 patients with heart

failure and coronary artery disease. *J Am Coll Cardiol.* 2004;44:1587–1592.

26. Jessup M, Brozena S. Heart failure. *N Engl J Med.* 2003;348:2007–2018.

27. Smith GL, Lichtman JH, Bracken MB, et al. Renal impairment and outcomes in heart failure: systematic review and meta-analysis. *J Am Coll Cardiol.* 2006;47:1987–1996.

28. Dries DL, Exner DV, Domanski MJ, Greenberg B, Stevenson LW. The prognostic implications of renal insufficiency in asymptomatic and symptomatic patients with left ventricular systolic dysfunction. *J Am Coll Cardiol.* 2000;35:681–689.

29. Akhter MW, Aronson D, Bitar F, et al. Effect of elevated admission serum creatinine and its worsening on outcome in hospitalized patients with decompensated heart failure. *Am J Cardiol.* 2004;94:957–960.

30. McClellan WM, Flanders WD, Langston RD, Jurkovitz C, Presley R. Anemia and renal insufficiency are independent risk factors for death among patients with congestive heart failure admitted to community hospitals: a population-based study. *J Am Soc Nephrol.* 2002;13:1928–1936.

31. Marenzi G, Lauri G, Guazzi M, et al. Cardiac and renal dysfunction in chronic heart failure: relation to neurohumoral activation and prognosis. *Am J Med Sci.* 2001;321:359–366.

32. McAlister FA, Ezekowitz J, Tonelli M, Armstrong PW. Renal insufficiency and heart failure: prognostic and therapeutic implications from a prospective cohort study. *Circulation.* 2004;109:1004–1009.

33. Shlipak MG, Katz R, Fried LF, et al. Cystatin-C and mortality in elderly persons with heart failure. *J Am Coll Cardiol.* 2005;45:268–271.

34. Gottlieb SS, Abraham W, Butler J, et al. The prognostic importance of different definitions of worsening renal function in congestive heart failure. *J Card Fail.* 2002;8:136–141.

35. Forman DE, Butler J, Wang Y, et al. Incidence, predictors at admission, and impact of worsening renal function among patients hospitalized with heart failure. *J Am Coll Cardiol.* 2004;43:61–67.

36. Herzog CA, Muster HA, Li S, Collins AJ. Impact of congestive heart failure, chronic kidney disease, and anemia on survival in the Medicare population. *J Card Fail.* 2004;10:467–472.

37. Harris RP, Helfand M, Woolf SH, et al. Current methods of the U.S. Preventive Services Task Force: a review of the process. *Am J Prev Med.* 2001;20: 21–35.

38. Levine M, Walter S, Lee H, Haines T, Holbrook A, Moyer V. Evidence-Based Medicine Working Group Users' guides to the medical literature. IV. How to use an article about harm. *JAMA.* 1994;271:1615–1619.

39. Katz S, Downs TD, Cash HR, Grotz RC. Progress in development of the index of ADL Gerontologist 1970;10:20–3018. The Cochrane Collaboration. Available at: www.cochrane.org. Accessed July 20, 2005.

40. Mahon NG, Blackstone EH, Francis GS, Starling RC III, Young JB, Lauer MS. The prognostic value of estimated creatinine clearance alongside functional capacity in ambulatory patients with chronic congestive heart failure. *J Am Coll Cardiol.* 2002;40:1106–1113.

41. Al-Ahmad A, Rand WM, Manjunath G, et al. Reduced kidney function and anemia as risk factors for mortality in patients with left ventricular dysfunction. *J Am Coll Cardiol.* 2001;38: 955–962.

42. Smilde TD, Hillege HL, Voors AA, Dunselman PH, Van Veldhuisen DJ. Prognostic importance of renal function in patients with early heart failure and mild left ventricular dysfunction. *Am J Cardiol.* 2004;94:240–243.

43. Krumholz HM, Chen YT, Vaccarino V, et al. Correlates and impact on outcomes of worsening renal function in patients > or = 65 years of age with heart failure. *Am J Cardiol.* 2000;85:1110–1113.

44. Smith GL, Vaccarino V, Kosiborod M, et al. Worsening renal function: what is a clinically meaningful change in creatinine during hospitalization with heart failure? *J Card Fail.* 2003;9:13–25.

45. Smilde TD, Hillege HL, Navis G, Boomsma F, de Zeeuw D, van Veldhuisen DJ. Impaired renal function in patients with ischemic and nonischemic chronic heart failure: association with neurohormonal activation and survival. *Am Heart J.* 2004;148:165–172.

46. Lee DS, Austin PC, Rouleau JL, Liu PP, Naimark D, Tu JV. Predicting mortality among patients hospitalized for heart failure: derivation and validation of a clinical model. *JAMA.* 2003;290:2581–2587.

47. Fonarow GC, Adams KF Jr, Abraham WT, Yancy CW, Boscardin WJ. Risk stratification for in-hospital mortality in acutely decompensated heart failure classification and regression tree analysis. *JAMA.* 2005;293:572–580.

48. Ljungman S, Kjekshus J, Swedberg K. Renal function in severe congestive heart failure during treatment with enalapril (the Cooperative North Scandinavian Enalapril Survival Study [CONSENSUS] Trial). *Am J Cardiol.* 1992;70:479–487.

49. Masoudi FA, Rathore SS, Wang Y, et al. National patterns of use and effectiveness of angiotensin-converting enzyme inhibitors in older patients with heart failure and left ventricular systolic dysfunction. *Circulation.* 2004;110:724–731.

50. Sackner-Bernstein JD, Skopicki HA, Aaronson KD. Risk of worsening renal function with nesiritide in patients with acutely decompensated heart failure. *Circulation.* 2005;111:1487–1491.

51. Sarnak MJ, Katz R, Stehman-Breen CO, et al. Cystatin C concentration as a risk factor for heart failure in older adults. *Ann Intern Med.* 2005;142:497–505.

52. Sarnak MJ, Coronado BE, Greene T, et al. Cardiovascular disease risk factors in chronic renal insufficiency. *Clin Nephrol.* 2002;57:327–335.

53. Heywood JT, Fonarow GC, Costanzo MR, et al. High prevalence of renal dysfunction and its impact on outcome in 118,465 patients hospitalized with acute decompensated heart failure: a report from the ADHERE database. *J Cardiac Fail.* 2007;13;422–430.

54. Klein L, Massie BM, Leimberger JD, et al. Admission or changes in renal function during hospitalization for worsening heart failure predict postdischarge survival: results from the Outcomes of a Prospective Trial of Intravenous Milrinone for Exacerbations of Chronic Heart Failure (OPTIME-CHF). *Circ Heart Fail.* 2008;1:25–33.

55. Schrier RW. Blood urea nitrogen and serum creatinine: not married in heart failure. *Circ Heart Fail.* 2008;1:2–5.

56. Mullens W, Abrahams Z, Francis GS, et al. Importance of venous congestion for worsening renal function in advanced decompensated heart failure. *J Am Coll Cardiol.* 2009;53:589–596.

57. Jessup M, Costanzo MR. The cardiorenal syndrome: do we need a change in strategy or a change of tactics? *J Am Coll Cardiol.* 2009;53:597–599.

58. Nohria A, Hasselblad V, Stebbins A, et al. cardiorenal interaction: insights from the ESCAPE trial. *J Am Coll Cardiol.* 2008;51:1268–1274.

59. Owan TE, Hodge DO, Herges RM, et al. Secular trends in renal dysfunction and outcomes in heart failure patients. *J Card Fail.* 2006;12:257–262.

60. Butler J, Forman DE, Abraham WT, et al. Relationship between heart failure treatment and development of worsening renal function among hospitalized heart failure patients. *Am Heart J.* 2004;147:331–338.

61. Hasselblad V, Gattis Stough W, Shah M, et al. Relation between dose of loop diuretics and outcomes in a heart failure population: results of the ESCAPE trial. *Eur J Heart Fail.* 2007;9:1064–1069.

62. Cotter G, Weissgarten J, Metzkor E, et al. Increased toxicity of high-dose furosemide versus low-dose dopamine in the treatment of refractory congestive heart failure. *Clin Pharmacol Ther.* 1997;62:187–193.

63. Cotter G, Metzkor E, Kaluski E, et al. Randomised trial of high-dose isosorbide dinitrate plus low-dose furosemide versus high-dose furosemide plus low-dose isosorbide dinitrate in severe pulmonary oedema. *Lancet.* 1998;351:389–393.

64. Peacock WF, Costanzo MR, De Marco T, et al. Impact of intravenous diuretics on outcomes of patients hospitalized with acute decompensated heart failure: insights from the ADHERE registry. *Cardiology.* 2008;113:12–19.

65. Metra M, Nodari S, Parrinello G, et al. Worsening renal function in patients hospitalised for acute heart failure: clinical implications and prognostic significance. *Eur J Heart Fail.* 2008;10: 188–195.

Epidemiology of Cardiorenal Syndrome

4

Kalkidan G. Bishu
Margaret M. Redfield

Cardiorenal syndrome has been variably defined in the clinical literature, and a clear standardized definition is currently lacking. It is generally described as a disorder of the heart and kidneys in which an acute or chronic dysfunction in one organ may result in acute or chronic dysfunction in the other organ.[1] Liang et al[2] notes 3 features: concomitant renal and heart disease, worsening renal function during acute heart failure (HF) treatment, and diuretic resistance. Ronco et al[1] proposed 5 types characterizing the chronology of the pathophysiologic interactions between the kidney and the heart. In this chapter we describe the epidemiology of chronic kidney disease (CKD) and HF initially and then describe studies on the prevalence and incidence of several types of

cardiorenal syndrome. We will describe risk factors that have been identified for CKD, HF, and cardiorenal syndrome and discuss the implication of the projected prevalences for associated risk factors on the prevalence of cardiorenal syndrome.

Epidemiology of Chronic Kidney Disease and End-Stage Renal Disease

CKD is defined as glomerular filtration rate (GFR) < 60 mL/min/1.73 m^2 for at least 3 months or evidence of kidney damage for at least 3 months manifested by abnormalities of markers of kidney damage in the composition of blood or urine or abnormalities in imaging studies).[3] CKD is classified into 5 stages depending on the degree of loss of renal function as measured by GFR (Table 4.1).[3]

The Cardiorenal Syndrome: A Clinician's Guide to Pathophysiology and Management, 1st ed. © 2012 J. Thomas Heywood and John C. Burnett Jr., eds. Cardiotext Publishing, ISBN: 978-0-9790164-7-9.

Table 4.1 Chronic Kidney Disease Classification[3]

Stage 1   Abnormalities of kidney studies with GFR $\geq$ 90 mL/min/1.73 m^2

Stage 2   Evidence of kidney damage and mild decrease in GFR to 60–89 mL/min/1.73 m^2

Stage 3   GFR 30–59 mL/min/1.73 m^2

Stage 4   GFR 15–29 mL/min/1.73 m^2

Stage 5/ESRD   Dialysis or GFR < 15 mL/min/1.73 m^2

Patients in all stages of CKD are considered to be among the highest risk group of patients for cardiovascular disease (CVD). These patients are ultimately more likely to die from cardiovascular causes than they are to require dialysis or renal transplantation.

The 2008 US Renal Data System (USRDS) report shows that Medicare patients with recognized CKD are 5 times more likely to die than to progress to end-stage renal disease (ESRD/stage 5 CKD). Death in this group of patients is highly correlated with advancing cardiovascular morbidity. At 2 years' follow-up, among those who die, 63% have congestive heart failure (CHF) and 57% have atherosclerotic heart disease (Figure 4.1). Among those who remain alive at 2 years, 70% carry a diagnosis for CVD.[4] A study by Keith et al[5] with a longitudinal follow-up of 27,998 patients with CKD stage 2, 3, or 4 in a large managed care organization showed that the rate of renal replacement therapy over a 5-year period was 1.1%, 1.3%, and 19.9%, respectively, for stage 2, 3, and 4 CKD, but mortality rates were 19.5%, 24.3%, and 45.7%. This study noted that CHF, coronary artery disease, diabetes, and anemia were more prevalent in the patients who died.

Prevalence and Incidence of Chronic Kidney Disease

ESRD accounts for a small proportion of the poor outcomes seen in patients with kidney disease. CKD patients are more likely to have poor cardiovascular outcomes and die than progress to ESRD. It is important to study the prevalence and incidence of CKD to understand its contribution to cardiovascular mortality and morbidity.

Prevalence of CKD and Associated Risk Factors

According to the National Health and Nutrition Examination Survey (NHANES) conducted from 1988 to 1994 and from 1999 to 2004, the prevalence of CKD stages 1 through 4 increased from 10% to 13%. In the meantime, the US population became older, body mass index (BMI) increased, the non-Hispanic white population decreased, and diabetes and hypertension prevalence rates increased. CKD prevalence showed a similar trend after stratified analysis by sex and race and adjustment for age. The increase in CKD prevalence noted in these surveys is partially due to the increase in the prevalence of risk factors for CKD.[6] The prevalence of the

Likelihood of Death vs. ESRD in the Medicare Population

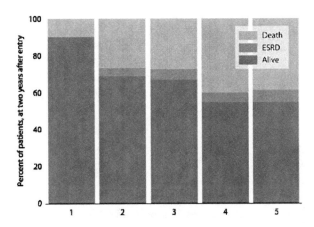

1: non-CKD, NDM, non-CHF 2: CKD only (NDM, non-CHF) 3: CKD + DM 4: CKD + CHF 5: CKD + DM + CHF

Figure 4.1. Likelihood of death vs ESRD in the Medicare population according to presence of CKD, CHF, and diabetes. US Renal Data System. *USRDS 2008 Annual Data Report: Atlas of Chronic Kidney Disease and End-Stage Renal Disease in the United States*, National Institutes of Health, National Institute of Diabetes and Digestive and Kidney Diseases, Bethesda, MD, 2008.

cardiovascular risk factors, diabetes, hypertension, heart disease (CHF, coronary heart disease, angina, stroke, or heart attack), and obesity also increases with increasing stage of renal dysfunction (Figure 4.2).[4]

Incidence of CKD and Associated Risk Factors

Among the Framingham Offspring Study participants free of CKD at baseline (mean age 43), after a mean follow-up of 18.5 years, 9.4% had developed CKD. Baseline age, GFR, BMI, diabetes, and smoking status were predictive of the development of CKD. Long-term, averaged risk factors associated with the development of CKD included hypertension, low HDL, and diabetes.[7] In a longitudinal cohort study of 17,375 apparently healthy volunteers of the general Viennese popula-

tion, age 20 to 89, after a median follow-up of 7 years, in 1.62% of patients GFR had decreased to < 60 mL/min/1.73 m². Age, female sex, baseline GFR, presence of proteinuria, BMI, smoking status, lack of involvement in sports, elevated uric acid, low HDL, hypertension, and diabetes mellitus were independent predictors of decline in GFR.[8]

Prevalence and Incidence of End-Stage Renal Disease

The USRDS collects, analyzes, and distributes information about ESRD in the United States. In ESRD the native kidney cannot function normally on its own and renal replacement therapy with hemodialysis, peritoneal dialysis, or renal transplantation is necessary.

GFR and the Prevalence of Cardiovascular Risk Factors

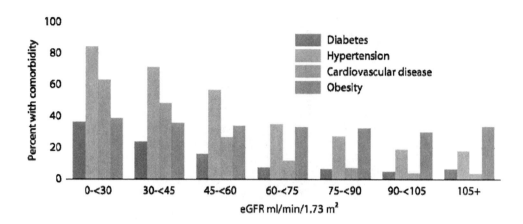

Figure 4.2. GFR and the prevalence of CVD risk factors based on NHANES 1999–2006 participants age 20 and older. U S Renal Data System. *USRDS 2008 Annual Data Report: Atlas of Chronic Kidney Disease and End-Stage Renal Disease in the United States*, National Institutes of Health, National Institute of Diabetes and Digestive and Kidney Diseases, Bethesda, MD, 2008.

The number of patients who are on dialysis or who receive renal transplantation has been steadily increasing over the past few decades.

Prevalence of ESRD

In 1995 there were 291,855 patients on renal replacement therapy.[9] This number increased to 506,256 in 2006 (Figure 4.3).[10] The number of patients on renal replacement therapy is projected to increase to 784,613 by year 2020.[4]

Incidence of ESRD and Associated Risk Factors

The incidence rate of renal replacement therapy in 2004 was 339 per million.[9] The USRDS 2008 Annual Data Report showed from data through 2006 that the incidence rate, adjusted for age, gender, and race, had increased to 360 per million, an annual increase of 2.1%, the highest in 5 years.[10] There had been an

epidemic growth in ESRD until 1999–2001 with more recent stabilization in the annual percent changes of incident ESRD. It is not clear if the annual increase of 2.1% seen from 2005 to 2006 will be sustained; more data are required to establish a clear trend.

The 3 leading causes of incident ESRD in 2004 were diabetes (44%), hypertension (27%), and glomerulonephritis (8%); the proportions were 39%, 31%, and 12%, respectively, in 2004.[11] The number of patients with diabetes as the primary cause of ESRD reached 48,157 in 2006, 4.6% greater than in the previous year, and 17.2% higher than in 2000. Incident rates for these patients have grown 3.7% since 2000, to reach 159 per million population.[4]

It appears that there has been dissociation between the increase in ESRD incidence and the prevalence of CKD over the past few decades. The extent of increase in ESRD

Adjusted Prevalent Rates and Annual Percent Change

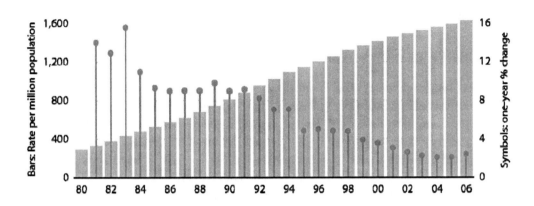

Figure 4.3. Adjusted ESRD prevalent rates and annual percent change through 2006. U S Renal Data System. *USRDS 2008 Annual Data Report: Atlas of Chronic Kidney Disease and End-Stage Renal Disease in the United States*, National Institutes of Health, National Institute of Diabetes and Digestive and Kidney Diseases, Bethesda, MD, 2008.

treatment initiation could not be accounted for using the recorded increments in CKD prevalence.[12,13] A longitudinal follow-up of 320,252 individuals who had a health check-up in Northern California between 1964 and 1985 found that individuals entering the cohort study in later years had a higher probability of initiating ESRD treatment, independent of the prevalence of CKD or risk factors for renal failure. They found an 8% per year increase in risk of starting ESRD therapy after adjustment for multiple ESRD risk factors including age, race, diabetes, blood pressure, proteinuria, and serum creatinine levels. One proposed hypothesis for the apparent discordance between incidence of ESRD and CKD is that renal replacement therapy has been more liberally offered in later years and likely reflects changing practice patterns.[12] ESRD treatment was observed to be initiated at higher levels of renal func-

tion (lower creatinine and higher GFR) concordant with increased access.

Future Trends

It is clear that there has been a significant increase in the prevalence of ESRD and CKD in the US population in the last few decades. Due to a continued increase in the prevalence of risk factors for CKD, it does not appear that there will be any respite in the prevalence of kidney disease. One in 3 US adults has high blood pressure.[14] The total population prevalence of diabetes mellitus in the United States is projected to double from 2005 to 2050 (from 5.6% to 12.0%) if current trends continue.[14] The number of people 65 years of age and above is projected to increase from 39 million to 69 million (20% of the population) in 2030.[15] Thus, a significant proportion of the US population remains at risk for CKD/ESRD, which will likely continue to be a major chronic health problem with substantial cardiovascular mortality and morbidity.

Epidemiology of Heart Failure

Heart failure is a major chronic public health problem in the United States. In 2006, there were 1,106,000 hospital discharges and 3,390,000 ambulatory care visits for HF.[14] The cost of caring for HF in the United States in 2009 was estimated at $37.2 billion.[14] In this section we discuss trends in the prevalence and incidence of HF and its associated risk factors.

Prevalence of Heart Failure and Secular Trends

Several studies have estimated the prevalence of HF in the community. A cross-sectional survey of Olmsted County, Minnesota, residents over 45 years old found a prevalence of symptomatic HF of 2.2%; of these, 44% had and ejection fraction (EF) above 50%.[16] In an English study of adults over 45 years old, left ventricular (LV) systolic dysfunction defined as EF < 40% was detected in 1.8%, half of whom had no symptoms. Definite HF that was symptomatic was noted in 2.3% of the population, out of which 41% had an EF < 40%.[17] In the Framingham Heart Study, among those aged 45 or above, the age-adjusted prevalence of CHF was 24 per 1000 men and 25 per 1000 women.[18] In the Rotterdam Study the point prevalence for HF among those older than 55 years, in 1997, 1998, and 1999, was 6.4%, 6.7%, and 7.0%, respectively. Prevalence was higher in men than in women (1998, 8% vs 6%). Prevalence estimates rose sharply with age (0.9%, age 55–64; 4.0%, age 65–74; 9.7%, age 75–84; 17.4%, above age 85).[19] A national survey of the prevalence of HF in Scotland showed a prevalence of 7.1 per 1000, increasing with age to 90.1 per 1000 among patients over 85 years old.[20]

Incidence of Heart Failure and Associated Risk Factors

The Framingham Study showed that for individuals over 65 years of age the incidence of HF is 1% per year. This rate doubles with each decade of life, reaching an incidence of 2% to 3% per year in individuals 85 to 94 years of age.[21] Another study from Framingham found that at age 40, the lifetime risk of incident HF is 21.0% for men and 20.3% for women. This risk did not change with advancing age, despite much shorter life expectancies, due to rapidly increasing incidence rates. Thus, at age 80 the lifetime risk was 20.2% for men and 19.3% for women. The lifetime risk doubled for blood pressure ≥ 160/100 mm Hg compared to < 140/90 mm Hg. The lifetime risk for HF in women free of historical myocardial infarction (MI) was similar to the risk for all women (1 in 6 vs 1 in 5), indicating an important role for factors other than MI. On the other hand, the lifetime risk for men free of MI is half the risk for all men (1 in 9 vs 1 in 5), indicating that antecedent MI plays a major role in men.[22] Another Framingham Study noted that the hazard for developing HF was 2-fold higher in men and 3-fold higher in women with hypertension. The population-attributable risk of hypertension for CHF in a multivariable model was 39% in men and 59% in women, making it the most important risk factor. MI, diabetes, LV hypertrophy, and valvular heart disease were also predictive of HF.[23]

Studies from multiple populations indicate that HF incidence is associated with male gender, older age, and black race (Figure 4.4).[19,24-27]

The studies described so far show that hypertension is the most important pre-

Incident heart failure by sex and race

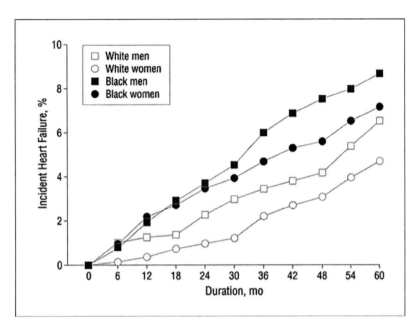

Figure 4.4. Incident cases of HF by sex and race from Health-ABC Study of elderly individuals. Kalogeropoulos A, Georgiopoulou V, Kritchevsky SB, Psaty BM, Smith NL, Newman AB, et al. Epidemiology of incident heart failure in a contemporary elderly cohort: The health, aging, and body composition study. *Arch Intern Med.* 2009;169:708–715. Copyright © 2009 American Medical Association. All rights reserved.

dictor for the development for HF, whereas diabetes, coronary artery disease, hyperlipidemia, CKD, and obesity also contribute to its development. As noted previously, these risk factors are similar to those associated with CKD.

Secular Trend in Heart Failure Incidence

The age- and sex-adjusted incidence of HF does not appear to be declining despite advances in the diagnosis and treatment of hypertension, coronary artery disease, diabetes, hyperlipidemia, and other forms of CVD. Data from the Framingham Heart Study cohort and from Olmsted County, Minnesota, document no major decline in age- and sex-

adjusted HF incidence in recent decades.[28,29] A retrospective cohort study of elderly patients in the Kaiser Permamente Northwest Region found increased HF incidence rates from 1970 to the 1990s, which were driven primarily by an increased incidence in the very elderly.[30] In contrast, a subsequent study evaluated a nationally representative sample of 3 million Medicare beneficiaries from 1994 to 2003 and noted a slight decline in age- and sex-adjusted HF incidence from 32 per 1000 person years in 1994 to 29 per 1000 person years in 2003.[31]

Heart failure survival has also improved, likely a result of advances in therapy over the last few decades. Increases in survival with HF contribute to increased prevalence.[29,30,32]

Accurately determining changes in incidence and prevalence over time is difficult. Differences in the studies cited may be influenced by study population and by methods of case ascertainment. Nonetheless, no dramatic decrease in incidence has been noted in recent decades. Increasing prevalence of HF risk factors (obesity, diabetes mellitus) may result in increasing HF incidence in coming decades. Continued improvement in survival with non–CVDs and the dramatic increases in the number of elderly persons will guarantee an increase in the number of persons with HF; even if age- and sex-adjusted incidence and prevalence are stable.

Heart Failure Hospitalizations

Data from the United States document a persistent climb in HF hospitalization rates in the past few decades. Hospitalization discharges for HF in the United States rose from 877,000 in 1996 to 1,106,000 in 2006.[14] Most of the increase in hospitalization rates appears to be among older persons (Figure 4.5).

A study of the National Hospital Discharge Survey of HF hospitalization rates documented an increased number of hospitalizations from 1985 to 1983.[33] A subsequent study from the same survey noted a tripling of HF hospitalization rates from 1.3 million to 3.9 million from 1979 to 2004; more than 80% of the patients admitted were older than 65 years of age.[34] The findings from multiple European studies, on the other hand, appear to indicate declining HF hospitalization rates. Age-adjusted rates increased until a peak in 1994 and have been steadily declining ever since in Scotland (Figure 4.6). This change was associated with improvements in rehospitalization rates and in the prescribing patterns of HF medications in primary care.[35] A national Swedish registry of hospital discharges also showed that after 1993 there was a yearly decrease in HF discharge rates.[36] The reasons for the disparate experiences in Europe and the United States are not clear.

Heart failure with preserved EF appears to account for an increasingly larger

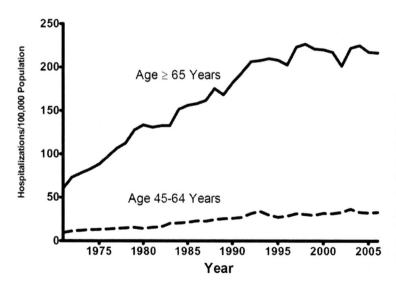

Figure 4.5. Hospitalization rates for HF, ages 45 to 64 and 65 and older, United States, 1971–2006. National Hospital Discharge Survey, NCHS. National Heart, Lung, and Blood Institute. National Institutes of Health and the U.S. Department of Health and Human Services.

Age-adjusted trends in discharges for a first hospitalization for HF according to sex

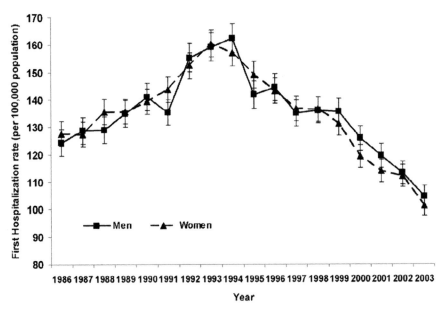

Figure 4.6. Age-adjusted trends in discharge for a first hospitalization for HF according to sex. Jhund PS, Macintyre K, Simpson CR, Lewsey JD, Stewart S, Redpath A, et al. Long-term trends in first hospitalization for heart failure and subsequent survival between 1986 and 2003: A population study of 5.1 million people. *Circulation.* 2009;119:515–523. With permission.

proportion of HF admissions. Owan et al[32] studied consecutive HF admissions in Olmstead County, Minnesota, over a 15-year period from 1987 to 2001. Fifty-three percent had a decreased EF (< 50%) and 47% had preserved EF (≥ 50%). The proportion of patients with preserved EF increased in the 3 consecutive 5-year periods studied from 38% to 47% to 54%. The proportion of patients with hypertension, atrial fibrillation, and diabetes mellitus increased over time, whereas the prevalence of coronary artery disease remained stable. There was slightly lower mortality in the group of patients with preserved EF compared to those with reduced EF (29% vs 32% at 1 year and 65% vs 68% at 5 years) (Figure 4.7). The roughly sim-

ilar outcomes in the 2 types of HF were also noted in a study of all patients with HF from Olmsted County, Minnesota, by Bursi et al[37] and in a Canadian community–based study of patients hospitalized with HF.[38] A recent meta-analysis of pooled studies adjusting for comorbidities noted better survival in HF with preserved EF.[39]

Importantly, the Owan study also showed that survival for HF with reduced EF improved over the years but remained stable in HF with preserved EF.[32] The lack of any effective, outcome–modulating treatment for HF with a preserved EF probably accounts for the lack of improvement of survival seen in this group of patients compared to those with a reduced EF.

Kaplan-Meier Survival Curves for Patients with Heart Failure and Preserved or Reduced Ejection Fraction

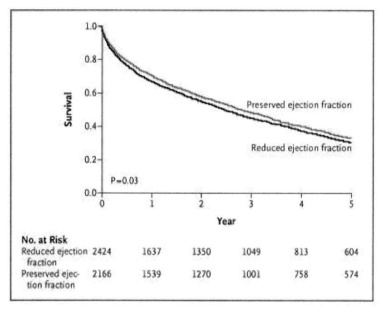

Figure 4.7. Survival according to presence or absence of LV systolic dysfunction and HF in patients hospitalized with HF in Mayo Clinic hospitals from 1987 to 2002. Owan TE, Hodge DO, Herges RM, Jacobsen SJ, Roger VL, Redfield MM. Trends in prevalence and outcome of heart failure with preserved ejection fraction. *N Engl J Med.* 2006;355:251–259. With permission. Copyright © (2006) Massachusetts Medical Society. All rights reserved.

Epidemiology of Cardiorenal Syndrome

Prevalence of Chronic Kidney Disease in Heart Failure

Several studies have defined the prevalence of renal dysfunction in patients with HF. The prevalence of renal insufficiency, defined as a GFR < 60 mL/min/1.73 m². has ranged from 26% to 57% in the major clinical trials that have enrolled ambulatory HF patients. This prevalence is high despite the fact that most clinical trials excluded patients with elevated creatinine. Moderate renal insufficiency predicted poor outcomes in all the trials (Table 4.2).[40–48]

Studies conducted in communities and registries of HF in a variety of settings place the prevalence of renal impairment defined as a GFR <60 mL/min between 35% and 56%. These studies also show that renal insufficiency predicts poor outcomes (Table 4.3).[49–54]

Studies of renal insufficiency in the hospital setting similarly show a high prevalence of moderate renal insufficiency, GFR < 60 mL/min, in 23.5% to 67.0% of patients. Most of the studies showed that poorer outcomes, including prolonged hospital stays, and increased in-hospital mortality were associated with renal impairment at baseline (Table 4.4).[55–60] A retrospective study of Medicare patients hospitalized with a diagnosis of HF in the National Heart Care project

Table 4.2: Prevalence of Renal Impairment
in the Major Ambulatory Heart Failure Clinical Trials

Clinical Trial	EF	Inclusion Serum Creatinine	% GFR < 60	n	Outcomes
Hillege et al[40] (CHARM)	All	< 3.0	36	2680	Increased all-cause mortality and combined end point of cardiovascular death or HF hospitalization
Al-Ahmad et al[43] (SOLVD)	≤ 35%	≤ 2.5	32	6630	Increased all-cause mortality
Bibbins-Domingo et al[46] (HERS) (women)	All	All	57	702	Increased mortality
Hillege et al[41] (PRIME-2)	< 35%	All	50	1906	Increased mortality
Ghali et al[44] (MERIT-HF)	< 40%	All	37	3965	Increased all-cause mortality and hospitalization for HF
Verma et al[45] (VALIANT-Echo)	HF or asymptomatic LV systolic dysfunction	< 2.5	29.9	603	Increase in combined end point of asymptomatic all-cause mortality or HF hospitalization LV systolic dysfunction
Shlipak et al[47] (DIG)	< 45%	≤ 3.0	46	6800	Increase in combined end point of all-cause mortality or HF hospitalization
Cohen-Solal et al[48] (SENIORS)	All	< 2.83	42	2112	Increased mortality of cardiovascular hospital admission

CHARM = Candesartan in Heart Failure Assessment of Reduction in Mortality and Morbidity; SOLVD = Studies of Left Ventricular Dysfunction; HERS = Heart and Estrogen/progestin Replacement Study; PRIME-2 = Second Prospective Randomized study of Ibopamine on Mortality and Efficacy; MERIT-HF = Metoprolol CR/XL Controlled Randomized Intervention Trial in Chronic HF; VALIANT-Echo = VALsartan In Acute myocardial iNfarcTion Trial-Echo; DIG = digoxin intervention group trial; SENIORS = Study of Effects of Nebivolol Intervention on Outcomes and Rehospitalization in Seniors with Heart Failure.

Table 4.3: Studies of Renal Impairment in the Community Setting

Studies	n	EF	GFR < 60	Factors Associated with Renal Impairment	Outcomes
Go et al[49] (ANCHOR)	59,772	All	47%	Not reported	Increased mortality and HF hospitalization
Ezekowitz et al[51] (APPROACH)	6427	HF Dx and coronary artery disease	39%	More comorbidities, greater coronary atherosclerotic burden, and lower EF; less likely to be prescribed ACE inhibitors, beta-blockers, statins, or aspirin	Increased 1-year mortality
de Silva et al[50]	955	< 45	54%	Anemia	Increased mortality
McAlister et al[52]	754	All	56%	Older, more likely to be female, had more symptomatic HF, were more likely to have coronary artery disease or hypertension, and were less likely to receive ACE inhibitors, beta-blockers, or spironolactone	Increased 1-year mortality
Mullens et al[53]	784	All	35%	Not reported	Increased all-cause mortality
Maeder et al[54]	196	LV systolic dysfunction	47%	Increased age, loop diuretic use, and tricuspid regurgitation severity associated; less likely to be on ACE inhibitors/ARB	Not reported

ANCHOR = Anemia in Chronic Heart Failure: Outcomes and Resource Utilization;
APPROACH = Alberta Provincial Project for Outcome Assessment in Coronary Heart Disease

Table 4.4: Studies on Prevalence of Renal Impairment in Heart Failure Hospitalizations

Study	n	EF	GFR Cutoff Value	Prevalence	Factors Associated with Renal Impairment	Outcome
Heywood et al[57] (ADHERE)	118,465	All	<60	64%	Hypertension, diabetes, coronary artery disease, peripheral vascular disease, older, female, and white	Increased in-hospital mortality
Smith et al[61] (NHC)	53,640	All	<60	67%	Black race, older, women, coronary artery disease, less likely to be on ACE inhibitors	Increased mortality, more pronounced in whites
Amsalem et al[58]	4102	All	<60	57%	Not reported	Increased in-hospital mortality
O'Connor et al[59] (IMPACT-HF)	567	All	<60	23.5%	Not reported	GFR did not predict outcomes
Nohria et al[55] (ESCAPE)	433	<30%	<60	31%	Baseline right atrial pressure correlates with baseline GFR and serum creatinine	Increased death, rehospitalizations
Akhter et al[56]	481	All	Serum creatinine > 1.5 mg/dL	45%	Old age, male sex, diabetes coronary artery disease, implantable cardioverter defibrillator, pacemakers	Prolonged length of stay and readmission, increased 6-month mortality
Mullens et al[60]	145	All	<60	64%	Baseline cardiac index	WRF

ADHERE = Acute Decompensated Heart Failure National Registry; NHC = National Heart Care Project; IMPACT-HF = Initiation Management Pre-discharge Assessment of Carvedilol Heart Failure; ESCAPE = Evaluation Study of Congestive Heart Failure and Pulmonary Artery Catheterization Effectiveness; VMAC = Vasodilation in the Management of Acute Congestive Heart Failure

(53,460 patients) suggested that the preva-lence of CKD among HF patients was lower in blacks.[61] A meta-analysis of 16 studies char-acterized the association of renal insufficien-cy and mortality in 80,098 hospitalized and nonhospitalized HF patients. Mild renal im-pairment was defined as creatinine > 1.0 mg/dL, creatinine clearance (CrCl) or GFR < 90 mL/min or cystatin C > 1.03 mg/dL, whereas moderate to severe impairment was defined as creatinine ≥ 1.5 mg/dL, CrCl or GFR < 53 mL/min or cystatin C ≥ 1.56 mg/dL. Sixty-three percent of HF patients were found to have renal impairment and 29% were noted to have moderate to severe impairment. Ad-justed all-cause mortality after a year was increased with renal impairment.[62]

In general, studies have shown that the prevalence of CKD is similar in patients with HF and preserved EF as compared to HF pa-tients with reduced EF.[40,45,48] However, the ADHERE registry suggested that HF with a preserved EF was more common in patients with CKD stage 5 (ESRD).[57]

Secular Trends in the Prevalence of Chronic Kidney Disease in Heart Failure

The severity of CKD present in patients with HF appears to be increasing. Owan et al studied secular trends in severity of CKD in 6440 patients hospitalized with acute de-compensated HF over the years 1987–2002.[63] As shown in Figure 4.8, age and creatinine increased while GFR decreased over the years. The proportion of patients with hy-pertension, atrial fibrillation, and diabetes mellitus all increased while the proportion with coronary artery disease remained the same. In the Evaluation Study of Conges-tive Heart Failure and Pulmonary Artery Catheterization Effectiveness (ESCAPE), an increase in average discharge diuretic dose compared to earlier studies was noted indi-cating worsening diuretic resistance.[64] While this was not a formal comparison, it is con-sistent with the increasing severity of CKD in HF patients over time in the study of Owan et al. The ESCAPE authors hypothesized that medical and device therapy improves mor-tality in HF but that chronic renal hypoper-fusion results in progressive CKD such that the CKD more patently contributes to the pathophysiology of HF now than in the past.

Incidence of WRF During Acute HF Therapy

Acute cardiorenal syndrome (type 2 cardio-renal syndrome) or worsening renal function (WRF) during HF exacerbation is of particular interest for clinicians. The pathophysiologic mechanisms causing WRF during acute HF therapy remain poorly defined. However, the development of renal dysfunction during HF therapy may limit use of proven HF thera-pies and is clearly a poor prognostic factor. Many studies have evaluated the prevalence, associations, and prognostic significance of WRF during HF treatment.

Studies have shown that WRF develops in approximately 25% of acute HF hospital-izations. In different studies, WRF was asso-ciated with male gender, older age, severity of renal dysfunction on admission, lower hemo-globin on admission, hypertension, diabe-tes, coronary artery disease, thiazide use in-hospital, loop diuretic use at baseline, calcium channel blocker use at baseline, diuretic dose, pulmonary edema, heart rate > 100 bpm, elevated central venous pressure, high-er NYHA class, and low LV ejection fraction (LVEF) (Table 4.5).[56,60,65–75] However, Forman et al[71] noted that the incidence of WRF was similar in patients with high and low EF.

A meta-analysis of 8 studies with 18,634 hospitalized and nonhospitalized patients assessed the relationship between WRF and mortality in HF. WRF was defined as an in-crease in serum creatinine of ≥ 0.2 mg/dL or a corresponding decrease in estimated GFR

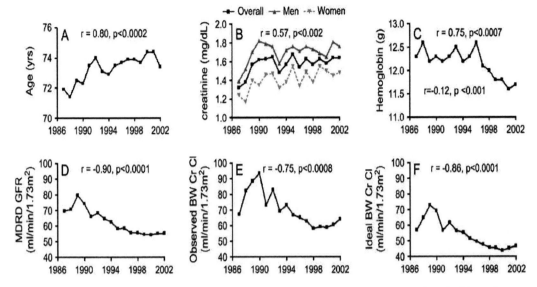

Figure 4.8. Secular trends in the severity of renal dysfunction present in hospitalized HF patients in Olmsted County, Minnesota, from 1987 to 2002. Trends for mean age (a), mean admission creatinine (b), mean admission hemoglobin (c), GFR (MDRD in D), CrCl (Cockroft-Gault equation entering observed body weight (e), and ideal body weight, (f) are shown. Pearson correlation coefficients and the P values for association with year of admission are shown. Owan TE, Hodge DO, Herges RM, Jacobsen SJ, Roger VL, Redfield MM. Secular trends in renal dysfunction and outcomes in hospitalized heart failure patients. *J Card Fail.* 2006;12:257–262. With permission from Elsevier.

of ≥ 5 mL/min/1.73 m². WRF developed in 25% of patients and was associated with an associated risk of mortality.[77]

Secular Trends in WRF During Acute HF Therapy

In the study of Owan et al[63] the incidence of WRF during hospitalization for acute decompensated HF was studied in 6440 consecutive patients in Rochester, Minnesota, over a period of 16 years. As outlined previously, while the severity of baseline renal dysfunction increased over time, surprisingly, the incidence of WRF remained stable over the course of the study. Patients who developed WRF had higher admission creatinine, lower GFR and hemoglobin, and a higher prevalence of hypertension, coronary disease, and diabetes. WRF also predicted 3-month and 5-year mortality in this study.

Conclusion

Regrettably, most studies indicate that the age- and sex-adjusted incidence of HF has not declined in recent decades despite marked improvements in treatment of CVD. A growing number of patients at risk will ensure that the number of persons with HF increases even if age- and sex-adjusted prevalence is stable. The prevalence of CKD is increasing in tandem with an increase in obesity and diabetes mellitus. Importantly, the severity of CKD in HF patients is increasing for complex reasons. Renal disease plays an increasing role in the epidemiology, pathophysiology, and treatment of HF.

Table 4.5: Studies on Worsening Renal Function During Heart Failure Hospitalization

Authors	n	Definition of WRF	% WRF	Factors Associated with WRF	Outcomes
Owan et al[63]	6440	> 0.3 mg/dL	23%	Higher admission creatinine, lower GFR and hemoglobin, higher prevalence of hypertension, coronary disease, and diabetes	Increased 3-month and 5-year mortality
Logeart et al[66]	416	≥ 0.28 mg/dL	37%	Old age, diabetes, hypertension, acute coronary syndrome	Increased 6-month mortality or readmission
Nohria et al[55] (ESCAPE)	433	≥ 0.3 mg/dL	29.50%	Hypertension and in-hospital thiazide use	No increase in death/hospitalization
Gottlieb et al[65]	1002	≥ 0.3 mg/dL	39%	Not reported	Increased mortality and length of stay
Akhter et al[56] (VMAC)	480	> 0.5 mg/dL	25%	Elevated baseline creatinine	Increased 6-month mortality and length of stay
Butler et al[67]	382	> 0.3 mg/dL	NA	Calcium channel blocker and loop diuretic use, high baseline creatinine, uncontrolled hypertension, hx of HF and diabetes	Not reported
Krumholz et al[68] (age >65)	1681	> 0.3 mg/dL	28%	Male gender, hypertension, rales > basilar, heart rate >100, systolic blood pressure >200, admission serum creatinine > 1.50	Increased length of stay, increased in-hospital mortality
Weinfeld et al[69]	48	≥ 25% increase to ≥ 2 mg/dL	21%	Old age, lower baseline CrCl, atrial fibrillation	Increased length of stay and mortality

Study	N	Definition	Predictors	Outcome
Cioffi et al[70]	79	≥ 25% increase to ≥ 2 mg/dL	Lower baseline CrCl and furosemide dose	Increased death and rehospitalization for heart failure
Forman et al[71]	1004	> 0.3 mg/dL	Diabetes mellitus, baseline creatinine > 1.5, systolic blood pressure > 160	Increased length of hospital stay and in-hospital mortality
Cowie et al[72] (POSH)	299	> 0.3 mg/dL	High baseline creatinine and pulmonary edema. Decreased in patients with atrial fibrillation	Increased length of stay; no effect in 6-month mortality or rehospitalization
Smith et al[73]	412	≥ 0.3 mg/dL	Not reported	Increased mortality only with the stricter definition ≥ 0.4 mg/dL
Klein et al[74] (OPTIME-CHF)	949	BUN increase > 25	Not reported	Increased 60-day mortality
Metra et al[74]	318	≥ 0.3 mg/dL and ≥ 25% increase	Baseline CKD, admission furosemide, NYHA class, low LVEF	Increased death and HF hospitalization
Mullens et al[60]	145	≥ 0.3 mg/dL	High admission and posttreatment central venous pressure, baseline renal insufficiency	Not reported
Damman et al[75] (COACH)	1023	≥ 0.3 mg/dL and ≥ 25%	Baseline GFR, age, diabetes, and anemia	Increased HF hospitalization and all-cause mortality

ESCAPE = Evaluation Study of Congestive Heart Failure and Pulmonary Artery Catheterization Effectiveness; VMAC = Vasodilation in the Management of Acute Congestive Heart Failure; POSH, Prospective Outcomes Study in Heart Failure; OPTIME-CHF = Outcomes of a Prospective Trial of Intravenous Milrinone for Exacerbations of Chronic Heart Failure; COACH = Outcomes of Advising and Counselling in Heart Failure.

References

1. Ronco C, House AA, Haapio M. Cardiorenal syndrome: refining the definition of a complex symbiosis gone wrong. *Intensive Care Med.* 2008; 34:957-962.

2. Liang KV, Williams AW, Greene EL, Redfield MM. Acute decompensated heart failure and the cardiorenal syndrome. *Crit Care Med.* 2008;36(1 suppl):S75-88.

3. K/DOQI clinical practice guidelines for chronic kidney disease: evaluation, classification, and stratification. *Am J Kidney Dis.* 2002;39(2 suppl 1):S1-266.

4. US Renal Data System, USRDS 2008 Annual Data Report: Atlas of Chronic Kidney Disease and End-Stage Renal Disease in the United States, National Institutes of Health, National Institute of Diabetes and Digestive and Kidney Disease, Bethesda, MD, 2008. The data reported here have been supplied by the US Renal Data System (USRDS). The interpretation and reporting of these data are the responsibility of the author(s) and in no way should be seen as an official policy or interpretation of the US government. 2008; Bethesda, Maryland.

5. Keith DS, Nichols GA, Gullion CM, Brown JB, Smith DH. Longitudinal follow-up and outcomes among a population with chronic kidney disease in a large managed care organization. *Arch Intern Med.* 2004;164:659-663.

6. Coresh J, Selvin E, Stevens LA, et al. Prevalence of chronic kidney disease in the United States. *JAMA.* 2007;298: 2038-2047.

7. Fox CS, Larson MG, Leip EP, Culleton B, Wilson PW, Levy D. Predictors of new-onset kidney disease in a community-based population. *JAMA.* 2004;291:844-850.

8. Obermayr RP, Temml C, Knechtelsdorfer M, et al. Predictors of new-onset decline in kidney function in a general middle-European population. *Nephrol Dial Transplant.* 2008;23:1265-1273.

9. Foley RN, Collins AJ. End-stage renal disease in the United States: an update from the United States Renal Data System. *J Am Soc Nephrol.* 2007;18: 2644-2648.

10. Collins AJ, Foley RN, Herzog C, et al. United States Renal Data System 2008 Annual Data Report Abstract. *Am J Kidney Dis.* 2009;53(1 suppl):vi-vii, S8-374.

11. Centers for Disease Control and Prevention (CDC). Racial differences in trends of end-stage renal disease, by primary diagnosis—United States, 1994-2004. *MMWR Morb Mortal Wkly Rep.* 2007;56:253-256.

12. Hsu CY, Go AS, McCulloch CE, Darbinian J, Iribarren C. Exploring secular trends in the likelihood of receiving treatment for end-stage renal disease. *Clin J Am Soc Nephrol.* 2007;2:81-88.

13. Hsu CY, Vittinghoff E, Lin F, Shlipak MG. The incidence of end-stage renal disease is increasing faster than the prevalence of chronic renal insufficiency. *Ann Intern Med.* 2004;141:95-101.

14. Lloyd-Jones D, Adams R, Carnethon M, et al; American Heart Association Statistics Committee and Stroke Statistics Subcommittee. Heart disease and stroke statistics—2009 update: a report from the American Heart Association Statistics Committee and Stroke Statistics Subcommittee. *Circulation.* 2009;119: 480-486.

15. United States Bureau of the Census. Current population reports. Series P-25, population estimates and projections. 1996, US Dept. of Commerce [For sale by the Supt. of Docs., U.S. G.P.O.]: Washington, D.C.

16. Redfield MM, Jacobsen SJ, Burnett JC Jr, Mahoney DW, Bailey KR, Rodeheffer RJ. Burden of systolic and diastolic ventricular dysfunction in the community: appreciating the scope of the heart failure epidemic. *JAMA*. 2003;289:194-202.

17. Davies M, Hobbs F, Davis R, et al. Prevalence of left-ventricular systolic dysfunction and heart failure in the Echocardiographic Heart of England Screening study: a population based study. *Lancet*. 2001;358:439-344.

18. Ho KK, Pinsky JL, Kannel WB, Levy D. The epidemiology of heart failure: the Framingham Study. *J Am Coll Cardiol*. 1993;22(4 suppl A):6A-13A.

19. Bleumink GS, Knetsch AM, Sturkenboom MC, et al. Quantifying the heart failure epidemic: prevalence, incidence rate, lifetime risk and prognosis of heart failure. The Rotterdam Study. *Eur Heart J*. 2004;25:1614-1619.

20. Murphy NF, Simpson CR, McAlister FA, et al. National survey of the prevalence, incidence, primary care burden, and treatment of heart failure in Scotland. *Heart*. 2004;90:1129-1136.

21. Kannel WB, Ho K, Thom T. Changing epidemiological features of cardiac failure. *Br Heart J*. 1994;72(2 suppl):S3-9.

22. Lloyd-Jones DM, Larson MG, Leip EP, et al; Framingham Heart Study. Lifetime risk for developing congestive heart failure: the Framingham Heart Study. *Circulation*. 2002;106:3068-3072.

23. Levy D, Larson MG, Vasan RS, Kannel WB, Ho KK. The progression from hypertension to congestive heart failure. *JAMA*. 1996;275:1557-1562.

24. Kalogeropoulos A, Georgiopoulou V, Kritchevsky SB, et al. Epidemiology of incident heart failure in a contemporary elderly cohort: the health, aging, and body composition study. *Arch Intern Med*. 2009;169:708-715.

25. Bibbins-Domingo K, Pletcher MJ, Lin F, et al. Racial differences in incident heart failure among young adults. *N Engl J Med*. 2009;360:1179-1190.

26. Bahrami H, Kronmal R, Bluemke DA, et al. Differences in the incidence of congestive heart failure by ethnicity: the multi-ethnic study of therosclerosis. *Arch Intern Med*. 2008;168:2138-2145.

27. Loehr LR, Rosamond WD, Chang PP, Folsom AR, Chambless LE. Heart failure incidence and survival (from the Atherosclerosis Risk in Communities study). *Am J Cardiol*. 2008;101:1016-1022.

28. Roger VL, Weston SA, Redfield MM, et al. Trends in heart failure incidence and survival in a community-based population. *JAMA*. 2004;292:344-350.

29. Levy D, Kenchaiah S, Larson MG, et al. Long-term trends in the incidence of and survival with heart failure. *N Engl J Med*. 2002;347:1397-1402.

30. Barker WH, Mullooly JP, Getchell W. Changing incidence and survival for heart failure in a well-defined older population, 1970-1974 and 1990-1994. *Circulation*. 2006;113:799-805.

31. Curtis LH, Whellan DJ, Hammill BG, et al. Incidence and prevalence of heart failure in elderly persons, 1994-2003. *Arch Intern Med*. 2008;168:418-424.

32. Owan TE, Hodge DO, Herges RM, Jacobsen SJ, Roger VL, Redfield MM. Trends in prevalence and outcome of heart failure with preserved ejection fraction. *N Engl J Med*. 2006;355:251-259.

33. Haldeman GA, Croft JB, Giles WH, Rashidee A. Hospitalization of patients with heart failure: National Hospital Discharge Survey, 1985 to 1995. *Am Heart J*. 1999;137:352-360.

34. Fang J, Mensah GA, Croft JB, Keenan NL. Heart failure-related hospitalization in

the U.S., 1979 to 2004. *J Am Coll Cardiol.* 2008;52:428–434.

35. Jhund PS, Macintyre K, Simpson CR, et al. Long-term trends in first hospitalization for heart failure and subsequent survival between 1986 and 2003: a population study of 5.1 million people. *Circulation.* 2009;119:515–523.

36. Schaufelberger M, Swedberg K, Köster M, Rosén M, Rosengren A. Decreasing one-year mortality and hospitalization rates for heart failure in Sweden; data from the Swedish Hospital Discharge Registry 1988 to 2000. *Eur Heart J.* 2004; 25:300–307.

37. Bursi F, Weston SA, Redfield MM, et al. Systolic and diastolic heart failure in the community. *JAMA.* 2006;296:2209–2216.

38. Bhatia RS, Tu JV, Lee DS, et al. Outcome of heart failure with preserved ejection fraction in a population-based study. *N Engl J Med.* 2006;355:260–269.

39. Somaratne JB, Berry C, McMurray JJ, Poppe KK, Doughty RN, Whalley GA. The prognostic significance of heart failure with preserved left ventricular ejection fraction: a literature-based meta-analysis. *Eur J Heart Fail.* 2009;11:855–862.

40. Hillege HL, Nitsch D, Pfeffer MA, et al; Candesartan in Heart Failure: Assessment of Reduction in Mortality and Morbidity (CHARM) Investigators. Renal function as a predictor of outcome in a broad spectrum of patients with heart failure. *Circulation.* 2006;113: 671–678.

41. Hillege HL, Girbes AR, de Kam PJ, et al. Renal function, neurohormonal activation, and survival in patients with chronic heart failure. *Circulation.* 2000;102:203–210.

42. Dries DL, Exner DV, Domanski MJ, Greenberg B, Stevenson LW. The prognostic implications of renal insufficiency in asymptomatic and symptomatic patients with left ventricular systolic dysfunction. *J Am Coll Cardiol.* 2000;35:681–689.

43. Al-Ahmad A, Rand WM, Manjunath G, et al. Reduced kidney function and anemia as risk factors for mortality in patients with left ventricular dysfunction. *J Am Coll Cardiol.* 2001;38: 955–962.

44. Ghali JK, Wikstrand J, Van Veldhuisen DJ, et al; MERIT-HF Study Group. The influence of renal function on clinical outcome and response to beta-blockade in systolic heart failure: insights from Metoprolol CR/XL Randomized Intervention Trial in Chronic HF (MERIT-HF). *J Card Fail.* 2009;15:310–318.

45. Verma A, Anavekar NS, Meris A, et al. The relationship between renal function and cardiac structure, function, and prognosis after myocardial infarction: the VALIANT Echo Study. *J Am Coll Cardiol.* 2007;50:1238–1245.

46. Bibbins-Domingo K, Lin F, Vittinghoff E, Barrett-Connor E, Grady D, Shlipak MG. Renal insufficiency as an independent predictor of mortality among women with heart failure. *J Am Coll Cardiol.* 2004;44:1593–1600.

47. Shlipak MG, Smith GL, Rathore SS, Massie BM, Krumholz HM. Renal function, digoxin therapy, and heart failure outcomes: evidence from the digoxin intervention group trial. *J Am Soc Nephrol.* 2004;15:2195–2203.

48. Cohen-Solal A, Kotecha D, van Veldhuisen DJ, et al; SENIORS Investigators. Efficacy and safety of nebivolol in elderly heart failure patients with impaired renal function: insights from the SENIORS trial. *Eur J Heart Fail.* 2009;11:872–880.

49. Go AS, Yang J, Ackerson LM, et al. Hemoglobin level, chronic kidney

disease, and the risks of death and hospitalization in adults with chronic heart failure: the Anemia in Chronic Heart Failure: Outcomes and Resource Utilization (ANCHOR) study. *Circulation*. 2006;113:2713–2723.

50. de Silva R, Rigby AS, Witte KK, et al. Anemia, renal dysfunction, and their interaction in patients with chronic heart failure. *Am J Cardiol*. 2006;98: 391–398.

51. Ezekowitz J, McAlister FA, Humphries KH, et al; APPROACH Investigators. The association among renal insufficiency, pharmacotherapy, and outcomes in 6,427 patients with heart failure and coronary artery disease. *J Am Coll Cardiol*. 2004;44:1587–1592.

52. McAlister FA, Ezekowitz J, Tonelli M, Armstrong PW. Renal insufficiency and heart failure: prognostic and therapeutic implications from a prospective cohort study. *Circulation*. 2004;109:1004–1009.

53. Mullens W, Abrahams Z, Skouri HN, et al. Prognostic evaluation of ambulatory patients with advanced heart failure. *Am J Cardiol*. 2008;10: 1297–1302.

54. Maeder MT, Holst DP, Kaye DM. Tricuspid regurgitation contributes to renal dysfunction in patients with heart failure. *J Card Fail*. 2008;14:824–830.

55. Nohria A, Hasselblad V, Stebbins A, et al. Cardiorenal interactions: insights from the ESCAPE trial. *J Am Coll Cardiol*. 2008;51:1268–1274.

56. Akhter MW, Aronson D, Bitar F, et al. Effect of elevated admission serum creatinine and its worsening on outcome in hospitalized patients with decompensated heart failure. *Am J Cardiol*. 2004;94:957–960.

57. Heywood JT, Fonarow GC, Costanzo MR, Mathur VS, Wigneswaran JR, Wynne J; ADHERE Scientific Advisory Committee and Investigators. High prevalence of renal dysfunction and its impact on outcome in 118,465 patients hospitalized with acute decompensated heart failure: a report from the ADHERE database. *J Card Fail*. 2007;13:422–430.

58. Amsalem Y, Garty M, Schwartz R, et al. Prevalence and significance of unrecognized renal insufficiency in patients with heart failure. *Eur Heart J*. 2008;29:1029–1036.

59. O'Connor CM, Stough WG, Gallup DS, Hasselblad V, Gheorghiade M. Demographics, clinical characteristics, and outcomes of patients hospitalized for decompensated heart failure: observations from the IMPACT-HF registry. *J Card Fail*. 2005;11:200–205.

60. Mullens W, Abrahams Z, Francis GS, et al. Importance of venous congestion for worsening of renal function in advanced decompensated heart failure. *J Am Coll Cardiol*. 2009;53:589–596.

61. Smith GL, Shlipak MG, Havranek EP, et al. Race and renal impairment in heart failure: mortality in blacks versus whites. *Circulation*. 2005;111:1270–1277.

62. Smith GL, Lichtman JH, Bracken MB, et al. Renal impairment and outcomes in heart failure: systematic review and meta-analysis. *J Am Coll Cardiol*. 2006;47:1987–1996.

63. Owan TE, Hodge DO, Herges RM, Jacobsen SJ, Roger VL, Redfield MM. Secular trends in renal dysfunction and outcomes in hospitalized heart failure patients. *J Card Fail*. 2006;12:257–262.

64. Binanay C, Califf RM, Hasselblad V, et al; ESCAPE Investigators and ESCAPE Study Coordinators. Evaluation study of congestive heart failure and pulmonary artery catheterization effectiveness: the ESCAPE trial. *JAMA*. 2005;294:1625–1633.

65. Gottlieb SS, Abraham W, Butler J, et al. The prognostic importance of different

definitions of worsening renal function in congestive heart failure. *J Card Fail.* 2002;8:136–141.

66. Logeart D, Tabet JY, Hittinger L, et al. Transient worsening of renal function during hospitalization for acute heart failure alters outcome. *Int J Cardiol.* 2008;127:228–232.

67. Butler J, Forman DE, Abraham WT, et al. Relationship between heart failure treatment and development of worsening renal function among hospitalized patients. *Am Heart J.* 2004;147:331–338.

68. Krumholz HM, Chen YT, Vaccarino V, et al. Correlates and impact on outcomes of worsening renal function in patients > or = 65 years of age with heart failure. *Am J Cardiol.* 2000;85:1110–1113.

69. Weinfeld MS, Chertow GM, Stevenson LW. Aggravated renal dysfunction during intensive therapy for advanced chronic heart failure. *Am Heart J.* 1999;138(2 Pt 1):285–290.

70. Cioffi G, Tarantini L, Pulignano G, et al. Prevalence, predictors and prognostic value of acute impairment in renal function during intensive unloading therapy in a community population hospitalized for decompensated heart failure. *J Cardiovasc Med.* (Hagerstown) 2007;8:419–427.

71. Forman DE, Butler J, Wang Y, et al. Incidence, predictors at admission, and impact of worsening renal function among patients hospitalized with heart failure. *J Am Coll Cardiol.* 2004;43:61–67.

72. Cowie MR, Komajda M, Murray-Thomas T, Underwood J, Ticho B; POSH Investigators. Prevalence and impact of worsening renal function in patients hospitalized with decompensated heart failure: results of the prospective outcomes study in heart failure (POSH). *Eur Heart J.* 2006;27:1216–1222.

73. Smith GL, Vaccarino V, Kosiborod M, et al. Worsening renal function: what is a clinically meaningful change in creatinine during hospitalization with heart failure? *J Card Fail.* 2003;9:13–25.

74. Klein L, Massie BM, Leimberger JD, et al. Admission or changes in renal function during hospitalization for worsening heart failure predict postdischarge survival. *Circ Heart Fail.* 2008;1:25–33.

75. Metra M, Nodari S, Parrinello G, et al. Worsening renal function in patients hospitalised for acute heart failure: clinical implications and prognostic significance. *Eur J Heart Fail.* 2008;10:188–195.

76. Damman K, Jaarsma T, Voors AA, Navis G, Hillege HL, van Veldhuisen DJ; COACH investigators. Both in- and out-hospital worsening of renal function predict outcome in patients with heart failure: results from the Coordinating Study Evaluating Outcome of Advising and Counseling in Heart Failure (COACH). *Eur J Heart Fail.* 2009;11:847–854.

77. Damman K, Navis G, Voors AA, et al. Worsening renal function and prognosis in heart failure: systematic review and meta-analysis. *J Card Fail.* 2007;13:599–608.

Hemodynamic Considerations in Cardiorenal Syndrome

5

W. H. Wilson Tang
Gary S. Francis

Cardiorenal syndrome is often encountered when therapy to relieve congestion in heart failure (HF) is limited by a significant decline in renal function. It is important to emphasize that the majority of our understanding regarding hemodynamic derangements that contribute to cardiorenal syndrome stems from observations made in the "acute" phase of cardiorenal compromise. Despite the heterogeneity of its presentation, worsening renal function (WRF) typically occurs within days after hospitalization, particularly in the setting of aggressive diuretic therapy. Since glomerular filtration and tubular function rely heavily on adequate renal perfusion, these observations imply a potential relation of renal compromise to the hemodynamic derangement resulting from cardiac insuf-

ficiency. This chapter discusses the "classic" hemodynamic considerations and the interplay between the failing heart and kidney compromise, which can play important roles in the development of cardiorenal syndrome.

Arterial Underfilling of the Kidneys: The Heart's Perspective

The prevailing concept of arterial underfilling of the kidneys focuses on the inability of the failing heart to generate sufficient output, leading to hypoperfusion of the kidneys (or impaired renal "preload," Figure 5.1). Often, the reduced cardiac output (CO) is exacerbated by redistribution of blood flow to vital organs (such as the brain), which can lead to a relatively diminished perfusion of the kidneys. Persistent hypoperfusion may even result in renal parenchymal and corti-

The Cardiorenal Syndrome: A Clinician's Guide to Pathophysiology and Management, 1st ed. © 2012 J. Thomas Heywood and John C. Burnett Jr., eds. Cardiotext Publishing, ISBN: 978-0-9790164-7-9.

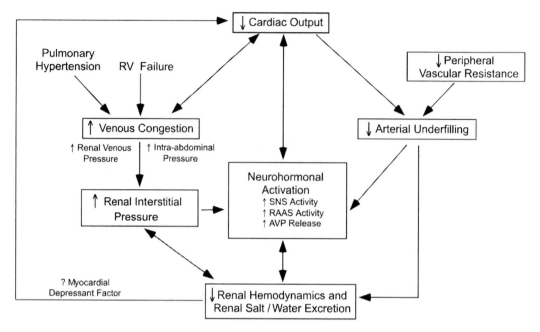

Figure 5.1. Hemodynamic determinants of acute cardiorenal syndrome. Tang WH, Mullens W. Cardio-renal syndrome in decompensated heart failure. *Heart.* 2010;96:(4)255-260. With permission from BMJ Publishing Group Ltd.

cal ischemia (or infarction) and progressive renal insufficiency. Indeed, insufficient CO can directly lead to a reduced renal perfusion despite all the compensatory mechanisms, requiring inotropic support[1-3] or mechanical circulatory support[4] to restore adequate renal blood flow.

To better understand the impact of cardiac insufficiency on the kidney, we should revisit a fundamental concept in cardiovascular physiology. The Frank–Starling mechanism is based on the length–tension relationship within the ventricle. If ventricular end diastolic volume (preload) is increased, the ventricular fiber length will correspondingly increase, resulting in an increased tension of myocytes (Figure 5.2). Hence, CO is directly related to venous return at a given heart rate in the normal physiologic setting, and such a relationship may be shifted downward in the setting of impaired cardiac contractility (meaning, a low

augmentation in CO as a result of increased end–diastolic volume). This relationship may even plateau or dip as a consequence of diminished efficiency, when no further increase in CO can be achieved by raising end–diastolic volume (see Figure 5.1). Hence, removal of excessive congestion (ie, "unloading") may sometimes achieve a higher level of myocardial efficiency and CO to generate adequate renal perfusion.

Although attractive, the concept of "low-output" state being the *sole* culprit does not fully explain cardiorenal syndrome. Mechanistic studies have indicated that in the setting of cardiac dysfunction the kidneys can tolerate a relatively low CO (as low as 1.5 L/min/m²) in order to maintain adequate renal perfusion pressures.[5] Recent data from large registries indicate that the proportion of patients with acute decompensated heart failure (ADHF) presenting with low CO is relatively small,[6,7] far less than those experi-

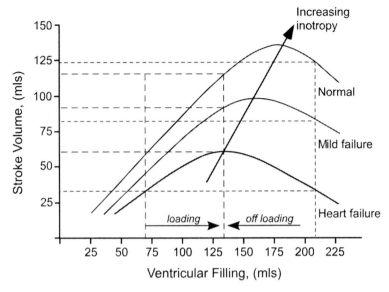

Figure 5.2. Frank-Starling relationship in normal and failing hearts.

encing cardiorenal syndrome. Furthermore, the majority of congested patients appeared to have relatively preserved (or even high) blood pressures,[6] and the incidence of WRF was similar amongst patients with decompensated HF and reduced versus preserved systolic function (the latter often presents with increased left ventricular impedance rather than impaired CO).[8]

In the setting of congestion, redistribution of blood from the arterial to the venous circulation can lead to an effective reduction in renal arterial blood flow. Such diminished flow or volume can also be detected by various sensors, which will then lead to enhanced sodium and water absorption via stimulation of the sympathetic nervous system, the renin-angiotensin-aldosterone system (RAAS), and vasopressin secretion, leading to a vicious cycle of further congestion. An obvious temporal factor distinguishes what is improvement specific to regional hemodynamic environment versus what is a product of improvement in the overall cardiac status. Early studies on vasodilator

drugs have also provided some intriguing insights into how improving cardiac physiology (such as with the use of hydralazine) may not provide immediate improvement in renal hemodynamics, but potential subsequent improvement after prolonged use;[9] this may imply that hemodynamic decongestion or neurohumoral improvement of the failing myocardium may have indirect and profound long-term consequences in improving renal hemodynamics.

Arterial Underfilling of the Kidneys: The Kidney's Perspective

Excessive and persistent salt and water retention in the setting of congestive heart failure (CHF) is counterintuitive to the concept of relative "hypoperfusion" of the kidneys. However, renal hemodynamics are complex.[10] In the normal kidney, reduced renal blood flow caused by circulatory impairment promptly leads to a compensatory increase in filtration fraction, a consequence of renal glomerular efferent arteriolar vasoconstriction and increased intraglomerular hydraulic pressure. This in turn leads to preservation of GFR, but also more than offsets any reduction in renal blood flow. In the setting of HF, several factors come into play. First, aggressive diuresis can lead to intravascular volume depletion. Second, profound activation of neurohumoral systems either as a result of such intravascular volume depletion or underlying neurohumoral up-regulation of HF state can lead to high renovascular resistance. In particular, studies have shown that angiotensin II-mediated vasoconstriction of the efferent arteriole is one important such mechanism in preserving adequate filtration fraction.[11] Impairment in tubuloglomerular feedback mechanisms between the flow of the renal tubules and the renal vasculature to achieve a salt and water balance may also occur as a consequence of tubular injury. All can result in inadequate blood "volume" across the capillary bed (glomeruli), leading to diminished renal blood flow and hence reduction in filtration fraction without adequate compensation. Therefore, drugs that produce afferent arteriole vasoconstriction (such as nonsteroidal anti-inflammatory drugs or cyclosporine) or efferent arteriole vasodilation (such as ACE inhibitors or angiotensin II receptor blockers) may directly impact the delicate balance of renal hemodynamics. Hence in patients with limited renal reserve, administration of these medications may directly lead to WRF.[12,13] Several drug classes have been developed (eg, adenosine receptor antagonists) to specifically improve renal hemodynamics, but to date clinical trials with them have been disappointing.

The dynamics of how these factors interplay are poorly understood at the bedside. Nevertheless, a proof of concept of the importance of renovascular perfusion has been demonstrated by direct injection of vasoactive drugs to the renal vasculature. In particular, intrarenal infusion of fenoldopam[14] and dopamine,[15] as well as nesiritide,[16] all produced impressive renal arterial vasodilation and improvement in glomerular filtration and natriuresis without systemic hypotension. Needless to say, renal perfusion pressures can be directly affected by systemic blood pressure, which can diminish the potential benefits of these agents when administered systemically.[17]

In the clinical context, direct obstruction of the major renal vessels leading to a physical blockage to blood flow to the glomeruli needs to be excluded. Often, renal artery stenosis or fibromuscular dysplasia can present with clinical presentations of difficult-to-control secondary hypertension, which can directly lead to hypertensive HF and renal function worsened by drugs targeting the RAAS. Diminished flow as a result of such renovascular diseases may occur in the absence of cardiac insufficiency, and can often be relieved by percutaneous revascularization.

Venous Congestion of the Kidneys

In animal models, an increase in renal vein pressure leads to renal insufficiency independent of arterial perfusion of the kidneys.[18] This seemed to be, to a certain extent, a reversible phenomenon as lowering of renal vein pressure immediately improved urine output and glomerular filtration (Figure 5.3). Temporary renal vein compression may result in reduced sodium excretion, increased renal interstitial pressure, and reduced glomerular filtration.[18-21] These concepts have been now confirmed in humans. In larger and more contemporary clinical

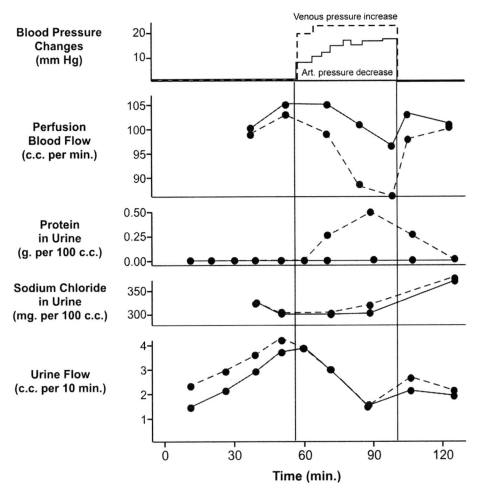

Figure 5.3. Interplay between arterial and venous pressure changes in renal blood flow and function. Winton FR. The influence of venous pressure on the isolated mammalian kidney. *J Physiol.* 1931;72:49-61. With permission.

experience, increased central venous pressure (CVP) had the strongest association with reduced GFRs in patients with pulmonary hypertension as well as in those with cardiovascular diseases, particularly in those with evidence of low renal blood flow.[22,23] In the ADHF setting, WRF is better predicted by preexisting elevated CVP than impaired CO (Figure 5.4).[24]

The exact mechanism of how venous congestion contributes to cardiorenal syndrome is debated. With the kidney being an encapsulated organ, it was thought that in-creased venous pressure might distend the venules surrounding the distal ends of the tubules so that the lumen of the tubule could be obliterated until the pressure of the fluid within it exceeded that in the vein.[18] Others simply postulated that increased CVP could be transmitted backwards to the renal veins and cause an increase in renal interstitial pressure.[20] This may lead to a hypoxic state (ischemia) of the renal parenchyma. Furthermore, intrarenal but also systemic angiotensin II concentrations may increase with increasing renal venous pressure. This will

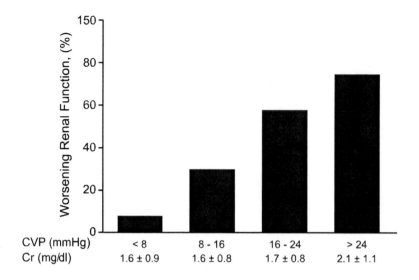

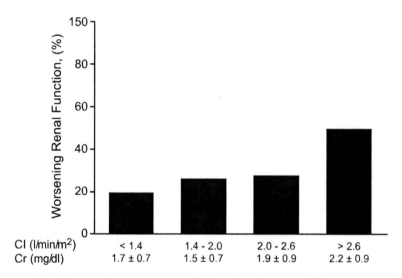

Figure 5.4. Impact of baseline central venous pressure (CVP) and cardiac index (CI) on prevalence of WRF during hospitalization. Adapted from Mullens W, Abrahams Z, Francis GS, et al. Importance of venous congestion for worsening of renal function in advanced decompensated heart failure. *J Am Coll Cardiol.* 2009;53:589–596. With permission from Elsevier.

lead to a further fall in glomerular filtration and increase sympathetic system activity. Finally, counterregulatory mechanisms to decrease sensitivity of the tubuloglomerular feedback may be blunted in HF, thereby compromising the maintenance of filtration fraction. The combination of such hemodynamic and neurohormonal alterations induced by venous congestion will ultimately lead to a downward spiraling of renal function as a result of reduction in *net* filtration pressure across the glomeruli (Figure 5.5).

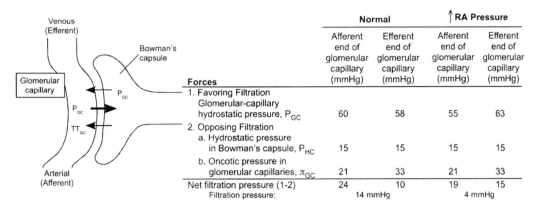

		Normal		↑RA Pressure	
		Afferent end of glomerular capillary (mmHg)	Efferent end of glomerular capillary (mmHg)	Afferent end of glomerular capillary (mmHg)	Efferent end of glomerular capillary (mmHg)
	Forces				
	1. Favoring Filtration				
	Glomerular-capillary hydrostatic pressure, P_{GC}	60	58	55	63
	2. Opposing Filtration				
	a. Hydrostatic pressure in Bowman's capsule, P_{HC}	15	15	15	15
	b. Oncotic pressure in glomerular capillaries, π_{GC}	21	33	21	33
	Net filtration pressure (1-2)	24	10	19	15
	Filtration pressure:		14 mmHg		4 mmHg

Figure 5.5. Impact of increased venous pressure on renal filtration in an example of normal and increased CVP. P_{bc} = hydrostatic pressure in Bowman's capsule; P_{GC} = glomerular capillary hydrostatic pressure; Π_{gc} = oncotic pressure in glomerular capillaries. Jessup M, Costanzo MR. The cardiorenal syndrome: do we need a change of strategy or tactics? *J Amer Coll Cardiol.* 2009;53:597–599. With permission from Elsevier.

Raised Intra-Abdominal Pressure

Abdominal symptoms are not uncommon in patients with CHF, particularly in those with significant "right-sided" failure where extensive edema is present, sometimes with accompanying increased abdominal girth. Although frank ascites can be found in a subset of cases, many patients simply have what is postulated as "visceral edema." Extensive surgical literature has highlighted the contribution of raised intra-abdominal pressure leading to "abdominal compartment syndrome" as a possible explanation of WRF in that significant accumulation of edema forces external compression to the kidneys (often up to 15–20 mm Hg). Like the hepatojugular reflex, raised intra-abdominal pressure may also raise CVP and produce venous congestion. The prevalence of raised intra-abdominal pressure in patients with HF is not well described, although a recent survey found up to 40% of patients admitted to the HF intensive care unit demonstrated this hemodynamic derangement despite the lack of severe abdominal complaints. Elevated intra-abdominal pressure was directly associated with more impaired renal function at baseline, and improvement in renal function following intensive medical therapy was associated with a reduction of intra-abdominal pressure in most patients.[25] In those with persistently elevated intra-abdominal pressure, treatment either by manually removing ascites fluid (via paracentesis) or mechanical removal of venous congestion by ultrafiltration can reduce intra-abdominal pressure and correspondingly improve renal function.[26] Thus, reducing intra-abdominal pressure or right atrial pressure in addition to improving renal arterial perfusion may play an important role in our therapeutic strategies.[28] These findings warrant further investigations.

Conclusion

The intrinsic imbalance between central and renal hemodynamic derangements and compensatory mechanisms combined with extrinsic alterations by inappropriate interventions (particularly with vasoactive drug therapies) in the setting of HF likely contributes to the development of cardiorenal syndrome. There is unlikely any "single" etiology, and over the past century there have been various competing (yet complementary) hypotheses that attempt to explain the interplay between cardiac and renal hemodynamics. Many of the mechanisms described remain poorly understood at the bedside, and will likely warrant future investigations using better measurement techniques and better drug or device interventions.

References

1. Klein L, Massie BM, Leimberger JD, et al. Admission or changes in renal function during hospitalization for worsening heart failure predict postdischarge survival: results from the Outcomes of a Prospective Trial of Intravenous Milrinone for Exacerbations of Chronic Heart Failure (OPTIME-CHF). *Circ Heart Fail.* 2008;1:25-33.

2. Al-Hesayen A, Parker JD. The effects of dobutamine on renal sympathetic activity in human heart failure. *J Cardiovasc Pharmacol.* 2008;51:434-436.

3. Yilmaz MB, Yalta K, Yontar C, et al. Levosimendan improves renal function in patients with acute decompensated heart failure: comparison with dobutamine. *Cardiovasc Drugs Ther.* 2007;21:431-435.

4. Khot UN, Mishra M, Yamani MH, et al. Severe renal dysfunction complicating cardiogenic shock is not a contraindication to mechanical support as a bridge to cardiac transplantation. *J Am Coll Cardiol.* 2003;41:381-385.

5. Ljungman S, Laragh JH, Cody RJ. Role of the kidney in congestive heart failure. Relationship of cardiac index to kidney function. *Drugs.* 1990;39:10-21; discussion 22-14.

6. Adams KF Jr, Fonarow GC, Emerman CL, et al. Characteristics and outcomes of patients hospitalized for heart failure in the United States: rationale, design, and preliminary observations from the first 100,000 cases in the Acute Decompensated Heart Failure National Registry (ADHERE). *Am Heart J.* 2005;149:209-216.

7. Nohria A, Hasselblad V, Stebbins A, et al. Cardiorenal interactions: insights from the ESCAPE trial. *J Am Coll Cardiol.* 2008;51:1268-1274.

8. Yancy CW, Lopatin M, Stevenson LW, De Marco T, Fonarow GC. Clinical presentation, management, and in-hospital outcomes of patients admitted with acute decompensated heart failure with preserved systolic function: a report from the Acute Decompensated Heart Failure National Registry (ADHERE) Database. *J Am Coll Cardiol.* 2006;47:76-84.

9. Mathey D, Hanrath P, Polster J, Witte G, Montz R, Bleifeld W. Acute and chronic effects of oral hydralazine on left ventricular pump function and renal hemodynamics in chronic left heart failure. *Eur Heart J.* 1980;1:25-29.

10. Rea ME, Dunlap ME. Renal hemodynamics in heart failure: implications for treatment. *Curr Opin Nephrol Hypertens.* 2008;17:87-92.

11. Textor SC, Tarazi RC, Novick AC, Bravo EL, Fouad FM. Regulation of renal hemodynamics and glomerular filtration in patients with renovascular hypertension during converting enzyme inhibition with captopril. *Am J Med.* 1984;76:29-37.

12. Kittleson M, Hurwitz S, Shah MR, et al. Development of circulatory-renal limitations to angiotensin-converting

enzyme inhibitors identifies patients with severe heart failure and early mortality. *J Am Coll Cardiol.* 2003;41: 2029-2035.

13. Weinfeld MS, Chertow GM, Stevenson LW. Aggravated renal dysfunction during intensive therapy for advanced chronic heart failure. *Am Heart J.* 1999;138:285-290.

14. Grube E, Baim D, Burkhoff D, Mueller R, Buellesfeld L, Teirstein P. Local intra-renal fenoldopam infusion causes greater increases in renal artery flow velocity than systemic intravenous fenoldopam infusion: a pilot study. *Euro Intervention.* 2005;1:305-308.

15. Elkayam U, Ng TM, Hatamizadeh P, Janmohamed M, Mehra A. Renal vasodilatory action of dopamine in patients with heart failure: magnitude of effect and site of action. *Circulation.* 2008;117:200-205.

16. Chen HH, Cataliotti A, Schirger JA, Martin FL, Harstad LK, Burnett JC Jr. Local renal delivery of a natriuretic peptide a renal-enhancing strategy for B-type natriuretic peptide in overt experimental heart failure. *J Am Coll Cardiol.* 2009;53:1302-1308.

17. Elkayam U, Akhter MW, Liu M, Hatamizadeh P, Barakat MN. Assessment of renal hemodynamic effects of nesiritide in patients with heart failure using intravascular Doppler and quantitative angiography. *JACC Cardiovasc Imaging.* 2008;1:765-771.

18. Winton FR. The influence of venous pressure on the isolated mammalian kidney. *J Physiol.* 1931;72:49-61.

19. Blake WD, Wegria R, Keating RP, Ward HP. Effect of increased renal venous pressure on renal function. *Am J Physiol.* 1949;157:1-13.

20. Burnett JC Jr, Knox FG. Renal interstitial pressure and sodium excretion during renal vein constriction. *Am J Physiol.* 1980;238:F279-282.

21. Firth JD, Raine AE, Ledingham JG. Raised venous pressure: a direct cause of renal sodium retention in oedema? *Lancet.* 1988;1:1033-1035.

22. Damman K, Navis G, Smilde TD, et al. Decreased cardiac output, venous congestion and the association with renal impairment in patients with cardiac dysfunction. *Eur J Heart Fail.* 2007;9:872-878.

23. Damman K, van Deursen VM, Navis G, Voors AA, van Veldhuisen DJ, Hillege HL. Increased central venous pressure is associated with impaired renal function and mortality in a broad spectrum of patients with cardiovascular disease. *J Am Coll Cardiol.* 2009;53:582-588.

24. Mullens W, Abrahams Z, Francis GS, et al. Importance of venous congestion for worsening of renal function in advanced decompensated heart failure. *J Am Coll Cardiol.* 2009;53:589-596.

25. Mullens W, Abrahams Z, Skouri HN, et al. Elevated intra-abdominal pressure in acute decompensated heart failure: a potential contributor to worsening renal function? *J Am Coll Cardiol.* 2008; 51:300-306.

26. Mullens W, Abrahams Z, Francis GS, Taylor DO, Starling RC, Tang WH. Prompt reduction in intra-abdominal pressure following large-volume mechanical fluid removal improves renal insufficiency in refractory decompensated heart failure. *J Card Fail.* 2008;14:508-514.

27. Tang WH, Mullens W. Cardio-renal syndrome in decompensated heart failure. *Heart.* 2010;96(4):255-260.

28. Jessup M, Costanzo MR. The cardiorenal syndrome: do we need a change of strategy or tactics? *J Am Coll Cardiol.* 2009;53:597-599.

Diuretic Use in Heart Failure Patients with Renal Dysfunction

6

Jeremy S. Bock
Stephen S. Gottlieb

Diuretic medications form the cornerstone of therapy for patients with congestive heart failure (CHF) who are hospitalized for symptoms of volume overload. This class of medications is also important for maintenance of euvolemia in the outpatient setting. However, these drugs may have other effects; it is currently unknown if diuretics exacerbate the underlying pathophysiology of CHF as they treat volume overload. In particular, the effects of diuretics on renal function are complex and incompletely understood.

Renal dysfunction is common and often progressive in patients with CHF. Because impaired clearance of sodium and water are features of both heart failure (HF) and renal dysfunction, patients with these comorbidities have a profound tendency toward

The Cardiorenal Syndrome: A Clinician's Guide to Pathophysiology and Management, 1st ed. © 2012 J. Thomas Heywood and John C. Burnett Jr., eds. Cardiotext Publishing, ISBN: 978-0-9790164-7-9.

volume overload and effective diuretic management is essential. A unique set of challenges is encountered when using diuretics in patients with CHF and renal disease, as these agents can cause further neurohormonal activation and direct and indirect nephrotoxicity. Such adverse consequences can lead to progression of both diseases.

Basic Physiology of Diuretic Agents When Renal Dysfunction Is Present

Loop Diuretics

Loop diuretics are among the most potent agents for stimulating diuresis and natriuresis. Agents such as furosemide, torsemide, bumetanide, and ethacrynic acid inhibit the $Na^+/K^+/2Cl^-$ cotransporter on the luminal side of the thick ascending limb of the loop of Henle (LOH). Because 25% of the filtered load of sodium chloride (NaCl) is normally reabsorbed here, loop diuretics can cause profound diuresis and natriuresis. When functioning normally, the $Na^+/K^+/2Cl^-$ cotransporter increases intracellular potassium concentration, creating a driving force for passive recycling of potassium into the tubule lumen; this generates a net positive electrical potential within the lumen that drives paracellular transport of divalent cations. Thus, when the cotransporter is inhibited by loop diuretics, the net positive potential is blunted and heightened excretion of magnesium and calcium ensues.

Increased delivery of NaCl to distal portions of the nephron would typically stimulate a commensurate decrease in glomerular filtration rate (GFR) via tubuloglomerular feedback (TGF), probably via adenosine. However, this phenomenon does not occur following loop diuretic administration, which partially explains its potent diuretic effect. Nevertheless, loop diuretics often lower GFR.[1] The mechanisms are unclear but may involve adenosine release[1-3] and stimulation of the renin-angiotensin-aldosterone system (RAAS).[4] Because serum creatinine and worsening renal function are important predictors of in-hospital mortality in patients admitted for symptomatic CHF,[5,6] factors that worsen renal function need to be investigated.

Loop diuretics decrease pulmonary congestion and lower left ventricular (LV) filling pressures prior to the onset of their diuretic effects. This decrease is probably related to increased synthesis and release of prostaglandins by the kidney in response to these agents.[7] In this way, loop diuretics can be effective in the treatment of acute pulmonary congestion and edema even in cases of advanced or end-stage renal disease.

However, they also cause hypomagnesemia, which may negatively impact myocardial performance and is associated with reduced survival in HF.[8]

Distal Convoluted Tubule Diuretics

Thiazide diuretics and metolazone (a thiazide-like agent) inhibit an electrically neutral sodium and chloride cotransporter in the early distal convoluted tubule. These drugs are rarely used as sole diuretic agents in HF as they are significantly less potent compared to loop diuretics. Renal clearance of thiazides is affected greatly in CHF or other disorders with impaired renal blood flow (RBF). Compared to loop diuretics, thiazides also carry a greater risk for hyponatremia and hypokalemia.[9]

Thiazide and thiazide-like agents have greatest utility in CHF when used concomitantly with loop diuretics.[10,11] In advanced HF the combination of decreased RBF, progressive renal dysfunction, and RAAS activation may render maximal doses of loop diuretic therapy ineffective. In the setting of acute and chronic loop diuretic therapy, functional adaptation of the distal tubule with compensatory increases in sodium reabsorption (or diuretic resistance) and the effects of extracellular fluid volume depletion (or braking phenomenon) have also been well described (see discussion that follows). Simultaneous use of high-dose loop diuretics and a thiazide or metolazone inhibits sodium transport in the ascending thick limb of the LOH as well as the compensatory sodium reabsorption in the early distal convoluted tubule. Most thiazide drugs also directly inhibit carbonic anhydrase, which minimizes compensatory sodium reabsorption in the proximal tubule. Diuresis and natriuresis can be greatly enhanced by combination diuretic therapy, though the risk of severe hyponatremia and hypokalemia can be significant.[11,12] In contrast to traditional thiazide agents, metolazone remains active at lower GFRs. This represents a considerable advantage of using metolazone over a thiazide diuretic in advanced HF with renal dysfunction.[13,14]

Potassium-Sparing Diuretics

The potassium-sparing diuretics spironolactone, eplerenone, triamterene, and amiloride inhibit sodium reabsorption by cells of the cortical collecting tubule. Spironolactone and eplerenone function as competitive inhibitors of the intracellular mineralocorticoid receptor, decreasing translocation of active sodium transporters to the luminal membrane. Triamterene and amiloride, on the other hand, directly inhibit these extracellular sodium channels. In the presence of open channels, sodium entry into tubular epithelial cells is passive due to low intracellular concentration. The net negative lumen potential that results from sodium reabsorption favors passive excretion of potassium into the tubule lumen. Thus, blockade of this mechanism leads to potassium retention.

Because only 1% to 2% of the filtered load of NaCl is normally absorbed at this location, the potassium-sparing diuretics have relatively low potency as diuretic and natriuretic agents. Their typical diuretic utility in HF is to counteract potassium wasting and hypokalemic metabolic alkalosis associated with loop and thiazide diuretic use. Unlike loop or thiazide diuretics, spironolactone and eplerenone have also been shown to improve mortality at low doses in patients with advanced CHF who are already receiving maximal standard medical therapy.[15,16,17] This outcome is probably not mediated by any diuretic effect but rather is because of synergistic inhibition of the RAAS when used with

an angiotensin-converting enzyme (ACE) inhibitor. This inhibition decreases myocardial fibrosis and remodeling[18,19] and may have a modest effect on limiting sodium reabsorption. In general, high doses of potassium-sparing diuretics should be avoided or used with caution in patients with CHF and renal dysfunction as development of dose-dependent hyperkalemia is especially common in this setting.[16] Higher doses of spironolactone have been reported to improve natriuresis in diuretic-resistant patients.[20]

Effect of Diuretic Use on Morbidity and Mortality

According to the ADHERE database of more than 105,000 individuals admitted for acute CHF, 70% of patients took a diuretic as part of their outpatient medication regimen.[21] Thirty percent of these patients had a history of renal insufficiency and 20% had serum creatinine levels > 2.0 mg/dL. Among patients hospitalized for HF, loop diuretic use is associated with further deterioration of renal function and is observed more frequently among patients receiving combination loop diuretic and metolazone therapy.[22] Furthermore, higher doses of loop diuretics are associated with higher serum creatinine and reduced survival.[23] Individuals taking loop diuretics also have an increased risk of hospitalization and death related to CHF compared to those not taking these medications. Concomitant use of potassium-sparing diuretics may attenuate these risks.[24]

These observations regarding progression of renal disease and HF associated with diuretic use come from nonrandomized or retrospective studies and should be considered with extreme caution. Even though multivariate analyses of retrospective studies that have adjusted for possible confounders have observed disease progression associated with diuretics,[24] such studies cannot control for all the differences among patients. Individuals with more severe renal disease and HF are the most likely to be on diuretics, and thus the severity of baseline disease, rather than the diuretic therapy, may be the cause of the disease progression and death. However, one prospective, randomized controlled study of pigs with tachycardia–induced CHF demonstrated clear progression of systolic dysfunction and elevated neurohormonal concentrations in the animals given furosemide.[25] Further investigation of this issue is needed. Interestingly, among the loop diuretics, some evidence suggests that use of torsemide may be associated with reduced mortality as compared to furosemide.[26]

While the use of diuretics is essential for most patients with CHF, there are clear adverse outcomes associated with worsening renal and LV function. Spironolactone and eplerenone are currently the only diuretics that have been shown to reduce mortality in HF and this is probably not related to the agents' diuretic effect.[15]

Diuretics and Sodium and Water Restriction

Increased renal sodium reabsorption secondary to RAAS activation is marked in CHF and exacerbated further following the administration of diuretics.[4] Advanced stages of CHF are frequently associated with biventricular failure, hepatic congestion, and hypoalbuminemia. When low albumin is present in the setting of renal sodium avidity, interstitial volume expansion occurs and this may contribute to patient symptoms. Interstitial fluid is unavailable for renal clearance, as it does not contribute to arterial blood volume such that attempted diuresis

can result in further intravascular volume depletion, neurohormone elevation, and a worsening of renal function.

Because of the increased sodium retention in patients with HF, it is generally recommended that CHF patients, particularly those with renal dysfunction, observe a low-sodium diet. While it is well-known that pharmacologic diuresis and natriuresis can be completely abolished when high sodium intake persists between doses, some investigators believe adherence to a low-sodium diet may not be beneficial. Some studies show that CHF patients who observe low–sodium diets (1.8 g/day) in combination with high–dose diuretic therapy and fluid restriction have increased hospitalizations and elevated neurohormone concentrations compared to patients who consume normal sodium diets (2.8 g/day).[27,28] These studies theorize that low-sodium diets may be insufficient to maintain arterial blood volume, renal perfusion, and suppression of the RAAS, and thus favor further deterioration of cardiac and renal function. Such conclusions have not been widely accepted, however, and low–sodium intake is not generally believed to cause the renal dysfunction associated with diuresis.

Dosing and Pharmacokinetic Considerations in the Presence of Renal Dysfunction

There is considerable patient-to-patient variability in the effective dose of diuretic when CHF and renal disease are present. In general, worsening LV systolic dysfunction and worsening GFR are associated with needing higher doses, blunted therapeutic responses, and increased relative impact of side effects of diuretics.

Heart Failure Effects

In CHF, effective doses of diuretics are influenced by (1) decrease in RBF, (2) postdiuretic sodium retention secondary to activation of the RAAS in the setting of intravascular volume depletion, (3) loop diuretic resistance, and (4) bowel edema, which may delay absorption and blunt peak concentration of oral formulations. Because loop diuretics act on the luminal side of the urinary tubule, diuretic elimination and activity strongly correlate with secretion by the proximal tubule and, to a much lesser extent, glomerular filtration (loop diuretics are highly bound to albumin and are not readily filtered). After a threshold dose of loop diuretic is given, there exists a classic dose–response curve between the rate of diuretic excretion and natriuresis. This dose–response curve is blunted (right-shifted) in CHF secondary to decreased RBF and increased distal sodium resorption associated with heightened activity of the RAAS.[29,30]

Renal Failure Effects

Tubular dysfunction is associated with decreased rate of secretion of loop diuretics and lower urinary tubule concentration of the drug. It is true that the acidemia associated with advanced renal disease tends to displace loop diuretics from serum proteins, resulting in higher unbound fraction of the drug and increased filtration at the glomerulus. However, increases in drug reaching the tubule lumen by this mechanism is significantly outweighed by displacement of loop diuretics from the organic acid secretory pump of the proximal tubule by other circulating organic acids. The net effect of worsening renal function is significantly decreased secretion of the diuretic, which outweighs increased glomerular filtration.

Decreased rate of secretion of furosemide markedly prolongs its half-life but not of torsemide or bumetanide, as the later agents are metabolized by the liver. Thus, renal dysfunction may be associated with prolonged but less intense effects of furosemide, which necessitates administration of higher doses to reach threshold activity in the urinary tubules. Like CHF, the dose-response curve (fractional excretion of sodium vs furosemide concentration) is right-shifted in individuals with renal dysfunction.

Pharmacodynamics

Maximum effective doses of diuretics in individuals with normal renal function are seen following administration of 40 mg of intravenous furosemide or 15 to 20 mg of intravenous or oral torsemide. Higher doses have not been shown to elicit any appreciable increase in diuresis or natriuresis and markedly increase the risk of side effects.[30] The maximum effective dose of loop diuretics is increased in HF and renal dysfunction for the reasons described (reduced RBF, RAAS activation, impaired proximal tubular secretion, delayed absorption). In general, sequential doubling of the ineffective dose until a therapeutic response is achieved is more efficacious than administering the original dose more frequently. Single oral doses of furosemide up to 400 mg have been used in patients with HF and advanced renal disease who are resistant to lower doses.

Continuous infusions of loop diuretics are often used in patients with severe CHF and renal dysfunction when bolus dosing fails to elicit appreciable diuresis. Dosing by this method theoretically favors maintenance of the threshold concentration of drug in the urinary tubule and also minimizes the periods of exaggerated sodium avidity that occur between bolus doses (see discussion that follows). A recent study evaluated bolus versus continuous as well as high- or low-dose diuretic infusions in acute heart failure. There was no significant difference in renal function between the strategies, although the high–dose group diuresed more.[31]

Pharmacokinetics

Absorption and bioavailability of oral furosemide is about 50% but can vary widely (10%–100%) among both normal individuals and patients with CHF and/or renal dysfunction.[30] Variability occurs both between individuals and within the same individual from day to day; this is probably related to variable absorption when ingested with food, a theoretical contribution from bowel edema, as well as changes in bioavailability secondary to inconsistent first-pass elimination. Because all loop diuretics are highly protein–bound, volume of distribution is limited to the intravascular space.

Changes in absorption of oral furosemide in CHF patients compared to normal individuals probably contribute little to the observed differences in response to diuretics between each of these states; the ratio of urinary furosemide concentration after oral dosing to the urinary furosemide concentration after intravenous dosing routes is similar.[32] Said differently, average absorption and bioavailability of oral furosemide appears to be 50% in both normal individuals and those with CHF. The advantages of administering intravenous furosemide is largely limited to a more rapid and predictable diuretic response, as the bioavailability of intravenous drugs is 100%.

Diminished delivery of loop diuretics in CHF contributes to the need for increased doses. Thus, impaired LV function and decreased RBF can increase the need for higher serum concentrations. Renal delivery and secretion of loop diuretics into the urinary tubule are delayed secondary to decreased renal perfusion in individuals with HF.[32] This delay leads to a blunting of proximal tubular secretion and peak concentration in the urine such that threshold concentration in the tubule may not be sufficient for therapeutic response. This phenomenon is treated by increasing the dose of the loop diuretic, either oral or intravenously given.

While it is commonly believed that absorption of furosemide is decreased significantly in volume-overloaded, hypoalbuminemic patients secondary to intestinal edema, there are limited data to support this supposition.[29,33] Some studies suggest that differences in absorption do not significantly affect response to loop diuretics, that total absorption is not affected, and that time to peak serum concentration may be delayed slightly in volume-overloaded states without being clinically important.[32,34]

In summary, individuals with CHF and renal disease are more likely to require higher doses of oral or intravenous loop diuretics for appreciable diuresis and natriuresis. This necessity for higher doses is probably not a reflection of impaired absorption secondary to bowel edema. Other factors seem to be more important. Higher serum concentrations are required to overcome diminished renal perfusion in the setting of worsening LV function. Moreover, higher doses and increased serum concentrations of loop diuretics may be necessary to overcome displacement of the drug from the organic acid secretory pump by accumulating organic acids associated with progressive renal dysfunction. Neurohormonal stimulation may also lead to decreased urine output.

Torsemide and Bumetanide

In contrast to oral furosemide, oral formulations of torsemide and bumetanide have consistent bioavailabilities of 80% to 100% and absorption does not appear to be changed by concomitant ingestion of food. Use of these agents affords a more predictable and consistent diuresis at a given dose.

Torsemide is absorbed and reaches peak serum concentrations more rapidly than furosemide and has a longer serum half-life in normal individuals.[35] On the other hand, furosemide has a markedly prolonged serum half-life compared to torsemide in individuals with renal dysfunction as torsemide is cleared by the liver. Because torsemide does not exhibit absorption-limited kinetics, bioavailability of oral formulations is not significantly different from intravenous forms. Diuresis and natriuresis following administration of torsemide does not appear to be different after an intravenous dose versus an oral dose, even when renal dysfunction is present.[36] Like furosemide, the presence of CHF and renal dysfunction also do not appear to be important predictors of absorption or bioavailability of torsemide.[34,35,37] In general, higher doses of torsemide are needed to elicit a therapeutic response in CHF because of reduced RBF. In most patients, the dose of furosemide may be adjusted to reflect the delayed absorption, obviating the need for the more expensive torsemide.

There is limited evidence to suggest that HF patients taking torsemide have fewer hospitalizations and better quality of life compared to those taking furosemide.[38] Unblinded studies suggest that patients taking torsemide exhibit lower all-cause mortality and improvement in NYHA functional class compared to furosemide.[26,39] These studies were small or nonrandomized, and the possible cause of this purported benefit is unclear. One suggested mechanism is that torsemide exerts an antialdosterone effect, which may be beneficial in preventing progressive ventricular remodeling in CHF.

Diuretic Resistance in Chronic Heart Failure and Renal Dysfunction

The kidney's intrinsic short-term and chronic adaptations to diuretic therapy often limit a sustained response to these agents, and these adaptations appear to be more robust when CHF or baseline renal disease is present. Profound diuresis and natriuresis result after initial administration of diuretic medications. Over the span of several days to several weeks, however, the daily net negative sodium and fluid balance declines until a prediuretic steady state is again reached.

Immediate and Short-Term Adaptations

Sodium concentration of fluid entering the distal tubule increases markedly following loop diuretic administration. Because of increased delivery, there is a rapid rise in transcellular absorption of NaCl via the thiazide-sensitive NaCl cotransporter in the distal tubule, and this tends to attenuate net sodium and fluid losses after a single dose of loop diuretic.[40] Blocking this intrinsic compensatory mechanism with simultaneous administration of a thiazide or thiazide-like drug is the rationale behind coadministration of loop diuretics and metolazone described previously.[10,11]

Diuretic administration activates mechanisms that tend to minimize further sodium and fluid losses. Activation of the RAAS, suppression of natriuretic hormones, and stimulation of efferent renal sympathetic nerves collectively contribute to the phenomenon known as postdiuretic sodium retention.[4,28,41] Thus, after a period of natriuresis, concentration of diuretic in the urinary tubule falls below threshold needed for therapeutic response, sodium transporters are released from inhibition, and a period of sodium retention ensues. These short-term adaptations contribute to diuretic resistance. Because individuals with CHF and renal dysfunction have baseline alterations in renal hemodynamics and neurohormonal tone, the tendency toward diuretic resistance and the adverse consequences of resistance are greatly exaggerated in these disease states.

Chronic Adaptations and Diuretic Resistance

Diuretic resistance is a common component of cardiorenal syndrome. Ongoing or frequent use of diuretics can lead to depletion of the extracellular fluid volume. In this setting, there will be a progressive reduction in the magnitude of natriuresis following each diuretic dose, and this is related to activation of sodium-retaining neurohormones, stimulation of renal sympathetic nerves, and suppression of natriuretic peptides. This so-called braking phenomenon tends to occur earlier in the course of diuretic therapy in CHF and renal diseases marked by hypoalbuminemia because of baseline reductions in intravascular volume. The time course and degree of the braking phenomenon and decline in GFR following diuretic administration depend on NaCl intake; reduction in natriuresis is marked with low-sodium diets and can be abolished with high sodium intake.[42]

Adaptation in the proximal tubular segments of the nephron also appears be to important in limiting natriuresis with chronic diuretic administration. Volume contraction tends to stimulate RAAS-mediated increases in proximal tubular reabsorption of sodium. This limits sodium delivery to the distal nephron, blunting the effect of inhibiting the $Na^+/K^+/2Cl^-$ cotransporter in the ascending LOH and the thiazide-sensitive NaCl co-transporter in the distal convoluted tubule. Loop diuretics have also been shown to stimulate distal nephron epithelial cell hypertrophy and hyperplasia and increase the luminal density of thiazide-sensitive NaCl cotransporters, which makes sodium reabsorption more efficient under these conditions and is thought to contribute to diuretic resistance.

Though all diuretics tend to stimulate the RAAS through extracellular volume contraction, only loop diuretics directly stimulate renin secretion at the macula densa.[4,43] Neurohormonal tone may be higher in CHF and renal disease secondary to renal hypoperfusion, and further direct and indirect stimulation of the RAAS by loop diuretics appears to be a critical factor in earlier resistance to these medicines and deterioration in renal function.

Conclusion

The cardiac and renal mechanisms responsible for maintaining adequate organ perfusion through salt and water homeostasis are extremely elegant. Sodium avidity leading to volume overload in CHF represents a maladaptive response to the abnormal hemodynamics of the circulation when LV systolic function is impaired. While diuretics are essential for maintenance of euvolemia and treating complications of hypervolemia in CHF, they may exacerbate the underlying pathophysiology through neurohormonal activation, effects on cardiac function, and further impairment in renal function. Optimal use of diuretics in CHF necessitates controlling volume overload without further triggering the very mechanisms responsible for sodium avidity. Continued investigation into the optimal means of controlling volume is needed. Meanwhile, diuresis should be used judiciously to treat symptoms, knowing that excessive use has the potential to be detrimental.

References

1. Gottlieb SS, Brater DC, Thomas I, et al. BG9719 (CVT-124), an A1 adenosine receptor antagonist, protects against the decline in renal function observed with diuretic therapy. *Circulation.* 2002;105:1348–1353.

2. Gottlieb SS, Skettino SL, Wolff A, et al. Effects of BG9719 (CVT-124), an A1-adenosine receptor antagonist, and furosemide on glomerular filtration rate and natriuresis in patients with congestive heart failure. *J Am Coll Cardiol.* 2000;35:56–59.

3. Elkayam U, Mehra A, Cohen G, et al. Renal circulatory effects of adenosine in patients with chronic heart failure. *J Am Coll Cardiol.* 1998;32:211–215.

4. Broqvist M, Dahlström U, Karlberg BE, Karlsson E, Marklund T. Neuroendocrine response in acute heart failure and the influence of treatment. *Eur Heart J.* 1989;10:1075–1083.

5. Gottlieb SS, Abraham W, Butler J, et al. The prognostic importance of different definitions of worsening renal function in congestive heart failure. *J Card Fail.* 2002;8:136–141.

6. Fonarow GC, Adams KF Jr, Abraham WT, Yancy CW, Boscardin WJ; ADHERE Scientific Advisory Committee, Study Group, and Investigators. Risk stratification for in-hospital mortality in acutely decompensated heart failure: classification and regression tree analysis. *JAMA.* 2005;293:572–580.

7. Bourland WA, Day DK, Williamson HE. The role of the kidney in the early nondiuretic action of furosemide to reduce elevated left atrial pressure in the hypervolemic dog. *J Pharmacol Exp Ther.* 1977;202:221–229.

8. Gottlieb SS, Baruch L, Kukin ML, Bernstein JL, Fisher ML, Packer M. Prognostic importance of the serum magnesium concentrations in patients with congestive heart failure. *J Am Coll Cardiol.* 1990;16:827–831.

9. Sonnenblick M, Friedlander Y, Rosin AJ. Diuretic-induced severe hyponatremia. Review and analysis of 129 reported patients. *Chest.* 1993;103:601–606.

10. Ghose RR, Gupta SK. Synergistic actions of metolazone with loop diuretics. *BMJ.* 1981;812:1432–1433.

11. Dormans TP, Gerlag PG. Combination of high-dose furosemide and hydrochlorothiazide in the treatment of refractory congestive heart failure. *Eur Heart J.* 1996;17:1867–1874.

12. Rosenberg J, Gustafsson F, Galatius S, Hildebrandt PR. Combination therapy with metolazone and loop diuretics in outpatients with refractory heart failure: an observational study and review of the literature. *Cardiovasc Drugs Ther.* 2005;19:301–306.

13. Kiyingi A, Field MJ, Pawsey CC, Yiannikas J, Lawrence JR, Arter WJ. Metolazone in treatment of severe refractory congestive heart failure. *Lancet.* 1990;335:29–31.

14. Dormans TP, Gerlag PG, Russel FG, Smits P. Combination diuretic therapy in severe congestive heart failure. *Drugs.* 1998;55:165–172.

15. Pitt B, Zannad F, Remme WJ, et al. The effect of spironolactone on morbidity and mortality in patients with severe heart failure. *N Engl J Med.* 1999;341:709–717.

16. Pitt B, Remme W, Zannad F, et al; Eplerenone Post-Acute Myocardial Infarction Heart Failure Efficacy

and Survival Study Investigators. Eplerenone, a selective aldosterone blocker, in patients with left ventricular dysfunction after myocardial infarction. *N Engl J Med.* 2003;348:1309–1321.

17. Zannad F, McMurray JJ, Krum H, et al. Eplerenone in patients with systolic heart failure and mild symptoms. *N Engl J Med.* 2010;364:11–21.

18. Izawa H, Murohara T, Nagata K, et al. Mineralocorticoid receptor antagonism ameliorates left ventricular diastolic dysfunction and myocardial fibrosis in mildly symptomatic patients with idiopathic dilated cardiomyopathy: a pilot study. *Circulation.* 2005;112: 2940–2945.

19. MacFadyen RJ, Barr CS, Struthers AD. Aldosterone blockade reduces vascular collagen turnover, improves heart rate variability and reduces early morning rise in heart rate in heart failure patients. *Cardiovasc Res.* 1997;35:30–34.

20. van Vliet AA, Donker AJ, Nauta JJ, Verheugt FW. Spironolactone in congestive heart failure refractory to high-dose loop diuretic and low-dose angiotensin-converting enzyme inhibitor. *Am J Cardiol.* 1993; 71:21A–28A.

21. Adams KF Jr, Fonarow GC, Emerman CL, et al; ADHERE Scientific Advisory Committee and Investigators. Characteristics and outcomes of patients hospitalized for heart failure in the United States: rationale, design, and preliminary observations from the first 100,000 cases in the Acute Decompensated Heart Failure National Registry (ADHERE). *Am Heart J.* 2005;149:209–216.

22. Butler J, Forman DE, Abraham WT, et al. Relationship between heart failure treatment and development of worsening renal function among hospitalized patients. *Am Heart J.* 2004;147:331–338.

23. Eshaghian S, Horwich TB, Fonarow GC. Relation of loop diuretic dose to mortality in advanced heart failure. *Am J Cardiol.* 2006;97:1759–1764.

24. Domanski M, Norman J, Pitt B, Haigney M, Hanlon S, Peyster E. Studies of left ventricular dysfunction. Diuretic use, progressive heart failure, and death in patients in the studies of left ventricular dysfunction (SOLVD). *J Am Coll Cardiol.* 2003;42:705–708.

25. McCurley JM, Hanlon SU, Wei SK, Wedam EF, Michalski M, Haigney M. Furosemide and the progression of left ventricular dysfunction in experimental heart failure. *J Am Coll Cardiol.* 2004;44:1301–1307.

26. Cosín J, Díez J; for the TORIC investigators. Torasemide in chronic heart failure: results study. *Eur J Heart Fail.* 2000;4:507–513.

27. Paterna S, Gaspare P, Fasullo S, Sarullo FM, Di Pasquale P. Normal-sodium diet compared with low-sodium diet in compensated congestive heart failure: is sodium an old enemy or a new friend? *Clin Sci.* 2008;114:221–230.

28. Paterna S, Parrinello G, Cannizzaro S, et al. Medium term effects of different dosage of diuretic, sodium, and fluid administration on neurohormonal and clinical outcome in patients with recently compensated heart failure. *Am J Cardiol.* 2009;103:93–102.

29. Brater DC, Day B, Burdette A, Anderson S. Bumetanide and furosemide in heart failure. *Kidney Int.* 1984;26:183–189.

30. Brater, DC. Pharmacology of diuretics. *Am J Med Sci.* 2000;319:38–50.

31. Felker GM, Lee KL, Bull DA, et al. Diuretic strategies in patients with acute decompensated heart failure. *N Engl J Med.* 2011;364:797–805.

32. Brater DC, Seiwell R, Anderson S, Burdette A, Dehmer GJ, Chennavasin P. Absorption and disposition of furosemide in congestive heart failure. *Kidney Int.* 1982;22:171–176.

33. Vasko MR, Cartwright DB, Knochel JP, Nixon JV, Brater DC. Furosemide absorption altered in decompensated congestive heart failure. *Ann Intern Med.* 1985;102:314–318.

34. Gottlieb SS, Khatta M, Wentworth D, Roffman D, Fisher ML, Kramer WG. The effects of diuresis on the pharmacokinetics of the loop diuretics furosemide and torsemide in patients with heart failure. *Am J Med.* 1998;104:533–538.

35. Vargo DL, Kramer WG, Black PK, Smith WB, Serpas T, Brater DC. Bioavailability, pharmacokinetics, and pharmacodynamics of torsemide and furosemide in patients with congestive heart failure. *Clin Pharmacol Ther.* 1995;57:601–609.

36. Rudy DW, Gehr TW, Matzke GR, Kramer WG, Sica DA, Brater DC. The pharmacodynamics of intravenous and oral torsemide in patients with chronic renal insufficiency. *Clin Pharmacol Ther.* 1994;56:39–47.

37. Gehr TW, Rudy DW, Matzke GR, Kramer WG, Sica DA, Brater DC. The pharmacokinetics of intravenous and oral torsemide in patients with chronic renal insufficiency. *Clin Pharmacol Ther.* 1994;56:31–38.

38. Murray MD, Deer MM, Ferguson JA, et al. Open-label randomized trial of torsemide compared with furosemide therapy for patients with heart failure. *Am J Med.* 2001;111:513–520.

39. Müller K, Gamba G, Jaquet F, Hess B. Torasemide vs. furosemide in primary care patients with chronic heart failure NYHA II to IV—efficacy and quality of life. *Eur J Heart Fail.* 2003;5:793–801.

40. Ellison DH, Velaquez H, Wright FS. Adaptation of the distal convoluted tubule of the rat: structural and functional effects of dietary salt intake and chronic diuretic infusion. *J Clin Invest.* 1989;83:113–126.

41. Petersen JS, Dibona GF. Effects of renal denervation on sodium balance and renal function during chronic furosemide administration in rats. *J Pharmacol Exp Ther.* 1992;262:1103–1109.

42. Wilcox CS, Mitch WE, Kelly RA. Response of the kidney to furosemide: effects of salt intake and renal compensation. *J Lab Clin Med.* 1983;102:450–458.

43. Martínez-Maldonado M, Gely R, Tapia E, Benabe JE. Role of macula densa in diuretics-induced renin release. *Hypertension.* 1990;16:261–268.

The Use of ACE Inhibitors and Angiotensin Receptor Blockers in Patients with Coexistent Renal Disease and Heart Failure

7

Domenic A. Sica

Compounds that interfere with activity of the renin–angiotensin–aldosterone system (RAAS) have been established as effective in the treatment of hypertension, as well as a variety of end-organ diseases including proteinuric chronic kidney disease (CKD), heart failure (HF), and stroke. Inhibitors of the RAAS either quantitatively reduce angiotensin II concentrations (angiotensin–converting enzyme [ACE] inhibitors and direct renin inhibitors [DRIs]) or limit the activity of angiotensin II at the receptor level (angiotensin receptor blockers [ARBs]). Although RAAS inhibitors typically increase renal blood flow (RBF) and sodium (Na^+) excretion rates in HF and reduce the rate at which renal injury progresses in CKD, their use can also be coupled to a syndrome of "functional

renal insufficiency" and/or hyperkalemia. This form of acute kidney injury (AKI) most commonly develops shortly after beginning ACE inhibitor, ARB, or DRI therapy but can occur at any time in the course of chronic therapy, even in the absence of obvious predisposing factors.[1,2]

Acute kidney injury with RAAS inhibitors typically occurs when renal perfusion pressure cannot be maintained because of a substantial decrease in mean arterial pressure (MAP) or when the glomerular filtration rate (GFR) is overly dependent on the postglomerular efferent arteriolar constricting effect of angiotensin II.[3,4] Conditions that predict an adverse renal hemodynamic effect of RAAS inhibitors in patients with HF are preexisting low MAP values (typically < 60–65 mm Hg) and/or extracellular fluid volume (ECFV) depletion to the extent that the lowered cardiac filling pressures lead to a reduction in cardiac output. Glomerular filtration rate is heavily dependent on angiotensin II during

The Cardiorenal Syndrome: A Clinician's Guide to Pathophysiology and Management, 1st ed. © 2012 J. Thomas Heywood and John C. Burnett Jr., eds. Cardiotext Publishing, ISBN: 978-0-9790164-7-9.

ECFV depletion, high–grade bilateral renal artery stenosis, stenosis of a dominant or single kidney (as in a renal transplant recipient), and/or extensive microvascular renal disease. Understanding the pathophysiological mechanisms and the common risk factors for RAAS inhibitor–induced functional AKI is of some particular importance, because preventive approaches for AKI exist, and when such strategies are brought into play, they may allow for use of these compounds in a less restrictive fashion.[1,4]

Systemic/Renal Effects of Angiotensin II Pertinent to Heart Failure

Under usual physiological conditions, renal vascular resistance is coupled to the process of renal autoregulation, which, in turn, is influenced by local and systemically produced angiotensin II (as well as sympathetic nervous system [SNS] activity and other neurohumoral systems). As renal perfusion pressure falls in HF, both the SNS and the RAAS activate and generous amounts of angiotensin II are produced. Angiotensin II so generated has a predominant constricting effect on the postglomerular circulation, and this vascular action increases upstream glomerular capillary pressures, thereby maintaining glomerular filtration despite the otherwise reduced renal perfusion pressures. Angiotensin II also promotes proximal tubular Na^+ reabsorption and acts as a central dipsogen (ie, an agent that induces thirst).[5,6] These latter 2 aspects of angiotensin II effect contribute to the occurrence of hyponatremia in untreated HF. Administration of a RAAS inhibitor increases serum Na^+ concentrations in the HF patient with

hyponatremia unless the GFR has significantly declined with this therapy.[7]

Benefits of Long-Term Use of ACE Inhibitors and Angiotensin Receptor Blockers in Heart Failure

In patients with both symptomatic and asymptomatic myocardial dysfunction, long–term administration of ACE inhibitors reduces symptoms from HF, as well as the morbidity and mortality that accompanies this disease.[8] This beneficial effect of ACE inhibitors was recognized as early as 1984 and more recently has been shown to be the case with ARB therapy. ACE inhibitor and/or ARB therapy favorably affects the progression rate of a number of proteinuric and nonproteinuric renal diseases (that are often associated with HF development), which results in their being commonly used in the patient with CKD.[9] The beneficial effects of ACE inhibitor and ARB therapy in chronic nephropathies (with or without HF) are related to their hemodynamic actions as well as a wide range of neurohumoral, cellular, and vascular actions. This positive effect of ACE inhibitor and/or ARB therapy in chronic nephropathies is marked by a transient/reversible fall in the GFR in the order of 10% to 20%.[10] In the patient with early stage HF and a reduced GFR (either of a primary or a secondary nature) given ACE inhibitor and/or ARB therapy, a similar degree of change in the GFR is an anticipated treatment consequence. Alternatively, in the more advanced stages of HF, wherein GFR is reduced in tandem with the HF state, the change in GFR with either ACE inhibitor and/or ARB therapy can be dramatic and therapy limiting.[1]

Renal Function and the Heart

The issue of change in renal function with ACE inhibitor and/or ARB therapy in patients with coexistent renal disease and HF is a confusing one and often requires careful deciphering based on the definitional terminology in use. Acute kidney injury (functional renal insufficiency) in HF is defined as a sudden reduction in renal function, usually heralded by a not insignificant rise in serum creatinine concentration. Although no precise increase in serum creatinine defines AKI, an increase of 0.5 mg/dL (44 μmol/L) if the serum creatinine was initially < 2.0 mg/dL, or 1.0 mg/dL if the serum creatinine was above 2.0 mg/dL, was offered as a practical working definition in an American Heart Association scientific statement published in 2001.[1] Since that time, there has been a revival of interest in how best to define a change in renal function in HF (with or without ACE inhibitor therapy) with attention directed to novel biomarkers other than creatinine and use of estimated change in GFR (eGFR) rather than change in serum creatinine.[11]

The fast-changing nature of this field is best exemplified in the area of acute decompensated heart failure (ADHF), where functional renal insufficiency is a not infrequent occurrence impacting overall prognosis. Therein, the term *worsening renal function* (WRF) has been employed to describe a treatment-related rise in serum creatinine with increases of ≥ 0.3 mg/dL being of short- and long-term prognostic significance.[12] WRI, if sufficiently extreme and accompanied by features such as diuretic resistance and anemia, has been termed *cardiorenal syndrome*.[13] Although the expression has quickly become a term of convenience used to mark a change in renal function in the HF patient, there has not been a consistent meaning to its use.

A recent classification of cardiorenal syndrome into categories, albeit arbitrary, provides needed perspective on the sorting of the confusing bidirectional nature of kidney-heart interactions. Five subtypes of cardiorenal syndrome have been proposed, which reflect the temporal nature of the organ interactions as well as the primary and secondary pathology of the kidney-heart exchange.

- **Type 1 cardiorenal syndrome** (acute cardiorenal syndrome) reflects an abrupt worsening of cardiac function, such as ADHF, leading to acute kidney injury.
- **Type 2 cardiorenal syndrome** (chronic cardiorenal syndrome) describes long-standing abnormalities in cardiac function, such as chronic advanced-stage HF causing progressive and permanent CKD.
- **Type 3 cardiorenal syndrome** (acute renocardiac syndrome) reflects an abrupt worsening of renal function, such as with the nephrotic syndrome, bringing about an acute cardiac disorder, such as HF or coronary ischemia.
- **Type 4 cardiorenal syndrome** (chronic renocardiac syndrome) describes CKD of any origin contributing to structural and functional cardiac abnormalities and an amplified risk of cardiovascular events.
- **Type 5 cardiorenal syndrome** (secondary cardiorenal syndrome) is a systemic condition, such as sepsis, leading to both cardiac and renal dysfunction.[13]

Acute Renal Failure Due to ACE Inhibitor or Angiotensin Receptor Blocker Therapy

The frequency with which renal function changes in HF patients treated chronically with ACE inhibitors has been reported in several studies. In the Studies of Left Ventricular Dysfunction (SOLVD) trials, 3379 patients were randomly assigned to enalapril (median follow-up of 974 days) and 3379 patients randomly assigned to placebo (mean follow-up of 967 days). Decreased renal function was defined as a rise in serum creatinine of ≥ 0.5 mg/dL (44–µmol/L) above baseline. Sixteen percent of patients randomly assigned to enalapril had a decrease in renal function compared with 12% in the placebo controls, indicating a 4% (16% minus 12%) greater likelihood of an episode of decreased renal function with ACE inhibitor therapy. By multivariate analysis, in both the placebo and enalapril groups, older age, diuretic therapy, and diabetes were associated with a greater likelihood of a negative renal function change, whereas beta–blocker therapy and a higher ejection fraction were renoprotective in all patients irrespective of therapy.[14]

The frequency with which renal function changes in both the enalapril and placebo-treated limbs of SOLVD offers at best a rough approximation of what can be expected in trials lasting several months or longer. As such, the variables that might increase the frequency with which renal function deteriorates include (1) what change in serum creatinine is defined as being a "renal" event, (2) higher administered doses of either an ACE inhibitor and/or an ARB, and (3) the frequency of sampling taken to detect a change in renal function, concomitant medications in use (concurrent beta–blocker use affords some renoprotection), and/or whether a predominantly renally or renally/hepatically cleared RAAS inhibitor is being used.[1,15]

Renal function can deteriorate suddenly when RAAS inhibitor therapy is first begun, or it can acutely change in patients receiving chronic therapy particularly in patients with systolic HF and a low pretreatment MAP value. In either instance there is typically a > 50% increase in the serum creatinine value. Chronic RAAS inhibitor therapy in the HF patient presents a different set of circumstances; therein, a small change (< 30%) in serum creatinine values often marks the initiation of therapy. Intercurrent events, such as dehydration and/or hypotension, may accentuate the unfavorable renal hemodynamic effects of RAAS inhibitors, with the result being a significant additional decline in function. In the patient receiving chronic RAAS inhibitor therapy, a change in renal function, as assessed by serum creatinine values, is a poor barometer of renal function. It should also be appreciated that situations exist in which a rise in creatinine occurs without a realized change in GFR. Such is the case when trimethoprim (a component of Bactrim) or cimetidine is administered. Both of these compounds are organic cations, known to compete with creatinine for its tubular secretion, and therein limit its utility as an effective marker of renal function.[16,17]

In most patients who experience AKI with RAAS inhibitor therapy, one or more of 4 mechanisms are typically implicated. First and most importantly, if MAP falls to levels that cannot maintain renal perfusion and/or that provoke substantial reflex renal sympathetic nerve activity, renal function can be expected to decline under such circumstances.[18-20] In addition to triggering a sudden and sometimes prolonged decline in angiotensin II levels, ACE inhibitor therapy may lower MAP by other mechanisms, including an increase in vasodilatory prostaglandins and/or a decline in total peripheral resistance in a setting in which there may be an inadequate compensatory change in cardiac output owing to underlying myocardial dysfunction.

ACE inhibitor–related hypotension is generally more common with long-acting agents or in situations in which the pharmacological half-life of an ACE inhibitor is inordinately prolonged, as occurs when the degree of renal insufficiency is underestimated and an ACE inhibitor cleared predominantly by renal mechanisms is being given.[20] Under similar clinical circumstances ARBs appear to reduce blood pressure (or cause frank hypotension) to a similar degree as what is seen with ACE inhibitor therapy.

Second, ACE inhibitors or ARBs are more likely to cause AKI in the patient with HF who becomes volume depleted, whether it be from overly aggressive diuresis and/or an intercurrent volume-depleting illness. Mandal et al[21] reported from a retrospective chart review of patients receiving an ACE inhibitor (for HF, hypertension, and/or diabetes) that AKI occurred in 33.0% of those receiving a diuretic together with an ACE inhibitor; alternatively, AKI occurred in only 2.4% of patients who received ACE inhibitor therapy absent concurrent diuretic therapy. Moreover, Packer et al[22] observed in patients with HF treated with ACE inhibitors that those whose serum creatinine levels increased had received higher doses of diuretics, had lost more weight, and had lower left ventricular/right atrial pressures than those whose creatinine levels remained stable (if not improved). In the former group of patients, when salt intake was liberalized and/or diuretic doses reduced serum creatinine levels returned to pretreatment levels.

Third, ACE inhibitors may induce AKI in patients with high-grade bilateral renal artery stenosis or stenosis of a dominant or a single kidney renal artery, in patients with extensive atherosclerotic disease in smaller preglomerular vessels, or in patients with significant luminal narrowing of afferent arterioles as may be seen in patients with long-standing, poorly treated hypertension or chronic calcineurin inhibitor use.[23]

Fourth, ACE inhibitors may precipitate AKI in patients who are taking nonsteroidal anti-inflammatory agents (NSAIDs) or cyclooxygenase-2-specific inhibitors. Therein, the decrease in vasodilatory prostaglandins that derives from NSAID use favors renal vasoconstriction, compounding the reduced renal perfusion that occurs with ACE inhibitor therapy.[24]

Lastly, the risk of ACE inhibitor–induced AKI is greater in patients with CKD of any cause than in those with normal renal function. Reversal of hyperfiltration in the CKD kidney with either ACE inhibitor or ARB therapy will generally lead to an initial fall in GFR in the order of 10% to 20%.[10] In the CKD patient with HF the fall in GFR can be greater than this dependent on the prevailing volume state/MAP of the patient. A corollary to these observations is that there is no serum creatinine level per se at which use of ACE inhibitor or ARB therapy is contraindicated unless therapy with either of these drug classes results in clinically significant hyperkalemia. Acute kidney injury in association with ACE inhibitor and/or ARB therapy typically reverses with drug discontinuation or volume repletion, although occasionally, recovery is delayed or does not occur in a meaningful fashion.[25]

Management of Acute Kidney Injury in RAAS Inhibitor-Treated Patients

If monitoring is sufficiently judicious, those patients prone to AKI with RAAS inhibitors can be pinpointed early, without having to withhold therapy out of fear of the possibility of renal functional deterioration subsequent to their use. Serum creatinine and electrolyte values should be assessed at the start of RAAS inhibitor therapy and 5 to 7 days thereafter in the patient with HF. There is little gain from checking serum creatinine levels earlier unless a significant decrease is blood pressure has occurred or is anticipated. Absent the capacity for a patient to check blood pressure at home, a noteworthy drop in urine output or a change in the usual responsiveness to diuretic therapy might underscore an early significant decline in GFR attributable to a RAAS inhibitor and the need for earlier assessment of renal function. This is particularly the case in the patient with HF and hyponatremia, in whom the RAAS is typically highly activated and renal function particularly sensitive to RAAS inhibition.[7,26]

It is prudent prior to beginning RAAS inhibitor therapy to consider what an acceptable upper-limit rise in serum creatinine should be, above which both discontinuation of the medication and possible diagnostic studies for reversible vascular disease should be considered. For example, a rise in serum creatinine > 0.5 mg/dL if the initial serum creatinine is < 2.0 mg/dL (or a rise > 1.0 mg/dL if the baseline creatinine exceeds 2.0 mg/dL), particularly if the level progressively increases thereafter, should prompt consideration for stopping the medication as evaluation for renovascular disease is undertaken. Of note, the relationship between serum creatinine values and creatinine clearance is that of a rectangular hyperbola. Thus, at steady state, a doubling of serum creatinine, as might be reflected in a serum creatinine increase from 0.8 to 1.6 mg/dL, represents at least a 50% decrease in creatinine clearance.

The process of stopping a RAAS inhibitor because of an "excessive" rise in serum creatinine remains, however, an empiric one as to when evaluation should occur for reversible renal vascular disease. Renal artery stenosis and microvascular renal disease are not uncommon in the HF patient.[23] A very high plasma renin activity value (> 10 ng/mL/h), a size differential between both kidneys (> 1- to 2-cm difference in kidney length), and existing vascular disease in other organ beds/periphery are clues of some considerable importance in determining whether renal imaging should be aggressively pursued. Identification and correction of such lesions can be followed by a substantially greater renal and blood pressure tolerance of RAAS inhibitor therapy.[27,28]

Acute kidney injury complicating RAAS inhibitor therapy is almost always reversible within a matter of days. The reversible nature of ACE inhibitor–associated AKI is explained by the fact that the decline in the GFR is due to lowered glomerular capillary pressures (low inflow based on reduced blood pressure and absent postglomerular vasoconstriction), which return to baseline as soon as angiotensin II production is restored. In instances where substantial hypotension accompanies RAAS therapy–related AKI, an element of ischemia may be added to the process and recovery, despite discontinuation of the RAAS inhibitor, may be slowed or nonexistent.[25,29] To date, no biomarkers are clinically available that might allow one to predict the time course for correction of AKI related to RAAS inhibitors.

When AKI occurs with an ACE inhibitor, an ARB or a DRI should not be substituted as a RAAS inhibitor with a presumably more benign renal safety profile since they would have similar adverse effects on renal hemodynamics. Extracellular fluid volume depletion, either secondary to diuretic therapy or as the result of an intercurrent illness, has an important permissive effect on the reduction in GFR that occurs in the patient with HF receiving RAAS inhibitor therapy.[29] Careful replacement of an ECFV deficit, along with discontinuation of diuretic therapy, and treatment of intercurrent illnesses are the most efficacious approaches to resolution of the AKI episode.[22] In the setting of volume depletion it is not known to what degree temporary withdrawal of a RAAS inhibitor speeds the rate of renal functional recovery, although this is a common clinical recommendation. In addition, withdrawal of interacting drugs, supportive management of fluid and electrolyte abnormalities, and temporary dialysis where indicated are the mainstays of therapy. It is not known whether the use of dialysis to remove dialyzable ACE inhibitors also influences the time course of the AKI episode. The ACE inhibitors enalapril, lisinopril, and captopril undergo significant cross-dialyzer clearance. None of the ARBs are dialyzable.[30]

Where CKD is present, and especially when renal function is variable (as with unstable HF), several options are available in selecting an ACE inhibitor. One is to select a drug that is eliminated in part by hepatic clearance rather than by renal excretion and is therefore less likely to accumulate in the presence of a reduced GFR. Alternatively, one can select a drug eliminated solely by renal clearance, in which case drug accumulation needs to be factored into the dose given. At this time, the significance or potential consequences of such accumulation in patients with CKD are unclear. Likewise, when a patient needs hemodialysis, therapy can be simplified if an ACE inhibitor is chosen that is not significantly dialyzed, such as fosinopril, so that therapy can proceed uninterrupted by issues of drug dialysance (Table 7.1).[30]

Unresolved Questions Regarding Acute Kidney Injury in RAAS Inhibitor-Treated Patients

A number of unanswered questions exist regarding ACE inhibitor–related functional renal insufficiency. For example, it is known that the *DD* genotype for ACE is associated with elevated serum and tissue ACE levels. However, whether this or the II or ID phenotypes affect the propensity for AKI after ACE inhibition is unclear[31,32]; differing ACE phenotypes would not be an issue with ARB therapy. In addition, no available information supports the use of ARBs in place of ACE inhibitors in the HF patient prone to deterioration in renal function with these drugs. It is not known whether the timing of ACE inhibitor administration influences the development of AKI. Diuretic action, especially that of loop diuretics, is critically dependent on a threshold MAP for delivery of both diuretic and filtrate to the kidney, particularly in the HF patient. Timing of administration of an ACE inhibitor so that its peak blood pressure–lowering effect does not coincide with diuretic administration may allow for more predictable diuresis.[33] Clinically, this variable may be important in maintaining an optimal state of salt and water balance and lessening the risk of ACE inhibitor–related renal dysfunction in the CHF patient. Finally, it is unclear as to the extent to which aspirin therapy makes the CHF patient more susceptible to ACE inhibitor–associated renal failure.[34]

Table 7.1: Elimination Characteristics
of ACE Inhibitors in Maintenance Hemodialysis

Drug	Dialyzable[*]	Route of Elimination
Captopril	Yes	Renal
Enalapril	Yes	Renal
Lisinopril	Yes	Renal
Perindopril	Yes	Renal
Ramipril	Yes	Renal
Fosinopril	No	Renal/hepatic
Quinapril	No	Renal
Benazepril	NA	Renal
Moexipril	NA	Renal
Trandolapril	NA	Renal/hepatic

* "Yes" indicates drug is removed during dialysis; NA, data not available. The extent to which dialyzable ACE inhibitors are cleared related to dialyzer size, inflow blood flow rate, and blood pressure considerations during the session.

Note: Postdialysis drug supplementation or administration within 4 hours after dialysis is considered when the drug is removed by dialysis or blood pressure control is necessary or blood pressure is high enough to allow for drug tolerance.

Modified from Sica DA, Gehr TW, Fernandez A. Risk-benefit ratio of angiotensin antagonists versus ACE inhibitors in end-stage renal disease. *Drug Saf.* 2000; 22:350-360. With permission from Adis, a Wolters Kluwer business (© Adis Data Information BV 2000. All rights reserved.)

Conclusion

The use of ACE inhibitors or ARBs in patients with HF, hypertension, and chronic nephropathies can be viewed as a double-edged sword. As long as renal perfusion pressure is adequate and volume depletion is not excessive, ACE inhibitors can improve the abnormal renal hemodynamics of HF. However, because angiotensin II is necessary for maintenance of GFR during states of significant volume depletion, these agents also can cause GFR to decrease rapidly, with consequent oliguric or anuric renal failure. ACE inhibitors or ARBs can generally be safely restarted after resolution of an AKI episode, particularly if the underlying conditions having predisposed to the episode can be rectified. The principles of RAAS inhibition therapy in HF are summarized in Table 7.2.

Table 7.2: Principles of RAAS Inhibitor Therapy: Renal Considerations

- ACE inhibitors and ARBs improve renal blood flow and stabilize glomerular filtration rate in most patients with HF unless they adversely affect cardiac hemodynamics.

- ACE inhibitor and ARB therapy is indicated in patients with diabetic nephropathy and in patients with nondiabetic nephropathies when protein excretion exceeds 1 g/day. Concurrent primary renal diseases are not uncommon in the HF patient.

- A rise in serum creatinine may occur after initiation of RAAS inhibitor therapy in patients with HF. This rise usually occurs shortly after initiation of therapy, is in the 10% to 20% range, is not progressive, and is of renal hemodynamic origin. Renal function often stabilizes and may decline thereafter.

- Although there is no serum creatinine level per se that contraindicates ACE inhibitor therapy, greater increases in serum creatinine occur more frequently when ACE inhibitors are used in patients with underlying CKD.

- The occurrence of AKI should prompt a search for systemic hypotension (MAP < 65 mm Hg), ECFV depletion, or nephrotoxin administration and attempts to correct/remove these factors. Consideration should also be given to searching for high-grade bilateral renal artery stenosis or stenosis in a solitary kidney.

- ACE inhibitors should be temporarily discontinued when AKI occurs and precipitating factors for AKI corrected; an ARB or a DRI is not an appropriate substitute under these conditions. Once AKI has resolved with correction of the precipitating factors, ACE inhibitor therapy can be cautiously reintroduced.

References

1. Schoolwerth AC, Sica DA, Ballermann BJ, Wilcox CS; Council on the Kidney in Cardiovascular Disease and the Council for High Blood Pressure Research of the American Heart Association. Renal considerations in angiotensin converting enzyme inhibitor therapy: a statement for healthcare professionals from the Council on the Kidney in Cardiovascular Disease and the Council for High Blood Pressure Research of the American Heart Association. Circulation. 2001;104:1985–1991.

2. Suki WN. Renal hemodynamic consequences of angiotensin–converting enzyme inhibition in congestive heart failure. Arch Intern Med. 1989;149:669–673.

3. Sica DA. Renal considerations in the use of angiotensin–converting enzyme inhibitors in the treatment of congestive heart failure. Clin Cardiol. 1997;20(suppl II):II20–II23.

4. Oster JR, Materson BJ. Renal and electrolyte complications of congestive heart failure and effects of therapy with angiotensin–converting enzyme

inhibitors. *Arch Intern Med.* 1992;152: 704–710.

5. Schuster VL. Effects of angiotensin on proximal tubular reabsorption. *Fed Proc.* 986;45:1444–1447.

6. Phillips MI, Sumners C. Angiotensin II in central nervous system physiology. *Regul Pept.* 1998;78:1–11.

7. Packer M, Medina N, Yushak M. Correction of dilutional hyponatremia in severe chronic heart failure by converting–enzyme inhibition. *Ann Intern Med.* 1984;100:782–789.

8. Garg R, Yusuf S; for the Collaborative Group on ACE Inhibitor Trials. Overview of randomized trials of angiotensin–converting enzyme inhibitors on mortality and morbidity in patients with heart failure. *JAMA.* 1995;273:1450–1456.

9. Taal MW, Brenner BM. Renoprotective benefits of RAS inhibition: from ACEI to angiotensin II antagonists. *Kidney Int.* 2000;57:1803–1817.

10. Bakris GL, Weir MR. Angiotensin–converting enzyme inhibitor-associated elevations in serum creatinine: is this a cause for concern? *Arch Intern Med.* 2000;160:685–693.

11. Patel PC, Ayers CR, Murphy SA, et al. Association of cystatin C with left ventricular structure and function: the Dallas Heart Study. *Circ Heart Fail.* 2009;2:98–104.

12. Hillege HL, Nitsch D, Pfeffer MA, et al; Candesartan in Heart Failure: Assessment of Reduction in Mortality and Morbidity (CHARM) Investigators. Renal function as a predictor of outcome in a broad spectrum of patients with heart failure. *Circulation.* 2006;113: 671–678.

13. Ronco C, Haapio M, House AA, Anavekar N, Bellomo R. Cardiorenal syndrome. *J Am Coll Cardiol.* 2008;52: 1527–1539.

14. Knight EL, Glynn RJ, McIntyre KM, Mogun H, Avorn J. Predictors of decreased renal function in patients with heart failure during angiotensin–converting enzyme inhibitor therapy: results from the Study Of Left Ventricular Dysfunction (SOLVD). *Am Heart J.* 1999;138:849–855.

15. Sica DA. Kinetics of angiotensin converting enzyme inhibitors in renal failure. *J Cardiovasc Pharmacol.* 1992;20(suppl 10):S13–S20.

16. Tangri N, Alam A, Giannetti N, Deedwardes MB, Cantarovich M. Predicting glomerular filtration rate in heart transplant recipients using serum creatinine-based equations with cimetidine. *J Heart Lung Transplant.* 2008;27:905–909.

17. Myre SA, McCann J, First MR, Cluxton RJ Jr. Effect of trimethoprim on serum creatinine in healthy and chronic renal failure volunteers. *Ther Drug Monit.* 1987;9:161–165.

18. Kostis JB, Shelton B, Gosselin G, et al. Adverse effects of enalapril in the Studies of Left Ventricular Dysfunction (SOLVD). *Am Heart J.* 1996;131:350–355.

19. Packer M, Medina N, Yushak M, Meller J. Hemodynamic patterns of response during long–term captopril therapy for severe chronic heart failure. *Circulation.* 1983;68:803–812.

20. Davidson NC, Coutie WJ, Webb DJ, Struthers AD. Hormonal and renal differences between low dose and high dose angiotensin converting enzyme inhibitor treatment in patients with chronic heart failure. *Heart.* 1996;75: 576–581.

21. Mandal AK, Markert RJ, Saklayen MG, Mankus RA, Yokokawa K. Diuretics potentiate angiotensin converting enzyme inhibitor–induced acute renal failure. *Clin Nephrol.* 1994;42:170–174.

22. Packer M, Lee WH, Medina N, Yushak M, Kessler PD. Functional renal insufficiency during long-term therapy with captopril and enalapril in severe chronic heart failure. *Ann Intern Med.* 1987;106:346–354.

23. de Mast Q, Beutler JJ. The prevalence of atherosclerotic renal artery stenosis in risk groups: a systematic literature review. *J Hypertens.* 2009;27:1333–1340.

24. Slørdal L, Spigset O. Heart failure induced by non-cardiac drugs. *Drug Saf.* 2006;29:567–586.

25. Al Shohaib S, Raweily E. Acute tubular necrosis due to captopril. *Am J Nephrol.* 2000;20:149–152.

26. Packer M. Identification of risk factors predisposing to the development of functional renal insufficiency during treatment with converting-enzyme inhibitors in chronic heart failure. *Cardiology.* 1989;76:50–55.

27. de Silva R, Loh H, Rigby AS, et al. Epidemiology, associated factors, and prognostic outcomes of renal artery stenosis in chronic heart failure assessed by magnetic resonance angiography. *Am J Cardiol.* 2007;100:273–279.

28. Balachandran KP, Oldroyd KG. Successful reintroduction of previously failed ACE inhibitor therapy following stenting of atherosclerotic renovascular disease. *Indian Heart J.* 2008;60:55–57.

29. Wynckel A, Ebikili B, Melin JP, Randoux C, Lavaud S, Chanard J. Long-term follow-up of acute renal failure caused by angiotensin converting enzyme inhibitors. *Am J Hypertens.* 1998;11: 1080–1086.

30. Sica DA, Gehr TW, Fernandez A. Risk-benefit ratio of angiotensin antagonists versus ACE inhibitors in end-stage renal disease. *Drug Saf.* 2000;22:350–360.

31. Isbir SC, Tekeli A, Ergen A, et al. Genetic polymorphisms contribute to acute kidney injury after coronary artery bypass grafting. *Heart Surg Forum.* 2007;10:E439–E444.

32. du Cheyron D, Fradin S, Ramakers M, et al. Angiotensin converting enzyme insertion/deletion genetic polymorphism: its impact on renal function in critically ill patients. *Crit Care Med.* 2008;36:3178–3183.

33. Sica DA. Edema mechanisms in the patient with heart failure and treatment options. *Heart Fail Clin.* 2008;4:511–518.

34. Juhlin T, Jönsson BA, Höglund P. Renal effects of aspirin are clearly dose-dependent and are of clinical importance from a dose of 160-mg. *Eur J Heart Fail.* 2008;10:892–898.

The Effect of Inotropes on Renal Function in Patients with Heart Failure

8

Tien M. H. Ng
Nudrat Khatri
Uri Elkayam

Information from the Acute Decompensated Heart Failure National Registry (ADHERE) demonstrates the use of intravenous inotropes in approximately 10% of patients hospitalized with acute decompensated heart failure (ADHF) in the United States.[1] These drugs are used to increase cardiac contractility and improve cardiac output (CO) and renal function.[2] Guidelines from the Heart Failure Society of America also recommend the use of these drugs in patients with evidence of fluid overload if they respond poorly to intravenous diuretics or manifest diminished or worsening renal function.[3] Although these guidelines are based on the clinical belief that inotropic drugs improve renal hemodynamics and function, the effects of these drugs on the kidney in patients with heart failure (HF) have not been clearly defined.

Dobutamine

Dobutamine is a catecholamine-derived inotrope that acts predominantly on beta-1- and beta-2-adrenergic receptors. Although dobutamine also binds to alpha-1-adrenergic receptors, the clinical effect of vasoconstriction appears to be mitigated by the beta-2-mediated vasodilation. The physiologic effects of dobutamine on renal vasculature also reflect this pharmacology.[4] Studies in animals report conflicting findings in regard to whether dobutamine can increase renal blood flow (RBF) and decrease renal vascular resistance.[5,6] Several studies in healthy human volunteers, using either fixed dosing of 2.5 to 10.0 µg/kg/min or dose titration to an increase in CO, have failed to

The Cardiorenal Syndrome: A Clinician's Guide to Pathophysiology and Management, 1st ed. © 2012 J. Thomas Heywood and John C. Burnett Jr., eds. Cardiotext Publishing, ISBN: 978-0-9790164-7-9.

show an increase in RBF measured by io-dohippurate clearance.[7-9] In fact, one study found a reduction in glomerular filtration rate (GFR), fractional excretion of sodium, and fractional free water clearance.[8] Another study utilizing Doppler ultrasonography also failed to find evidence of any effect of dobutamine on renal artery mean velocity or waveform pulsatility, which represent RBF and renal vascular resistance, respectively.[10] Dobutamine has also not been found to have a significant effect on renal function or urine output in the setting of critical illness despite favorable systemic hemodynamic effects.[11-14] In the setting of coronary artery bypass, do-butamine has been shown to improve RBF in patients with depressed cardiac index post-surgery.[15,16] Importantly, the increase in RBF is proportional (no change in RBF:CO ratio) to the improvement in CO, suggesting that dobutamine does not have measurable direct effects on renal vascular resistance.[16]

A crossover study in 13 severe HF patients was the first to define dobutamine's effects on systemic and regional hemodynamics in this syndrome.[17] Dobutamine, given at 2.5 to 10.0 µg/kg/min for 24 hours, was associated with significant increases in urine flow, urine sodium concentrations, and creatinine clearance, which were accompanied by increases in stroke volume and CO. However, subsequent studies in patients with HF have not replicated these original findings. A study of 8 severe HF patients demonstrated no significant effect on RBF with dobutamine 5 to 15 µg/kg/min despite dose-dependent effects on cardiac index, systemic vascular resistance, right atrial pressures, and pulmonary capillary wedge pressure.[18] In a randomized parallel-group study, 30 severe HF patients with reduced cardiac index (< 1.9 L/min/m²), NYHA functional class III and IV, received dobutamine initiated at 2.5 to 5.0 µg/kg/min and titrated to a 20% improvement in cardiac index for 7 days.[19] Dobutamine improved RBF as assessed by para-aminohippurate clearance but was not associated with an improvement in GFR. Similarly, a randomized, parallel-group study of 88 severe HF patients requiring inotropic support, NYHA functional class III and IV, compared dobutamine initiated at 5 µg/kg/min titrated to clinical effect for up to 72 hours to levosimendan.[20] Dobutamine was associated with an increase in urine output but no change in GFR at 24 or 72 hours.

Overall, dobutamine's ability to augment RBF appears to depend on the clinical setting and most likely only occurs when renal perfusion is improved secondary to an increase in CO, although this has not been a universal finding. Despite its potential to aid renal perfusion, clinical studies suggest dobutamine has little effect on renal vascular resistance and indices of renal function such as GFR. Notwithstanding the totality of the data, a more recent study in 11 HF patients has renewed interest in the need for more complete evaluation of dobutamine's renal effects in HF.[21] In this open-label study, dobutamine titrated to an increase in peak dP/dt of 25% was associated with a 50% reduction in efferent renal sympathetic activity, which may have prognostic implications considering what is known about cardiorenal pathophysiology.

Milrinone

Milrinone confers its positive inotropic effect through antagonism of the phosphodiesterase III enzyme, resulting in cyclic adenosine monophosphate (cAMP)–mediated increases in cardiomyocyte intracellular calcium concentrations. Milrinone also has profound vasodilatory effects, which have been demonstrated in peripheral, coronary, splanchnic, skeletal muscle, and renal arteries. Phosphodiesterase enzymes and cAMP are important mediators of renal vascular resistance.[22,23] Although conflicting data exist in terms of whether milrinone increases renal cAMP in isolated kidney preparations,[22,24,25] studies in intact dogs suggest milrinone reduces renal vascular resistance and increases RBF,[26,27] perhaps affecting medullary more than cortical blood flow.[26] In 2 studies of milrinone's effects on regional blood flow in rat and dog models of chronic HF, milrinone increased flow to renal vascular beds measured using radioactive microspheres.[28,29] This effect was achieved through a reduction in renal resistance and in conjunction with expected systemic hemodynamic effects.

Clinical studies of milrinone's renal effects in HF are limited. In an open-label study, 11 patients with severe chronic HF, NYHA functional class III or IV, and left ventricular ejection fraction (LVEF) < 20%, milrinone administered as a single oral dose of 7.5 mg was associated with a significant increase in RBF compared with baseline (417 ± 111 vs 289 ± 78 mL/min, $P < 0.05$) at 90 minutes postdose.[30] Another study evaluated the chronic effects of oral milrinone administered for 1 month in 13 severe HF patients.[31] This study found no overall change in RBF, renal vascular resistance, or estimated GFR rate at 1 month. However, there was heterogeneity in changes in RBF and GFR, with a significant correlation between these parameters and changes in cardiac index, suggesting individual responses to milrinone may vary. Whether intravenous milrinone has clinically relevant effects on renal physiology in HF remains undescribed.

Levosimendan

Levosimendan is an inodilator approved for ADHF in Europe and Scandinavia. Unlike catecholamine and phosphodiesterase III inhibitors, its inotropic effects are achieved without an increase in intracellular calcium. Levosimendan, at clinically relevant doses, is reported to be a calcium sensitizer, whereby the interaction between troponin C and calcium is enhanced during systole, leading to an increase in force generation. Levosimendan also activates ATP-dependent potassium channels, leading to significant vasodilatory effects. Levosimendan has been shown to dose-dependently increase CO, and decrease pulmonary capillary wedge pressure and systemic vascular resistance in HF patients. Levosimendan may also exhibit anti-inflammatory properties.

Experimental animal and human data demonstrate that levosimendan exerts effects on renal physiology. In a study assessing regional distribution of CO in anesthetized dogs, levosimendan infused for 15 minutes at doses of 0.75, 1.5, and 3.0 μg/kg/min increased renal medullary blood flow in a dose-dependent manner; this was accompanied by dose-dependent reductions in renal medullary and cortical vascular resistance.[26] These results were not reproducible in the setting of experimental septic shock in pigs and rabbits, where infusions of levosimendan 3.3 μg/kg/min failed to improve medullary or cortical renal artery blood flow.[32,33] However, despite these conflicting reports on renal perfusion, levosimendan was found to prevent endotoxin-induced acute renal failure in lipopolysaccharide-treated mice.[34] In one randomized, open-label study of levosimendan 0.2 μg/kg/min or dobutamine 5 μg/kg/min for 24 hours, in 28 patients with septic shock and preserved left ventricular function (LVEF ≥ 45%), levosimendan was associated with a 64% increase in creatinine clearance compared with baseline (72.1 ± 16.2 vs 43.9 ± 12.8 mL/min, $P < 0.05$).[14] Although the exact mechanism is unclear, the authors noted that a direct effect of levosimendan on renal perfusion was possible since mean arterial pressure was unchanged and cardiac index increased minimally.

Data on levosimendan and renal function in HF are limited to 2 small prospective studies and results from the Levosimendan Infusion versus Dobutamine (LIDO) study. In a study of 40 chronic HF patients awaiting transplantation, renal function was assessed 3 months after patients were randomized to receive levosimendan administered as a 12.0-μg/kg bolus followed by 0.1 μg/kg/min for 24 hours, or no levosimendan (control group).[35] The majority of patients were male (93%), with coronary artery disease (63%) and with a mean LVEF of 28%. Levosimendan was associated with a significant reduction in serum creatinine at 1 month compared with baseline (–0.32 ± 0.28 mg/dL, $P = 0.005$) whereas there was no change in the control group (–0.01 ± 0.13 mg/dL, $P = $ NS vs baseline). Calculated creatinine clearance was significantly higher with levosimendan than control at 1 month. The differences favoring levosimendan in serum creatinine (1.60 ± 0.26 vs 1.90 ± 0.14 mg/dL, $P = 0.005$) and creatinine clearance (53.6 ± 8.6 vs 44.0 ± 3.3 mL/min, $P = 0.005$) persisted through to 3 months. Univariate predictors of improved renal function at 3 months were levosimendan therapy, increase in LVEF, decrease in brain natriuretic peptide concentration, and ischemic etiology. However, only levosimendan therapy remained significant upon multivariate analysis, suggesting some of the benefit on renal preservation may be independent of its hemodynamic effects.

A second clinical trial evaluated renal function in 88 ADHF patients requiring inotropic therapy.[20] Patients were NYHA functional class III and IV with LVEF ≤ 40%. Patients were randomized in a 2:1 fashion to levosimendan 0.1 to 0.2 μg/kg/min for 24 hours or to dobutamine (initiated at 5 μg/kg/min and titrated to desired effect of primary physician) for a minimum of 24 hours.

Baseline serum creatinine for the levosimendan and dobutamine groups was 1.58 ± 0.56 and 1.41 ± 0.41 mg/dL, respectively. Median change in calculated GFR (using the MDRD equation) was higher with levosimendan than dobutamine at 24 hours (+15.3% vs –1.33%, $P < 0.001$). Levosimendan therapy was associated with improvement in calculated GFR compared with baseline at 24 hours (58.6 ± 21.9 vs 51.5 ± 22.1 mL/min/m², $P < 0.001$) and 72 hours (27 patients with follow-up data: 65.5 ± 30.4 vs 47.2 ± 24.1 mL/min/m², $P < 0.001$), whereas dobutamine was not associated with a significant effect. Urine output increased similarly in both treatment arms. These results may therefore suggest that levosimendan may exert renoprotective effects through multiple mechanisms.

The LIDO study was a phase 3 randomized, double-blind study comparing levosimendan to dobutamine in 203 hospitalized low-output HF patients.[36] Patients received either levosimendan (24-μg/kg bolus followed by 0.1 μg/kg/min) or dobutamine (5–10 μg/kg/min) for 24 hours. Serum creatinine was significantly reduced with levosimendan compared with dobutamine (–9 vs –1 μmol/L, $P = 0.03$).

Although experimental data are conflicting as to the effect of levosimendan on RBF, human studies suggest that it exerts clinically relevant effects on renal function and estimated GFR, and that it may confer renoprotective effects. The mechanism(s) of renoprotection are unknown but could include an augmentation of RBF via an increase in CO or reduction on vascular renal resistance, anti-inflammatory effects, and ATP-dependent potassium channel activation.

Dopamine

Dopamine is known to exhibit a graded pharmacological response with a dose-dependent predominant activation of dopaminergic receptors, beta-receptors, and alpha-receptors.[37,38] Generally, at doses < 3 μg/kg/min dopamine was found to activate dopamine A1 receptors, which cause vasodilatation of the renal arteries and other vascular beds, including mesenteric, coronary, and cerebral. In addition, there is stimulation of dopamine A2 receptors, which leads to inhibition of norepinephrine release from sympathetic nerve endings.[38] Activation of dopamine A1 and A2 receptors also leads to a decline in systemic vascular resistance and to an increase in RBF. Dopamine infused at approximately 3 to 5 μg/kg/min activates beta-1- and beta-2-adrenergic receptors, conferring a positive inotropic effect that is responsible for an increase in CO. At a dose of > 5 μg/kg/min dopamine has been reported to exert clinically relevant activation of alpha-1-adrenergic receptors, which may result in arterial vasoconstriction.

An early study by McDonald et al[39] described the renal effect of dopamine infusion at doses ranging from 1.3 to 3.6 μg/kg/min in 6 patients with HF and marked sodium retention. In all patients dopamine was associated with an increase in mean GFR, renal plasma flow, and urine flow. These changes were not statistically significant but were associated with a significant augmentation in sodium excretion. Beregovich et al[40] in 1974 studied the effect of dopamine 1.5 and 10.0 μg/kg/min in 9 patients with congestive heart failure (CHF) secondary to myocardial, coronary, or valvular heart disease. Cardiac output increased steadily and significantly with progressive doses of dopamine up to 87% over control values, with maximum increase achieved with a mean dose of 6.9 μg/kg/min. Other hemodynamic changes included a significant increase in heart rate and a decrease in systemic vascular resistance. There was a significant increase in urine flow with dopamine at a dose of 5 μg/

kg/min (1.5 ± 0.3 mL/min to 5.5 ± 1.3 mL/min) and 10 μg/kg/min (5.0 ± 1.4 mL/min). Dopamine was also associated with increases in sodium excretion (6.5 ± 3.4 mEq/min × 10^{-2} to 9.4 ± 3.5 mEq/min × 10^{-2} at 5 μg/kg/min) and creatinine clearance at 1, 5, and 10 μg/kg/min (from 59.0 ± 6.0 to 73.0 ± 4.7, 72.0 ± 3.6, and 90.0 ± 16.4 mL/min, respectively). Different results were reported by Good et al[41] in 1992. These investigators studied the effect of dopamine at a dose of 1 and 10 μg/kg/min in 6 men with HF and failed to find a significant effect on urine volume compared to placebo.

Varriale and Mossavi[42] in 1997 randomized 20 study patients with severe chronic CHF at the NYHA functional class III and IV and renal impairment represented by serum creatinine ≥ 1.5 mg/dL to either bumetanide 1 mg twice daily (group A) or the same diuretic regimen plus a continuous infusion of low-dose (2 μg/kg/min) dopamine (group B). All patients were placed on a low-sodium (2 g/day) diet and a fluid intake of 1.5 to 2.0 L daily. Both treatment groups showed a significant increase in urine flow rate (0.69 ± 0.20 mL/kg/h to 1.85 ± 0.24 mL/kg/h in group A and from 0.56 ± 0.16 to 2.02 ± 0.072 mL/kg/h in group B, both $P < 0.05$). However, patients who received low-dose dopamine in addition to bumetanide showed a significant improvement in the level of blood urea nitrogen (48.9 ± 10.3 mg/dL to 32.1 ± 14.4 mg/dL, $P < 0.05$) and an increase in creatinine clearance (35.6 ± 11.6 to 48.8 ± 12.3 mL/min, $P < 0.05$). Patients who did not received low-dose dopamine showed a nonsignificant deterioration in all indices of renal function after therapy.

Vargo et al[43] in 1996 examined whether the addition of low-dose (1-3 μg/kg/min) dopamine enhanced natriuresis in 6 patients with compensated CHF NYHA class II and III. The study was randomized, controlled, and open-label with crossover design. Infusion of dopamine alone caused a slight and statistically insignificant increase in natriuresis (from 6.7 ± 0.7 mEq/3 h to 36.7 ± 8.5 mEq/3 h). Furosemide alone markedly increased sodium excretion to 276.6 ± 47.2 mEq/3 h. The addition of dopamine to furosemide did not result in any further increase in natriuresis (253.8 ± 73.6 mEq/3 h).

Cotter et al[44] in 1997 evaluated the safety and efficacy of low-dose (4 µg/kg/min) dopamine combined with low-dose furosemide (80 mg/day given in 2 oral doses) compared with same-dose dopamine combined with medium-dose furosemide (5 mg/kg/day given as continuous intravenous administration) and to high-dose furosemide (10 mg/kg/day given as a continuous intravenous administration) alone in 20 patients with refractory CHF. All 3 groups were treated for 72 hours and showed a similar involvement in signs and symptoms of CHF and had similar urine output and weight loss. Mean blood pressure reduction was significantly smaller with low-dose furosemide as well as deterioration of renal function and development of hypokalemia. This study suggested that combined low-dose intravenous dopamine and oral furosemide has a similar effect on urine output but has less effect on blood pressure, less renal impairment, and less hypokalemia compared with a higher dose of furosemide either alone or in combination with low-dose dopamine.

Most recent evaluation of the renal circulation effect of dopamine in patients with HF was performed by Elkayam et al.[45] These investigators evaluated the renal effect of dopamine at a dose of 1, 2, 3, 5, and 10 µg/kg/min in 13 patients with chronic HF. Renal blood flow was calculated from a renal artery cross-sectional area measured with intravascular ultrasonography and RBF velocity–time integral measured by the intravascular Doppler technique. Renal blood flow increased, whereas renal vascular resistance decreased,

reaching statistical significance at 2 µg/kg/min through 10 µg/kg/min. Cardiac output gradually increased, reaching statistical significance at doses of 5 and 10 µg/kg/min, but the increase in RBF was proportionally larger than the corresponding increase in CO. This study, therefore, provided strong support to the direct vasodilatory effect of dopamine on both large conductance and small resistance renal blood vessel vascular resistance and thus to an increase in RBF. Ungar et al[46] studied short-term systemic and renal hemodynamic response to dopamine at 2.4 and 6.0 µg/kg/min in 16 patients with moderate to severe symptoms of HF. Effective renal plasma flow (ERPF) and GFR were determined by 131-labeled hippuran and iodine 125-labeled–iothalamate clearance techniques, respectively. Heart rate increased significantly with doses of 4 and 6 µg/kg/min, cardiac index was maximally enhanced (30%) at 4 µg/kg/min with no further increase at the higher dose, and systemic vascular resistance decreased at all dopamine doses. Dopamine infusion progressively increased ERPF and GFR with a maximum increase of 101% and 75%, respectively, occurring at 4 µg/kg/min. Renal vascular resistance was reduced at a dose of 2 µg/kg/min of dopamine with maximum effect achieved with 4 µg/kg/min. The beneficial effect of dopamine on RBF, GFR, and renal vascular resistance was decreased with the largest dose of 10 µg/kg/min used in this study.

Conclusion

In spite of a strong and favorable central hemodynamic effect of inotropes in patients with HF, the renal circulatory effect is incompletely defined and limited by a relatively small number of studies, including small number of patients. Available studies often present conflicting results. More information obtained by large, well-designed studies is needed to further explore the potential role of inotropic drugs in preservation or even improvement of renal function in patients hospitalized with decompensated HF.

References

1. Abraham WT, Adams KF, Fonarow GC, et al. In-hospital mortality in patients with acute decompensated heart failure requiring intravenous vasoactive medications: an analysis from the Acute Decompensated Heart Failure National Registry (ADHERE). *J Am Coll Cardiol.* 2005;46:57-64.

2. Felker GM, O'Connor CM. Inotropic therapy for heart failure: an evidence-based approach. *Am Heart J.* 2001;142:393-401.

3. Adams KF, Lindenfeld J, Arnold JMO, et al. Executive summary: HFSA 2006 comprehensive heart failure practice guideline. *J Card Fail.* 2006;12:10-38.

4. Ozaki N, Kawakita S, Toda N. Effects of dobutamine on isolated canine cerebral, coronary, mesenteric, and renal arteries. *J Cardiovasc Pharmacol.* 1982;4:456-461.

5. Robie NW, Goldberg LI. Comparative systemic and regional hemodynamic effects of dopamine and dobutamine. *Am Heart J.* 1975;90:340-345.

6. Fiser DH, Fewell JE, Hill DE, Brown AL. Cardiovascular and renal effects of dopamine and dobutamine in healthy, conscious piglets. *Crit Care Med.* 1988;16:340-345.

7. Mousdale S, Clyburn PA, Mackie AM, Groves ND, Rosen M. Comparison of the effects of dopamine, dobutamine, and dopexamine upon renal blood flow: a study in normal healthy volunteers. *Br J Clin Pharmacol.* 1988;25:555-560.

8. Westman L, Jarnberg PO. Effects of dobutamine on renal function in normal man. *Acta Anaesthesiol Scand.* 1986;30:72-75.

9. Olsen NV, Lund J, Jensen PF, et al. Dopamine, dobutamine, and dopexamine. A comparison of renal effects in unanesthetized human volunteers. *Anesthesiology.* 1993;79:685-694.

10. Yura T, Yuasa S, Fukunaga M, Badr KF, Matsuo H. Role for Doppler ultrasound in the assessment of renal circulation: effects of dopamine and dobutamine on renal hemodynamics in humans. *Nephron.* 1995;71:168-175.

11. Westman L, Jarnberg PO. Effects of dobutamine on haemodynamics and renal function in patients after major vascular surgery. *Acta Anaesthesiol Scand.* 1987;31:253-257.

12. Duke GJ, Briedis JH, Weaver RA. Renal support in critically ill patients: low-dose dopamine or low-dose dobutamine? *Crit Care Med.* 1994;22:1919-1925.

13. Ichai C, Soubielle J, Carles M, Giunti C, Grimaud D. Comparison of the renal effects of low to high doses of dopamine and dobutamine in critically ill patients: a single-blind randomized study. *Crit Care Med.* 2000;28:921-928.

14. Morelli A, De Castro S, Teboul JL, et al. Effects of levosimendan on systemic and regional hemodynamics in septic myocardial depression. *Intensive Care Med.* 2005;31:638-644.

15. MacGregor DA, Butterworth JF, Zaloga CP, Prielipp RC, James R, Royster RL. Hemodynamic and renal effects of dopexamine and dobutamine in patients with reduced cardiac output following coronary artery bypass grafting. *Chest.* 1994;106:835-841.

16. Sato Y, Matsuzawa H, Eguchi S. Comparative study of effects of adrenaline, dobutamine and dopamine

on systemic hemodynamics and renal blood flow in patients following open heart surgery. *Jpn Circ J.* 1982;46: 1059–1072.

17. Leier CV, Heban PT, Huss P, Bush CA, Lewis RP. Comparative systemic and regional hemodynamic effects of dopamine and dobutamine in patients with cardiomyopathic heart failure. *Circulation.* 1978;58(3 pt 1):466–475.

18. Thuillez C, Richard C, Teboul JL, et al. Arterial hemodynamics and cardiac effects of enoximone, dobutamine, and their combination in severe heart failure. *Am Heart J.* 1993;125:799–808.

19. Wimmer A, Stanek B, Kubecova L, et al. Effects of prostaglandin E1, dobutamine and placebo on hemodynamic, renal and neurohumoral variables in patients with advanced heart failure. *Jpn Heart J.* 1999;40:321–334.

20. Yilmaz MB, Yalta K, Yontar C, et al. Levosimendan improves renal function in patients with acute decompensated heart failure: comparison with dobutamine. *Cardiovasc Drugs Ther.* 2007;21:431–435.

21. Al-Hesayen A, Parker JD. The effects of dobutamine on renal sympathetic activity in human heart failure. *J Cardiovasc Pharmacol.* 2008;51:434–436.

22. Sandner P, Kornfeld M, Ruan X, Arendshorst WJ, Kurtz A. Nitric oxide/cAMP interactions in the control of rat renal vascular resistance. *Circ Res.* 1999;84:186–192.

23. Harris AL, Grant AM, Silver PJ, Evans DB, Alousi AA. Differential vasorelaxant effects of milrinone and amrinone on contractile responses of canine coronary, cerebral, and renal arteries. *J Cardiovasc Pharmacol.* 1989;13:238–244.

24. Jackson EK, Mi Z, Carcillo JA, Gillespie DG, Dubey RK. Phosphodiesterases in the rat renal vasculature. *J Cardiovasc Pharmacol.* 1997;30:798–801.

25. Lindgren S, Andersson KE. Effects of selective phosphodiesterase inhibitors on isolated coronary, lung and renal arteries from man and rat. *Acta Physiol Scand.* 1991;142:77–82.

26. Pagel PS, Hettrick DA, Warltier DC. Influence of levosimendan, pimobendan, and milrinone on the regional distribution of cardiac output in anaesthetized dogs. *Br J Pharmacol.* 1996;119:609–615.

27. Setoyama K, Ota H, Miura N, Fujiki M, Misumi K, Sakamoto H. Effects of milrinone on hemodynamics and regional blood flow in the hypoxic dog. *J Vet Med Sci.* 2002;64:499–503.

28. Liang CS, Thomas A, Imai N, Stone CK, Kawashima S, Hood WB Jr. Effects of milrinone on systemic hemodynamics and regional circulations in dogs with congestive heart failure: comparison with dobutamine. *J Cardiovasc Pharmacol.* 1987;10:509–516.

29. Drexler H, Hoing S, Faude F, Wollschlager H, Just H. Central and regional vascular hemodynamics following intravenous milrinone in the conscious rat: comparison with dobutamine. *J Cardiovasc Pharmacol.* 1987;9:563–569.

30. LeJemtel TH, Maskin CS, Mancini D, Sinoway L, Feld H, Chadwick B. Systemic and regional hemodynamic effects of captopril and milrinone administered alone and concomitantly in patients with heart failure. *Circulation.* 1985;72:364–369.

31. Cody RJ, Kubo SH, Covit AB, et al. Regional blood flow and neurohormonal responses to milrinone in congestive heart failure. *Clin Pharmacol Ther.* 1986;39:128–135.

32. Oldner A, Konrad D, Weitzberg E, Rudehill A, Rossi P, Wanecek M. Effects of levosimendan, a novel inotropic calcium–sensitizing drug, in experimental septic shock. *Crit Care Med.* 2001;29:2185–2193.

33. Faivre V, Kaskos H, Callebert J, et al. Cardiac and renal effects of levosimendan, arginine vasopressin, and norepinephrine in lipopolysaccharide-treated rabbits. *Anesthesiology.* 2005;103:514–521.

34. Zager RA, Johnson AC, Lund S, Hanson SY, Abrass CK. Levosimendan protects against experimental endotoxemic acute renal failure. *Am J Physiol Renal Physiol.* 2006;290:F1453–1462.

35. Zemljic G, Bunc M, Yazdanbakhsh AP, Vrtovec B. Levosimendan improves renal function in patients with advanced chronic heart failure awaiting cardiac transplantation. *J Card Fail.* 2007;13:417–421.

36. Follath F, Cleland JG, Just H, et al. Efficacy and safety of intravenous levosimendan compared with dobutamine in severe low–output heart failure (the LIDO study): a randomised double–blind trial. *Lancet.* 2002;360: 196–202.

37. Leier CV, Bambach D, Thompson MJ, Cattaneo SM, Goldberg RJ, Unverferth DV. Central and regional hemodynamic effects of intravenous isosorbide dinitrate, nitroglycerin and nitroprusside in patients with congestive heart failure. *Am J Cardiol.* 1981;48: 1115–1123.

38. Goldberg LI, Rajfer SI. Dopamine receptors: applications in clinical cardiology. *Circulation.* 1985;72:245–248.

39. McDonald RH Jr, Goldberg LI, McNay JL, Tuttle EP Jr. Effect of dopamine in man: augmentation of sodium excretion, glomerular filtration rate, and renal plasma flow. *J Clin Invest.* 1964;43: 1116–1124.

40. Beregovich J, Bianchi C, Rubler S, Lomnitz E, Cagin N, Levitt B. Dose-related hemodynamic and renal effects of dopamine in congestive heart failure. *Am Heart J.* 1974;87:550–557.

41. Good J, Frost G, Oakley CM, Cleland JG. The renal effects of dopamine and dobutamine in stable chronic heart failure. *Postgrad Med J.* 1992;68(suppl 2):S7–11.

42. Varriale P, Mossavi A. The benefit of low–dose dopamine during vigorous diuresis for congestive heart failure associated with renal insufficiency: does it protect renal function? *Clin Cardiol.* 1997;20:627–630.

43. Vargo DL, Brater DC, Rudy DW, Swan SK. Dopamine does not enhance furosemide–induced natriuresis in patients with congestive heart failure. *J Am Soc Nephrol.* 1996;7:1032–1037.

44. Cotter G, Weissgarten J, Metzkor E, et al. Increased toxicity of high–dose furosemide versus low–dose dopamine in the treatment of refractory congestive heart failure. *Clin Pharmacol Ther.* 1997;62:187–193.

45. Elkayam U, Ng TM, Hatamizadeh P, Janmohamed M, Mehra A. Renal vasodilatory action of dopamine in patients with heart failure: magnitude of effect and site of action. *Circulation.* 2008;117:200–205.

46. Ungar A, Fumagalli S, Marini M, et al. Renal, but not systemic hemodynamic effects of dopamine are influenced by the severity of congestive heart failure. *Crit Care Med.* 2004;32:1125–1129.

Novel Chimeric Natriuretic Peptides and Cardiorenal Syndrome

9

Paul M. McKie
Fernando L. Martin
John C. Burnett Jr.

Cardiorenal syndrome represents a complex syndrome of concomitant heart failure (HF) and renal dysfunction. Importantly, the syndrome is associated with greater cardiovascular mortality and morbidity than either HF or renal dysfunction alone. As such, there is an unmet need for novel therapeutics that enhance both cardiac and renal function and lead to improved outcomes. The natriuretic peptides represent a family of guanylyl cyclase (GC) activators that, via 2 distinct receptors (GC_A and GC_B), have cardiorenal-enhancing properties. In this chapter we review the design and clinical development of a first-in-class designer chimeric natriuretic peptide termed CD-NP. CD-NP, unlike the native natriuretic peptides (ANP and BNP, which bind to GC_A, and CNP, which binds to

GC_B), coactivates GC_A and GC_B. CD-NP, now in clinical trials, is therefore a dual activator of GC_A and GC_B ($GC_B > GC_A$) and possesses the strong antiproliferative and antifibrotic properties of CNP with the potently natriuretic and diuretic properties of DNP with less blood pressure–lowering effects than BNP. Thus, CD-NP has emerged as an appealing therapeutic strategy for cardiorenal syndrome.

An emerging focus of interest is the relationship between the heart and the kidney in both physiological regulation of cardiorenal homeostasis and the pathophysiology of HF and chronic kidney disease (CKD). This combination of renal dysfunction, either acute or chronic, and HF is termed *cardiorenal syndrome*. Importantly, cardiorenal syndrome portends a worse prognosis than either HF or renal dysfunction alone.[1-7] The high mortality and morbidity of the syndrome support an unmet need for novel therapeutics that enhance both heart and kidney organ

The Cardiorenal Syndrome: A Clinician's Guide to Pathophysiology and Management, 1st ed. © 2012 J. Thomas Heywood and John C. Burnett Jr., eds. Cardiotext Publishing, ISBN: 978-0-9790164-7-9.

systems and optimize cardiorenal function.

The mechanisms of cardiorenal syndrome are complex but are known to include decreased renal perfusion and hypoxia, increased sympathetic activity, increased intra–abdominal pressure, oxidative stress, endothelial dysfunction, and activation of the renin-angiotensin-aldosterone system (RAAS) and arginine vasopressin (AVP) system.[8-13] The ideal cardiorenal syndrome therapeutic would therefore (1) unload the heart and decrease venous pressure while minimizing reductions in blood pressure, thereby optimizing renal perfusion; (2) target the nephron to preserve or enhance glomerular filtration rate (GFR) and reduce sodium and water retention; and (3) suppress activation of the RAAS and AVP system.

The Natriuretic Peptide Family

The natriuretic peptide (NP) family consists of structurally similar although physiologically distinct peptides, including atrial natriuretic peptide (ANP), brain natriuretic peptide (BNP), and C–type natriuretic peptide (CNP) (Figure 9.1). A fourth NP, *Dendroaspis* natriuretic peptide (DNP), was initially isolated from the green mamba snake and is present in human atrial tissue and plasma.[14] The NPs exert their biologic activity primarily via binding to guanylyl cyclase receptor A and B (GC$_A$ and GC$_B$) and resultant activation of the intracellular second messenger molecule, cyclic guanosine monophosphate (cGMP) (Figure 9.2). ANP, BNP, and DNP bind preferentially to GC$_A$ and CNP to GC$_B$.[15,16] Via binding to GC$_A$ and GC$_B$ the NPs have multiple actions, which are natriuretic (via GC$_A$), renin and aldosterone inhibiting (via G$_A$), venodilating (G$_{B>A}$), antifibrotic (G$_{B>A}$), antihypertrophic (G$_{A>B}$), lusitropic (G$_A$), antiapoptotic (G$_A$), and vascular regenerating (G$_{A/B}$).[15-18] The NPs are degraded by binding to a third NP receptor, the non–guanylyl-cyclase-linked natriuretic peptide receptor C (NPR–C), as well as enzymatic degradation by neutral endopeptidase 24.11 (NEP), which is widely distributed in the kidney, lung, heart, and endothelial cells.

Of the native NPs the only approved for therapeutic use in the United States is BNP (nesiritide), which is specifically approved for acute decompensated heart failure (ADHF). BNP is a GC$_A$ receptor agonist with potent arterial vasodilating properties. It enhances renal function in conditions such as cardiopulmonary bypass surgery, but in ADHF

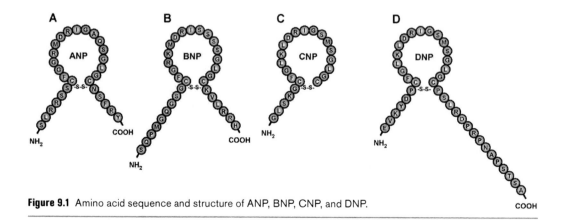

Figure 9.1 Amino acid sequence and structure of ANP, BNP, CNP, and DNP.

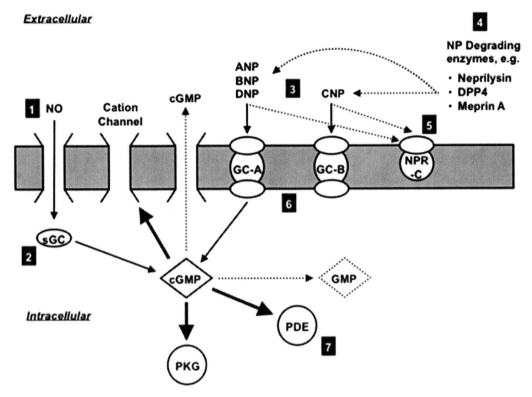

Figure 9.2 GC pathways; activation of cGMP as their second messenger. NO (nitric oxide) activates soluble GC. ANP, BNP, and DNP stimulate GC_A, while CNP stimulates GC_B. NPs also bind to the non-GC-linked NP clearance receptor (NPR-C). Cyclic GMP modulates cGMP-dependent protein kinase G (PKG), cGMP-regulated phosphodiesterases (PDEs), and cGMP-regulated cation channels. The cGMP signal is terminated by PDEs that hydrolyze cGMP to GMP. The NPs are degraded by peptidases such as neprilysin (also known as neutral endopeptidase 24.11), dipeptidyl peptidase IV (DPP4), and meprin A. Strategies to enhance cyclic GMP signaling therapeutically include (1) the use of NO mimetics such as nitro vasodilators, (2) direct sGC stimulators, (3) exogenous native and designer NPs, (4) inhibiting NP-degrading enzymes, (5) blocking NPR-C, (6) overexpressing GC_A or GC_B or both, and (7) inhibiting the activity of cGMP-hydrolyzing PDEs.

it may impair renal function secondary to excessive hypotension.[19,20] This effect has resulted in a controversy that it is hoped will be clarified soon by completion of the ASCEND–HF trial in patients with ADHF; the trial addresses the safety and efficacy of nesiritide in 7000 subjects randomized to BNP or standard care. It is important to note that several smaller studies suggest nesiritide improves renal function when administered at nonhypotensive doses.[21,22]

While the use of nesiritide in HF has meet significant challenges, the pleiotropic cardiorenal protective properties of the NP family continue to make them attractive HF treatment candidates. Efforts to optimize the beneficial cardiorenal actions of the NPs while minimizing undesirable effects such as hypotension have led to the design of the novel chimeric natriuretic peptide CD–NP (Figure 9.3). CD–NP is a designer peptide that integrates mature CNP with the C-terminus of DNP[23-25] and is currently being tested in phase 2 trials. The rationale for the design of CD–NP is based upon the vascular actions of CNP, which possesses venodila-

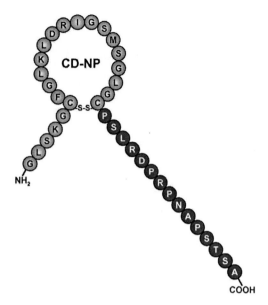

Figure 9.3 Amino acid (AA) sequence and structure of CD-NP composed of the complete 22-AA structure of C-type natriuretic peptide (shown in light gray) and the 18-AA COOH-terminus of DNP (shown in black).

tory properties but less hypotension than ANP or BNP.[24,26] CNP also accelerates endothelial repair, is potently antifibrotic, and inhibits hypertrophy in cardiomyocytes but is not natriuretic and does not suppress the RAAS.[27,28] CNP lacks a C-terminus, which makes it very susceptible to degradation by NEP. DNP, on the other hand,[14,29] binds to the GC_A receptor, giving it natriuretic and diuretic properties as well as aldosterone-suppressing actions.[30] Importantly, the 15 amino acid C-terminus of DNP confers high resistance to degradation. CD-NP is therefore a dual activator of GC_A and GC_B ($GC_B >$ GC_A),[23,24,31] and possesses the strong antiproliferative and antifibrotic properties of CNP with the potently natriuretic and diuretic properties of DNP with less blood pressure-lowering effects than BNP. Thus, CD-NP has emerged as an appealing therapeutic strategy for cardiorenal syndrome. Next we re-

view the biology of CNP and DNP followed by the latest data regarding CD-NP relevant to cardiorenal mechanisms in cardiorenal syndrome.

C-Type Natriuretic Peptide

CNP is a 22-AA peptide composed of a 17-AA disulfide-linked ring structure and a 5-AA amino–terminus (N-terminus). Unlike ANP and BNP, CNP does not possess a C-terminus. Originally discovered in the brain, CNP also is highly expressed in the vascular endothelium and kidneys and binds preferentially to GC_B, which is also highly expressed in the vasculature and in podocytes.[32-34] CNP plays an important role in the regulation of vascular tone, and it is well established that CNP is a vasodilator and potent venodilator whose actions are independent of nitric oxide (NO).[35] Indeed, infusion of CNP reduces cardiac-filling pressures primarily secondary to venodilation. Unlike other natriuretic peptides, CNP does not possess significant diuretic and natriuretic effects.[36] However, studies have established that CNP via GC_B is a potent activator of cGMP in podocytes compared to ANP, which may represent a mechanism for CNP-dependent renoprotection at the level of the glomerulus, especially in the control of the glomerular barrier and prevention of albuminuria. Studies also report that CNP is an endothelium–independent regulator of vascular smooth muscle tone involving activation of NPR-C, which has traditionally been thought to serve only as a clearance receptor.[37]

CNP also is known to be a regulator of the extracellular matrix, and it is established that CNP signaling plays an important antiproliferative and antifibrotic role in the heart and in the kidneys, where fibroblasts and endothelial cells secrete CNP.[38,39] Moreover, *in vitro* studies suggest CNP is a more potent antiproliferative and collagen-suppressing agent than ANP or BNP.[39] Indeed, infusion of CNP following acute ischemic insult to the heart results in a significant reduction in infarct size.[40] The mechanism by which CNP reduces infarct size has not been definitively elucidated and is likely multifactorial, including promoting angiogenesis and coronary dilation, reduction in heart rate, and antifibrotic signaling.

The biologic actions of endogenous CNP suggest that a CNP-based therapeutic may be beneficial in cardiorenal syndrome by promoting venodilation, cardiac unloading, and angiogenesis, and by inhibiting profibrotic remodeling of the heart and maintaining the glomerular barrier in the kidney. Indeed, recent studies suggest a CNP deficiency in HF where there is blunted renal secretion of CNP.[41] Further, a CNP-based therapeutic may have a role in rescuing the heart after ischemic injury, such as myocardial infarction or prophylactic in the case of surgeries that result in myocardial ischemia. Unfortunately, the limited natriuretic and diuretic actions and the short half-life of CNP limit its potential role in cardiorenal syndrome and other cardiovascular disease states.

Dendroaspis Natriuretic Peptide

DNP is a 38-AA NP with a 17-AA ring structure, 6-AA N-terminus, and 15-AA C-terminus. DNP shares structural similarities to other NPs and was first isolated from the venom of the green mamba.[14] DNP immunoreactivity is present in human atrial myocardium as well as plasma and appears to be elevated in congestive HF,[42] although its gene has not been reported in the human. Similar to ANP and BNP, DNP binds to GC_A and NPR-C, and reports suggest DNP binds to GC_A with a higher affinity in human car-

diomyocytes compared to ANP and BNP.[14] Of all the NPs, DNP possesses the longest C-terminus, which may account for its greater resistance to the degradative enzyme NEP compared to the other NPs.[43] DNP also binds less avidly to the clearance receptor NPR-C compared to ANP and BNP.[44] *In vivo* reports are that DNP possesses potent natriuretic, diuretic, renal-enhancing, cardiac-unloading, and hypotensive actions,[45] and administration of DNP in a canine model of HF results in significant cardiac unloading and enhancement of renal function.[46] The potent hypotensive actions of DNP, however, make it less suitable as a therapeutic for most cardiovascular disease states.

CD-NP: A Novel Chimeric Natriuretic Peptide

CD-NP represents a novel 37-AA chimeric NP designed at the Mayo Clinic that fuses the 15-AA C-terminus of DNP into the C-terminus position of the core 22-AA ring structure of CNP (Figure 9.3). As stated previously, the rationale for its design was to combine the cardiac unloading, antiproliferative, antifibrotic, and minimal hypotensive properties of CNP with the renal-enhancing and aldosterone-suppressing actions of DNP. It was thought that the extended C-terminus of DNP would render this fusion protein resistant to degradation by NEP and subsequently increase its half-life and biologic activity in circulation. The hope was to retain the GC_B agonism of CNP and the GC_A agonism of DNP, which would result in the first natriuretic peptide capable of dual GC_A and GC_B activation at physiologic doses. Next, we discuss the most up-to-date studies relating to the *in vitro* and *in vivo* actions of CD-NP as well as future directions.

CD-NP In Vitro *Studies*

Dickey and colleagues[31] assessed the ability of CD-NP to bind to specific NPRs compared to endogenous NPs (Figure 9.4). Using human embryonic kidney cells lacking endogenous GC receptors and then expressing a single GC receptor, the investigators assessed the ability of CD-NP to activate receptors in GC_A or GC_B expressing cells by measuring activation of cGMP. The addition of the C-terminus of DNP to CNP resulted in a 200-fold-greater GC_A activation compared to CNP, which is known to activate GC_A only minimally. Compared to saturated lev-

els of ANP and DNP, CD-NP resulted in less GC_A-generated cGMP activation, suggesting CD-NP is a partial agonist of GC_A. CD-NP was capable of activating the GC_B, but was a 5-fold-less potent activator of GC_B compared to CNP. To assess the affinity of CD-NP for the clearance receptor NPR-C (which does not activate cGMP), the investigators determined the ability of CD-NP to compete for 125I-ANP binding to NPR-C. Results suggest that CD-NP binds to NPR-C in a similar manner to CNP and DNP. Thus, CD-NP compared to CNP is a 200-fold-greater activator of GC_A and 5-fold-less potent activator of GC_B. These studies demonstrate that CD-NP is the first designer NP to activate both GC receptors at physiologic doses.

Increasing evidence suggests that an important component of worsening renal function (WRF) in HF may be secondary to structural remodeling of the kidney with podocyte injury and renal cortical and medullary fibrosis. It should be emphasized again that CNP has known antifibrotic and

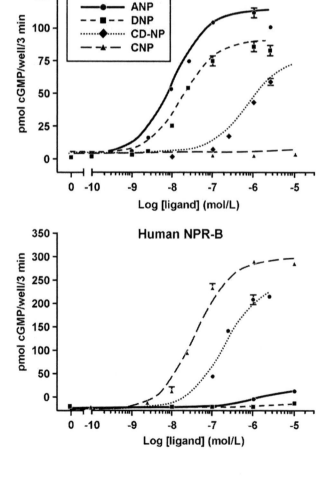

Figure 9.4 Chimeric peptide CD-NP, but not CNP, activates both GC_A and GC_B. Cells stably expressing either GC_A (NPR-A) (a) or GC_B (NPR-B) (b) were incubated with increasing concentrations of ligand for 3 minutes. Cellular cGMP concentrations were then measured by radioimmunoassay. Graphs are representative experiments from 3 separate assays; each point was assayed in triplicate. Dickey DM, Burnett JC Jr., Potter RL. Novel bifunctional natriuretic peptides as potential therapeutics. *J Biol Chem.* 2008;283:35003–35009. With permission from the American Society for Biochemistry and Molecular Biology.

antiproliferative effects in the absence of cardiovascular disease[39] and in models of acute myocardial ischemia and renal fibrosis.[40,47] Similar to CNP, in a model of cardiotrophin-1-induced fibrosis and hypertrophy, CD-NP suppressed cell proliferation in cultured human fibroblasts as measured by BrdU uptake to assess DNA synthesis and cellular proliferation.[25] Further, CD-NP significantly reduced TGF- 1–induced collagen–1 production in cultured human fibroblasts.[48] Overall, these *in vitro* results suggest that CD-NP, like CNP, is antifibrotic and antiproliferative.

CD-NP In Vivo *Studies*

Lisy and colleagues[25] first assessed the *in vivo* cardiorenal actions of CD-NP infusion in normal canines at 3 concentrations (10, 50, and 100 ng/kg/min). CD-NP markedly unloaded the heart with significant incremental reductions in pulmonary capillary wedge pressure (PCWP) and right atrial pressure (RAP) at 50 ng/kg/min and 100 ng/kg/min. Furthermore, there were potent diuretic and natriuretic responses following CD-NP. The natriuretic and diuretic effects were localized to the proximal and distal nephron where sodium reabsorption was decreased. The cardiac-unloading, natriuretic, and diuretic properties were associated with non-significant changes in mean arterial pressure (MAP) at 10 ng/kg/min and 50 ng/kg/min, and a significant, although modest, reduction in MAP at 100 ng/kg/min. Furthermore, at 100 ng/kg/min, CD-NP was associated with significant increases in GFR. There was no significant change in renal blood flow following CD-NP infusion. The hemodynamic actions of CD-NP in normal canines were associated with suppressed plasma renin activity (PRA) at 10 ng/kg/min and 50 ng/kg/min and significant increases in both plasma and urine cGMP at 50 ng/kg/min and 100 ng/kg/min.

To further support the rationale of using CD-NP as a therapeutic, CD-NP at 50 ng/kg/min was compared to equimolar recombinant BNP (nesiritide) in normal canines (Figure 9.5).[25] CD-NP was significantly less hypotensive than BNP and it significantly increased GFR, whereas BNP infusion did not change GFR. Taken together, these studies, performed in normal canines, suggest CD-NP has potent cardiac unloading

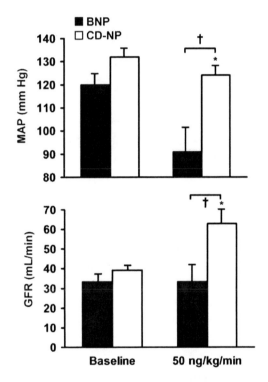

Figure 9.5 Effect of CD-NP and equimolar human BNP in 2 groups of normal dogs. Data are expressed as means ± SE. n = 6 in each group.

*$P < 0.05$ versus baseline; †$P < 0.05$ between groups.

Lisy O, Huntley BK, McCormick DJ, Kurlansky PA, Burnett JC Jr. Design, synthesis, and actions of a novel chimeric natriuretic peptide: CD-NP. *J Am Coll Cardiol.* 2008;52:60–68. With permission from Elsevier.

and renal enhancing, as well as a favorable neurohumoral profile.

The cardiorenal actions of CD-NP in a canine model of experimental HF induced by rapid ventricular pacing have been reported. CD-NP infusion (100 ng/kg/min) significantly increased renal blood flow, GFR, diuresis, and natriuresis.[49] There was significant unloading of the heart with reductions in RAP and PCWP, and a modest (9 mm Hg) reduction in MAP and a significant reduction in PRA following CD-NP infusion.

Most recently, CD-NP has been studied further in a rodent model of acute myocardial infarction (AMI) via coronary artery ligation, which was associated with renal injury and renal fibrosis.[50] Specifically, CD-NP was infused via osmotic pump for 2 weeks post-AMI. Compared to vehicle, CD-NP significantly lowered plasma aldosterone, increased renal blood flow, and decreased proteinuria. Further, ratio of heart weight to body weight and left ventricular fibrosis were lower in the CD-NP-treated group. Moreover, both renal medulla and cortex fibrosis was significantly reduced in the CD-NP-treated group compared to vehicle. These results from a rodent model of AMI suggest that CD-NP has potent antifibrotic and antiproliferative actions associated with renal-enhancing actions and a favorable neurohumoral profile.

CD-NP First-in-Human Studies

To translate the promising preclinical findings observed of these *in vitro* and animal studies, a first-in-human clinical trial of CD-NP in healthy patients was undertaken and published.[24] This study was a 2-stage trial: the first stage was a dose-escalation study to determine the maximum tolerated dose of CD-NP, and the second stage was a placebo-controlled study of the hemodynamics and neurohumoral actions of CD-NP. The maximum tolerated dose was determined to be 17 ng/kg/min with adverse reactions including flushing, orthostatic hypotension, dizziness, tachycardia, and dyspnea at 25 ng/kg/min. Overall, these events were transient and mild in nature. Analysis of anti-CNP and anti-CD-NP antibodies at days 7 and 28 following infusion did not suggest any significant immunogenicity.

While this proof-of-concept study was designed primarily to assess safety in healthy patients, the results also provide significant insight into the potential use of the results in HF and other cardiovascular disease states. Specifically, CD-NP significantly increased plasma and urinary cGMP compared to placebo (Figure 9.6). Thus, CD-NP was capable of interacting with human GC receptors and activating cGMP *in vivo* in humans. Activation of cGMP was associated with similar cardiorenal biologic actions as observed in the canine model. There was a significant diuretic and natriuretic response with preservation of GFR and a slight (although statistically significant) reduction in MAP. Moreover, in these healthy patients, CD-NP significantly suppressed aldosterone. The mechanism of aldosterone suppression is thought to be activation of GC_A, which is abundant in the adrenal glands. The ability to suppress aldosterone, despite natriuretic and diuretic effects, is a novel feature of the NPs when compared to conventional vasodilators, which tend to activate the RAAS. These results in healthy humans suggest CD-NP is a potent diuretic and natriuretic agent with a favorable neurohumoral profile but with only modest decreases in blood pressure and no change in GFR.

Initial results from an open-label dose-escalation study of CD-NP in HF (New York Heart Association class II/III) (n = 18) with ejection fraction < 40% have been reported.[51] In this study, CD-NP was compared to routine daily medications including furo-

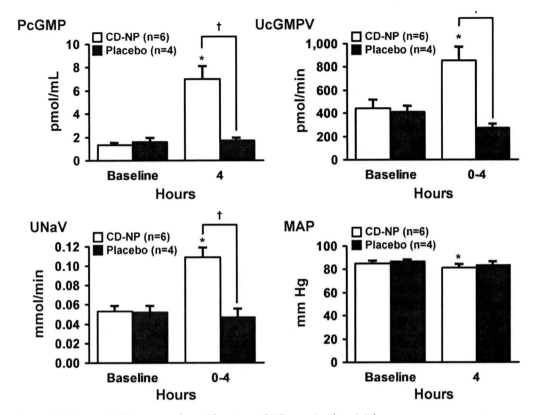

Figure 9.6 Plasma cGMP response (top left), urinary cGMP excretion (top right), natriuretic response (bottom left), and blood pressure response (bottom right). Mean ± SEM.

*$P < 0.05$ versus baseline; †$P < 0.05$ between groups.

cGMP = cyclic guanosine monophosphate; MAP = mean arterial pressure; UNaV = urinary sodium excretion; PcGMP = plasma cGMP; UcGMPV = urinary cGMP excretion.

Lee CY, Chen HH, Lisy O, Swan S, Cannon C, Lieu HD, Burnett JC Jr. Pharmacodynamics of a novel designer natriuretic peptide, CD-NP, in a first-in-human clinical trial in healthy subjects. *J Clin Pharmacol.* 2009;49:668–673. Reprinted by Permission of SAGE Publications.

semide. The diuretic actions of CD–NP were similar to furosemide, but CD–NP significantly improved renal function as measured by creatinine, Cockcroft–Gault creatinine clearance, and cystatin. These preliminary results suggest that CD–NP is an equally potent diuretic but, unlike furosemide, is also renal enhancing.

Future Research and Directions

Cardiorenal syndrome will continue to be a clinical challenge, as we still need to understand its mechanisms and seek more effective and safe therapies. The native NPs and their respective cGMP-linked GC receptors possess renal–enhancing actions but are limited by untoward effects on the kidney if associated with hypotension. Novel drug discovery and design taking key parts of native NPs and creating designer drugs like CD-NP may optimize renal-favorable effects such as renal protection and limit adverse actions such as excessive hypotension but still unload the heart and suppress aldosterone.

The observed renal-enhancing and cardiac-unloading properties of CD-NP in the absence of excessive hypotension or reductions in GFR in normal canine and healthy humans support the further development of CD-NP for the treatment of HF and other cardiovascular disease states. Indeed, the development of CD-NP continues to progress at a rapid pace, and several ongoing animal and human studies are advancing the use of CD-NP as a novel therapeutic in cardiovascular disease states[25,52]; these include ongoing phase 2 clinical trials in acute decompensated HF and stable chronic HF as well as *in vivo* experiment AMI studies. The results of these studies will be published in the near future. Further, delivery systems beyond intravenous administration, including conjugation technologies and oral administration using novel micelle, subcutaneous administrations, and polymer-based sustained-release systems, are being developed for chronic use.

Conclusion

CD-NP represents a novel therapeutic natriuretic peptide that is capable of dual GC_A and GC_B activation and subsequent cardiac-unloading, diuretic, natriuretic, antifibrotic, and aldosterone-inhibiting properties, while only minimally lowering blood pressure and with preservation of GFR. As such, CD-NP represents a novel peptide therapeutic for HF especially targeting the cardiorenal connection.

Disclosures

Dr. John Burnett is chair of the Scientific Advisory Board of Nile Therapeutics. No further potential conflicts of interest related to this article have been reported.

References

1. Coresh J, Astor B, Sarnak MJ. Evidence for increased cardiovascular disease risk in patients with chronic kidney disease. *Curr Opin Nephrol Hypertens.* 2004;13:73-81.

2. Culleton BF, Larson MG, Wilson PW, Evans JC, Parfrey PS, Levy D. Cardiovascular disease and mortality in a community-based cohort with mild renal insufficiency. *Kidney Int.* 1999;56:2214-2219.

3. Dries DL, Exner DV, Domanski MJ, Greenberg B, Stevenson LW. The prognostic implications of renal insufficiency in asymptomatic and symptomatic patients with left ventricular systolic dysfunction. *J Am Coll Cardiol.* 2000;35:681-689.

4. Garg AX, Clark WF, Haynes RB, House AA. Moderate renal insufficiency and the risk of cardiovascular mortality: results from the NHANES I. *Kidney Int.* 2002;61:1486-1494.

5. Go AS, Chertow GM, Fan D, McCulloch CE, Hsu C. Chronic kidney disease and the risks of death, cardiovascular events, and hospitalization. *N Engl J Med.* 2004;351:1296-1305.

6. Henry RM, Kostense PJ, Bos G, et al. Mild renal insufficiency is associated with increased cardiovascular mortality: the Hoorn Study. *Kidney Int.* 2002;62:1402-1407.

7. van Dokkum RP, Eijkelkamp WB, Kluppel AC, et al. Myocardial infarction enhances progressive renal damage in an experimental model for cardio-

renal interaction. *J Am Soc Nephrol.* 2004;15:3103–3110.

8. Doty JM, Saggi BH, Blocher CR, et al. Effect of increased renal venous pressure on renal function. *J Trauma.* 1999;47:1000–1003.

9. Malbrain ML, Cheatham ML, Kirkpatrick A, et al. Results from the International Conference of Experts on Intra-abdominal Hypertension and Abdominal Compartment Syndrome. I. Definitions. *Intensive Care Med.* 2006;32:1722–1732.

10. Damman K, van Deursen VM, Navis G, Voors AA, van Veldhuisen DJ, Hillege HL. Increased central venous pressure is associated with impaired renal function and mortality in a broad spectrum of patients with cardiovascular disease. *J Am Coll Cardiol.* 2009;53:582–588.

11. Schlaich MP, Sobotka PA, Krum H, Lambert E, Esler MD. Renal sympathetic-nerve ablation for uncontrolled hypertension. *N Engl J Med.* 2009;361: 932–934.

12. St. John Sutton M, Pfeffer MA, Moye L, et al; for the SAVE Investigators. Cardiovascular death and left ventricular remodeling two years after myocardial infarction: baseline predictors and impact of long-term use of captopril: information from the Survival and Ventricular Enlargement (SAVE) trial. *Circulation.* 1997;96:3294–3299.

13. Vaziri ND, Dicus M, Ho ND, Boroujerdi-Rad L, Sindhu RK. Oxidative stress and dysregulation of superoxide dismutase and NADPH oxidase in renal insufficiency. *Kidney Int.* 2003;63:179–185.

14. Schweitz H, Vigne P, Moinier D, Frelin C, Lazdunski M. A new member of the natriuretic peptide family is present in the venom of the green mamba (*Dendroaspis angusticeps*). *J Biol Chem.* 1992;267:13928–13932.

15. Martin FL, Chen HH, Cataliotti A, Burnett JC Jr. B-type natriuretic peptide: beyond a diagnostic. *Heart Fail Clin.* 2008;4:449–454.

16. Potter LR, Abbey-Hosch S, Dickey DM. Natriuretic peptides, their receptors, and cyclic guanosine monophosphate-dependent signaling functions. *Endocr Rev.* 2006;27:47–72.

17. Garbers DL, Chrisman TD, Wiegn P, et al. Membrane guanylyl cyclase receptors: an update. *Trends Endocrinol Metab.* 2006;17:251–258.

18. Boerrigter G, Lapp H, Burnett JC. Modulation of cGMP in heart failure: a new therapeutic paradigm. *Handb Exp Pharmacol.* 2009;191:485–506.

19. Mentzer RM Jr, Oz MC, Sladen RN, et al; NAPA Investigators. Effects of perioperative nesiritide in patients with left ventricular dysfunction undergoing cardiac surgery: the NAPA Trial. *J Am Coll Cardiol.* 2007;49:716–726.

20. Sackner-Bernstein JD, Kowalski M, Fox M, Aaronson K. Short-term risk of death after treatment with nesiritide for decompensated heart failure: a pooled analysis of randomized controlled trials. *JAMA.* 2005;293:1900–1905.

21. Burnett JC Jr, Korinek J. The tumultuous journey of nesiritide: past, present, and future. *Circ Heart Fail.* 2008;1:6–8.

22. Chen HH, Sundt TM, Cook DJ, Heublein DM, Burnett JC Jr. Low dose nesiritide and the preservation of renal function in patients with renal dysfunction undergoing cardiopulmonary-bypass surgery: a double-blind placebo-controlled pilot study. *Circulation.* 2007;116:I134–I138.

23. Lisy O, Huntley BK, McCormick DJ, Kurlansky PA, Burnett JC Jr. Design,

synthesis, and actions of a novel chimeric natriuretic peptide: CD-NP. *J Am Coll Cardiol.* 2008;52:60–68.

24. Lee CY, Chen HH, Lisy O, et al. Pharmacodynamics of a novel designer natriuretic peptide, CD-NP, in a first-in-human clinical trial in healthy subjects. *J Clin Pharmacol.* 2009;49:668–673.

25. McKie PM, Sangaralingham SJ, Burnett JC Jr. CD-NP: an innovative designer natriuretic peptide activator of particulate guanylyl cyclase receptors for cardiorenal disease. *Curr Heart Fail Rep.* 2010;7:93–98.

26. Wei CM, Aarhus LL, Miller VM, Burnett JC Jr. Action of C-type natriuretic peptide in isolated canine arteries and veins. *Am J Physiol.* 1993;264(1 pt 2): H71–H73.

27. Scotland RS, Ahluwalia A, Hobbs AJ. C-type natriuretic peptide in vascular physiology and disease. *Pharmacol Ther.* 2005;105:85–93.

28. Rubattu S, Sciarretta S, Valenti V, Stanzione R, Volpe M. Natriuretic peptides: an update on bioactivity, potential therapeutic use, and implication in cardiovascular diseases. *Am J Hypertens.* 2008;21:733–741.

29. Best PJ, Burnett JC, Wilson SH, Holmes DR Jr, Lerman A. Dendroaspis natriuretic peptide relaxes isolated human arteries and veins. *Cardiovasc Res.* 2002;55: 375–384.

30. Singh G, Kuc RE, Maguire JJ, Fidock M, Davenport AP. Novel snake venom ligand dendroaspis natriuretic peptide is selective for natriuretic peptide receptor-A in human heart: downregulation of natriuretic peptide receptor-A in heart failure. *Circ Res.* 2006;99:183–190.

31. Dickey DM, Burnett JC Jr, Potter RL. Novel bifunctional natriuretic peptides

as potential therapeutics. *J Biol Chem.* 2008;28:35003–35009.

32. Lewko B, Endlich N, Kriz W, Stepinski J, Endlich K. C-type natriuretic peptide as a podocyte hormone and modulation of its cGMP production by glucose and mechanical stress. *Kidney Int.* 2004;66: 1001–1008.

33. Stingo AJ, Clavell AL, Aarhus LL, Burnett JC Jr. Cardiovascular and renal actions of C-type natriuretic peptide. *Am J Physiol.* 1992;262(1 pt 2):H308–H312.

34. Sudoh T, Minamino N, Kangawa K, Matsuo H. C-type natriuretic peptide (CNP): a new member of natriuretic peptide family identified in porcine brain. *Biochem Biophys Res Commun.* 1990;168:863–870.

35. Wright RS, Wei CM, Kim CH, et al. C-type natriuretic peptide–mediated coronary vasodilation: role of the coronary nitric oxide and particulate guanylate cyclase systems. *J Am Coll Cardiol.* 1996;28:1031–1038.

36. Wright RS, Wei CM, Kim CH, et al. C-type natriuretic peptide: a selective cardiovascular peptide. *Am J Physiol.* 1993;264(2 pt 2):R290–R295.

37. Hobbs A, Foster P, Prescott C, Scotland R, Ahluwalia A. Natriuretic peptide receptor-C regulates coronary blood flow and prevents myocardial ischemia/reperfusion injury: novel cardioprotective role for endothelium-derived C-type natriuretic peptide. *Circulation.* 2004;110:1231–1235.

38. Surendran K, Simon TC. CNP gene expression is activated by Wnt signaling and correlates with Wnt4 expression during renal injury. *Am J Physiol Renal Physiol.* 2003;284:F653–F662.

39. Horio T, Tokudome T, Maki T, et al. Gene expression, secretion, and autocrine action of C-type natriuretic peptide in

cultured adult rat cardiac fibroblasts. *Endocrinology.* 2003;144:2279–2284.

40. Soeki T, Kishimoto I, Okumura H, et al. C-type natriuretic peptide, a novel antifibrotic and antihypertrophic agent, prevents cardiac remodeling after myocardial infarction. *J Am Coll Cardiol.* 2005;45:608–616.

41. Kalra PR, Clague JR, Coats AJ, Anker SD, Poole-Wilson PATIENTS, Struthers AD. C-type natriuretic peptide production by the human kidney is blunted in chronic heart failure. *Clin Sci.* 2010;118:71–77.

42. Schirger, JA, Heublein DM, Chen HH, et al. Presence of dendroaspis natriuretic peptide-like immunoreactivity in human plasma and its increase during human heart failure. *Mayo Clin Proc.* 1999;74:126–130.

43. Chen HH, Lainchbury JG, Burnett JC Jr. Natriuretic peptide receptors and neutral endopeptidase in mediating the renal actions of a new therapeutic synthetic natriuretic peptide dendroaspis natriuretic peptide. *J Am Coll Cardiol.* 2002;40:1186–1191.

44. Johns DG, Ao Z, Heidrich BJ, et al. Dendroaspis natriuretic peptide binds to the natriuretic peptide clearance receptor. *Biochem Biophys Res Commun.* 2007;358:145–149.

45. Lisy, O, Jougasaki M, Heublein DM, et al. Renal actions of synthetic dendroaspis natriuretic peptide. *Kidney Int.* 1999;56:502–508.

46. Lisy O, Lainchbury JG, Leskinen H, Burnett JC Jr. Therapeutic actions of a new synthetic vasoactive and natriuretic peptide, dendroaspis natriuretic peptide, in experimental severe congestive heart failure. *Hypertension.* 2001;37:1089–1094.

47. Canaan-Kühl S, Ostendorf T, Zander K, Koch KM, Floege J. C-type natriuretic peptide inhibits mesangial cell proliferation and matrix accumulation in vivo. *Kidney Int.* 1998;53:1143–1151.

48. Ichiki T, Huntley BK, Sangaralingham J, Chen HH, Burnett JC Jr. A novel designer natriuretic peptide CD-NP suppresses TGF-beta 1 induced collagen type I production in human cardiac fibroblasts. *J Card Fail.* 2009;15:S34.

49. Lisy O, Chen HH, Burnett J. Cardiorenal actions of new designer natriuretic peptide CD-NP in experimental heart failure. *J Am Coll Cardiol.* 2009;53:A149.

50. Martin FL, Sangaralingham SJ, McKie PM, et al. Prevention of cardiorenal fibrosis and suppression of proteinuria and aldosterone activation following experimental myocardial infarction with the novel natriuretic peptide CD-NP. *J Card Fail.* 2009;15:S3.

51. Lieu H, Goldsmith S, Neutal J, Massie B, Burnett J. Initial observations of intravenous CD-NP, chimeric natriuretic peptide, on renal functions in chronic heart failure patients. *J Card Fail.* 2009;15:S77.

52. Lee CY, Lieu H, Burnett HC Jr. Designer natriuretic peptides. *J Investig Med.* 2009;57:18–21.

New Therapies for Acute Heart Failure

Vasopressin Receptor Antagonists, Adenosine Receptor Antagonists

10

JOHN BLAIR

PETER S. PANG

MIHAI GHEORGHIADE

Congestion is the primary driver behind patients' presentation to the hospital with acute heart failure (HF) syndromes,[1] defined as new-onset or gradually or rapidly worsening HF signs and symptoms requiring urgent therapy. Increased left ventricular (LV) filling pressure is the common pathophysiology leading to congestion.[2]

Presently, intravenous non–potassium-sparing loop diuretics remain the cornerstone of therapy for relief from congestion in acute HF syndrome.[3] Although effective, loop diuretics have some detrimental effects, both in their acute and chronic use, by causing electrolyte disturbances and neurohormonal stimulation.[4-7] Retrospective studies in both acute and chronic HF have demon-

strated that higher doses of diuretics were associated with increased mortality, even after correcting for baseline clinical characteristics.[5,8] However, despite significant debate, no conclusive evidence exists to define loop diuretics as harmful and their sustained empiric use implies their benefits. Current studies are ongoing to provide greater evidence for loop diuretics in HF.

Given the lack of evidence, as well as the potential untoward drug effects of loop diuretics, new pharmacologic agents have been developed to remove fluid and relieve the signs and symptoms of congestion, without worsening cardiac or renal function. This chapter will discuss the vasopressin and adenosine receptor antagonists.

The Cardiorenal Syndrome: A Clinician's Guide to Pathophysiology and Management, 1st ed. © 2012 J. Thomas Heywood and John C. Burnett Jr., eds. Cardiotext Publishing, ISBN: 978-0-9790164-7-9.

Vasopressin Receptor Antagonists

Pathophysiology of Vasopressin in Heart Failure

Arginine vasopressin (AVP) is a nonapeptide hormone that plays an important role in maintaining serum osmolarity and central volume. AVP, also known as antidiuretic hormone (ADH), is synthesized in the hypothalamus and transported in secretory granules to the posterior pituitary, where it is stored until release after appropriate stimulation.[9] The most potent stimulus for AVP secretion is elevated serum osmolarity, through stimulation of osmoreceptors located in the hypothalamus.[10] Nonosmotic factors that stimulate AVP release include reduced cardiac output (CO), hypovolemia, or hemorrhage, which act through baroreceptors located in the carotid sinus, aortic arch, and left atrium.[11]

AVP acts primarily on 2 receptors (Table 10.1): the vasopressin 1a (V1a, also called V1) and V2 receptors. A third "pituitary-specific" vasopressin receptor has been identified (V1b or V3). V1a receptors are found primarily in smooth muscle cells and blood vessels. Stimulation results in vasoconstriction and a positive inotropic effect.[12] The V1a receptor is a G–protein–coupled receptor mediated by the inositol triphosphate pathway, releasing intracellular Ca^{2+} and stimulating protein kinase C. This receptor may also be responsible for myocardial and vascular hypertrophy and remodeling.[13-16] V2 receptors are found primarily in the kidneys. Stimulation of V2 receptors causes preformed cytoplasmic vesicles containing water channels called aquaporin-2 to fuse with the luminal membrane of the renal cortical collecting ducts, increasing permeability and reabsorption of water[17] (Figure 10.1). V2 receptors use adenylate cyclase as a secondary messenger and have also been implicated in endothelium–dependent vasodilation at high levels of vasopressin.[18] V1b receptors are present mostly in the anterior pituitary, and they play a major role in the regulation of adrenocorticotropic hormone (ACTH) during physiologic stress.[19]

AVP levels are high in both chronic and acute HF, although the mechanism by which this occurs is not fully understood.[20-24] When comparing newer HF trials with those before the routine use of ACE inhibitors

Table 10.1 Actions of Vasopressin

Receptor	Signaling Pathway	Location	Actions
V1a (V1)	G protein, IP3	Blood vessels, myocardium	Vasoconstriction, inotrope, mitogen
V2	Adenylate cyclase, cAMP	Renal tubules, endothelium	Water retention, vasodilation
V1b (V3)	G protein, IP3	Anterior pituitary	ACTH regulation

Adapted from Oghlakian G, Klapholz M. Vasopressin and vasopressin receptor antagonists in heart failure. *Cardiol Rev.* 2009;17(1):10-15.

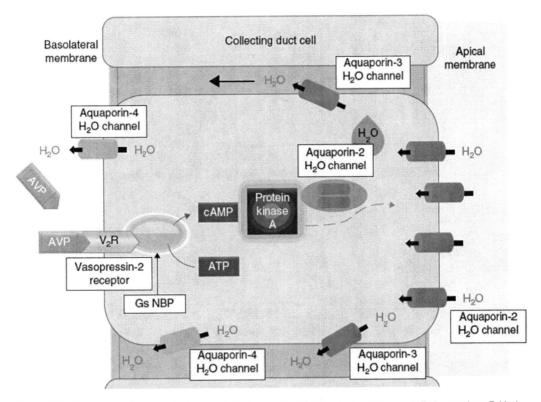

Figure 10.1. Mechanism of action of vasopressin in the renal collecting duct cell. Hoque MZ, Arumugham P, Huda N, Verma N, Afiniwala M, Karia DH. Conivaptan: promise of treatment in heart failure. *Expert Opin Pharmacother.* 2009;10(13):2161–2169. With permission of Informa Medical and Pharmaceutical Science.

(ACEIs), beta-blockers, and aldosterone receptor blockers, it appears that the levels of AVP are attenuated in the presence of neurohormonal blockade.[25] In patients with HF and hyponatremia, hypo-osmolality is associated with high plasma AVP levels, which suggests a nonosmotic mechanism for the release of AVP in some HF patients.[20] Activation of carotid baroreceptors due to arterial underfilling has been implicated as the predominant reflex in the release of AVP in HF.[26] To have elevated AVP levels, the carotid baroreceptor reflex must override the Henry-Gauer reflex, in which atrial stretch from increased atrial pressures leads to the suppression of AVP and water diuresis.[27] In addition to the effects on water retention, AVP has been demonstrated to cause a dose-

dependent reduction in CO and increase in mean arterial pressure (MAP), systemic vascular resistance, and pulmonary capillary wedge pressure in patients with chronic HF who received infusions of AVP (Figure 10.2).[28] In addition, AVP has been shown to be stimulated by angiotensin II and can lead to coronary vasoconstriction.

AVP release leads to free water retention. In states of hypovolemia or hemorrhage, AVP is important in maintaining adequate cardiac preload through stimulation of V1a and V2 receptors, and afterload through stimulation of V1a receptors, maintaining circulating volume. In HF, however, these effects are maladaptive, resulting in worsened HF and adverse ventricular remodeling. Vasopressin antagonists have been developed to remove

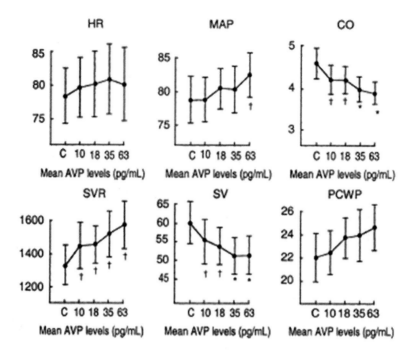

Figure 10.2. Hemodynamic effects of infused AVP in patients with chronic HF.

HR, = heart rate; MPA = mean arterial pressure; CO = cardiac output;
SVR = systemic vascular resistance; SV= stroke volume

* $P < 0.01$
† $P < 0.05$

Goldsmith SR, Gheorghiade M. Vasopressin antagonism in heart failure.
J Am Coll Cardiol. 2005;46(10):1785–1791. With permission from Elsevier.

fluid in patients with HF, while modulating the deleterious effects of vasopressin on LV function, and prevent and/or correct hyponatremia.

Vasopressin Receptor Antagonists and Heart Failure

V2 Antagonists

The only commercially available V2 antagonist is tolvaptan (OPC 41061, Otsuka Pharmaceuticals), with lixivaptan (VPA 459, Cardio-

kine) and SR 121463 (Sanofi–Aventis) in early stages of development.

Tolvaptan (OPC 41061)

In preclinical studies, tolvaptan exhibited potent V2 receptor selectivity, resulting in a dose-dependent aquaresis after single and multiple dosing, leading to increased serum sodium without affecting the renin-angiotensin-aldosterone system in conscious male rats.[29,30] After these and other promising preclinical and early clinical studies, tolvaptan was studied in a multicenter, randomized, double-blind, placebo-controlled trial of 254 patients with signs and at least 30 days of symptoms of HF (NYHA class I–III in 99.6% of patients), irrespective of left ventricular ejection fraction (LVEF), and on standard medical therapy including furosemide.[31] Patients were randomized in a 1:1:1:1 manner to either placebo or 1 of 3 doses of tolvaptan (30, 45, or 60 mg daily) for 25 days. The primary end point was change in body weight on day 14. Secondary end points were edema at the end of the study, and urine sodium excretion, urine osmolality, and urine volume measured on day 3. There was a decrease in body weight of between 0.79 and 0.96 kg, which did not appear to be dose-dependent in all 3 tolvaptan arms, compared with a body weight increase of 0.32 kg in the placebo arm at day 1 (Figure 10.3). This reduction was maintained throughout the study period and was significant compared

to placebo on all study days in all 3 tolvaptan doses. In addition, reduction in edema was observed in all tolvaptan arms but was significant compared to placebo only in the 45-mg group. Significant increases in urine sodium and decreases in urine osmolality and increases in urine volume were observed in all tolvaptan groups compared to placebo. Serum sodium concentrations generally increased approximately 3 mEq/L from baseline in all tolvaptan arms and decreased approximately 1 mEq/L in the placebo arm at day 1, drifting slowly toward baseline over time. Subanalysis of the group with baseline hyponatremia (serum sodium < 136 mEq/L) demonstrated a sustained increase in serum sodium throughout the study in all tolvaptan arms compared with placebo. By comparison, patients with normal baseline serum sodium (≥ 136 mEq/L) had an initial increase in serum sodium, fol-

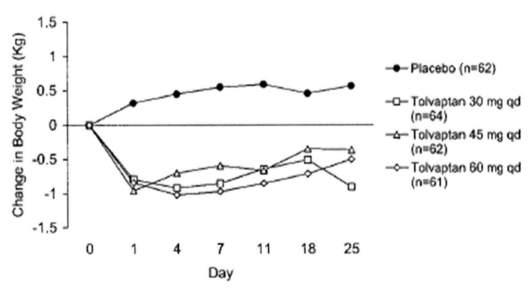

Figure 10.3. Changes in body weight in 254 patients with class I–III HF, randomized to 3 doses of tolvaptan or placebo. Gheorghiade M, Niazi I, Ouyang J, et al. Vasopressin V2-receptor blockade with tolvaptan in patients with chronic heart failure: results from a double-blind, randomized trial. *Circulation*. 2003;107(21):2690–2696. With permission.

lowed by eventual normalization over time in the tolvaptan arms. Complaints of dry mouth, thirst, and polyuria were observed more frequently in the tolvaptan arms compared to placebo, but there were no significant differences in quality-of-life score, renal function, serum potassium, blood pressure, or heart rate comparing all tolvaptan arms with placebo. The authors concluded that tolvaptan was a promising novel therapy that needed further investigation. In addition, the increase in urine sodium was hypothesized to be volume-driven, and the apparent differential effect on serum sodium based on baseline sodium was hypothesized to provide utility in patients with HF and hyponatremia.

Given the short-term efficacy of tolvaptan in mild chronic HF, the Acute and Chronic Therapeutic Impact of a Vasopressin Antagonist in Congestive Heart Failure (ACTIV in CHF) trial was designed to evaluate the clinical effects of tolvaptan in patients hospitalized for HF.[32] This was a randomized, multicenter, double-blind, placebo-controlled phase 2 trial of 319 patients hospitalized with worsening HF, LVEF < 40%, and signs of systemic congestion after initial in-hospital therapy for HF. Eligible patients were randomized in a 1:1:1:1 manner to either placebo or 1 of 3 doses of tolvaptan (30, 60, or 90 mg daily) in addition to standard HF therapy, including diuretics, and followed for 60 days both during the in-hospital and outpatient periods. Patients hospitalized for more than 10 days after the first dose of study drug were withdrawn in order to eliminate patients with significant comorbid conditions. The primary end points were change in body weight at 24 hours after drug administration, and worsening HF at 60 days after randomization, defined as hospitalization or unscheduled visit for HF, escalation of existing therapy or new therapy for HF, or death. Secondary end

points included changes in dyspnea, jugular venous distention (JVD), rales, edema, body weight (at discharge and outpatient), urine output (inpatient), serum electrolyte levels, length of hospital stay after randomization, use of diuretics, and patient- and physician-assessed symptom scales. Median body weight loss ranged from 1.8 to 2.1 kg in the tolvaptan group and again did not appear to be dose-dependent, compared to a weight loss of 0.6 kg in the placebo arm (Figure 10.4). There were no differences in worsening HF at 60 days (26.7% in patients in the tolvaptan vs 27.5% in the placebo group). Body weight was significantly lower at discharge in the groups receiving 30 and 60 mg of tolvaptan compared to placebo, but this difference disappeared at 1 week postdischarge and on the last clinic visit. Similar to the prior study, urine volume was significantly higher in the tolvaptan groups compared to placebo, serum sodium increased in the tolvaptan groups compared to placebo, and often normalized and was sustained in patients with hyponatremia, and there appeared to be no differences in potassium or vital signs in the tolvaptan groups compared to placebo. There was a nonsignificant trend toward reduction in JVD, rales, edema, and diuretic use, and a significant reduction in dyspnea in the tolvaptan groups compared to placebo. There were no differences in length of hospital stay or symptoms in the tolvaptan compared to placebo groups. There was a trend toward more thirst in patients in the tolvaptan groups compared to placebo. Although ACTIV in CHF trial failed to demonstrate a long-term clinical benefit with tolvaptan compared to placebo, posthoc analysis demonstrated a trend toward reduced mortality in patients with severe congestion or elevated blood urea nitrogen (BUN) treated with tolvaptan compared to placebo.[32]

While phase 3 clinical trials were planned or underway, 2 smaller studies

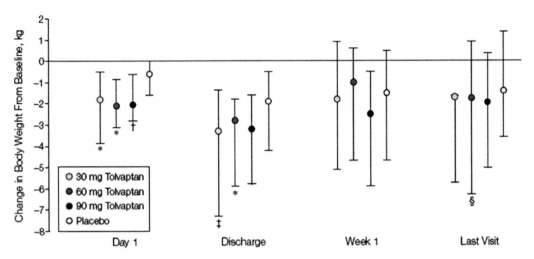

Figure 10.4. Changes in body weight in 319 patients hospitalized with worsening HF and reduced ejection fraction, randomized to 3 doses of tolvaptan or placebo.

* $P = 0.002$ ‡, $P = 0.006$

†, $P = 0.009$ §, $P = 0.008$ for comparisons with placebo group

of acute hemodynamics and the effects of long-term administration of tolvaptan on ventricular remodeling were also conducted. The Effect of Tolvaptan on Hemodynamic Parameters in Subjects with Heart Failure (ECLIPSE) study was designed to evaluate the hemodynamic effects of tolvaptan in severe chronic HF.[33] This study was a randomized, multicenter, double-blind, placebo-controlled trial of 181 patients with at least 3 months of severe (NYHA class III–IV) HF symptoms and LVEF ≤ 40%, on standard HF therapy. Patients were randomized in a 1:1:1:1 manner to either placebo or tolvaptan (15, 30, or 60 mg) given as a single dose, if the pulmonary capillary wedge pressure (PCWP) was > 18 mm Hg on 2 consecutive recordings at least 10 minutes apart after a 2- to 20-hour stabilization period. Hemodynamic and renal parameters were then measured

at multiple time points over an 8-hour assessment period, during which background diuretics and other cardiac medications were held, and fluid restricted to no more than 1 L over 8 hours. The primary end point was PCWP peak change from baseline within 3 to 8 hours after study drug administration, while secondary end points included the area under the curve (AUC) for the change in PCWP from baseline and other hemodynamic parameters, and renal and electrolyte parameters over the 8-hour assessment period. Peak PCWP reduction was significantly greater with tolvaptan (5.7–6.4 mm Hg in the tolvaptan groups compared with 4.2 mm Hg with the placebo group) (Figure 10.5). In addition, peak right atrial pressure and pulmonary arterial pressure reduction were significantly greater in the tolvaptan versus placebo groups. There was no significant

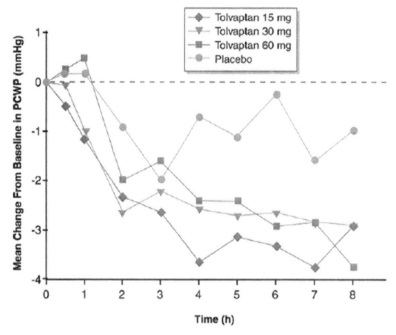

Figure 10.5. Acute hemodynamic effects of tolvaptan versus placebo in 181 patients with severe chronic HF and reduced ejection fraction. Udelson JE, Orlandi C, Ouyang J, et al. Acute hemodynamic effects of tolvaptan, a vasopressin V2 receptor blocker, in patients with symptomatic heart failure and systolic dysfunction: an international, multicenter, randomized, placebo-controlled trial. *J Am Coll Cardiol.* 2008;52(19):1540–1545. With permission from Elsevier

change in cardiac index, blood pressure, or systemic or pulmonary vascular resistances with tolvaptan compared to placebo. Urine output was significantly greater and urine osmolarity was significantly less than that of placebo as early as 1 hour after drug administration. Again, thirst and dry mouth were more common in the tolvaptan groups than in the placebo groups.

To determine the effects of long-term administration of tolvaptan on ventricular remodeling in chronic HF patients with mild systolic dysfunction, a multicenter, randomized, double-blind, placebo-controlled trial in 240 patients with NYHA class II or III chronic HF and LVEF ≤ 30% on optimal therapy for HF, randomized to either 30 mg tolvaptan or placebo, and followed for 1

year, was performed.[34] All patients underwent radionuclide ventriculography (RVG) at baseline and after 1 year of therapy, and repeated again approximately 1 week after withdrawal of the study drug. The primary outcome was change from baseline in left ventricular end diastolic volume index (LVEDVI) at the week 54 visit. The following prespecified secondary analyses were performed: comparison of the week 54 LVEDVI to that after drug withdrawal (week 55), Minnesota Living with Heart Failure Questionnaire results and symptom scales, vital signs, laboratory variables, and adverse events were compared between treatment groups. At 1 year, there was a small, nonsignificant reduction in LVEDVI in the tolvaptan versus placebo group (1.8 vs 0.0 mL/m²). There was also an overall slight increase in LVEDVI from baseline to week 55 in both groups. Symptom scores, blood pressure, and heart rate were not significantly different between treatment groups. Side effects of urinary frequency, thirst, and dry mouth were more commonly reported in the tolvaptan group compared to placebo. Posthoc nonprespecified time-to-event analysis of the composite end point of mortality or HF hospitalization demonstrated a significant favorable effect of tolvaptan over placebo.

The phase 3 Efficacy of Vasopressin Antagonist in Heart Failure Outcome Study with Tolvaptan (EVEREST) trials were designed to determine the short-term and long-term efficacy of tolvaptan when administered to patients hospitalized with worsened HF and LVEF ≤ 40% and continued postdischarge. Patients were well treated in regard to background medical therapy throughout the study.[35,36] EVEREST comprised 3 prospective, multicenter, randomized, double-blind, placebo-controlled trials: 2 identical short-term trials and a single long-term outcome study that combined all patients in the 2 short-term trials. Total enrollment for the EVEREST trials was 4133 patients followed for a median of 9.9 months. The 2 short-term trials were performed to fulfill regulatory requirements for establishing efficacy in at least 2 independent, adequately powered trials.[37] The short-term primary end point was a composite score of changes in body weight and improvement in patient-assessed global clinical status assessed at day 7 or discharge, while short-term secondary end points included changes in signs and symptoms during hospitalization. Long-term primary end points were all-cause mortality and the composite of cardiovascular death or hospitalization for HF, while secondary long-term end points included composite of cardiovascular mortality or cardiovascular hospitalization, incidence of cardiovascular

mortality, incidence of worsening HF (death, HF hospitalization, or unscheduled visit for HF), changes in body weight at day 1, edema at day 7 or discharge for those with baseline edema, patient-assessed dyspnea at day 1 for those with dyspnea at baseline, and Kansas City Cardiomyopathy Questionnaire (KCCQ) at outpatient week 1, and serum sodium at day 7 or discharge in patients with baseline serum sodium level of < 134 mEq/L.

The short-term trials demonstrated that tolvaptan resulted in significantly greater improvement in the composite primary end point, driven primarily by reduction in body weight. There was a mean reduction in body weight of 1.76 kg and 3.56 kg in the tolvaptan group compared with 0.97 and 2.76 kg with placebo at days 1 and day 7 or discharge, respectively, but no significant reduction in global clinical status with tolvaptan compared to placebo. There was a significantly greater improvement in dyspnea with tolvaptan versus placebo, and significantly greater improvement in edema only in 1 of the 2 short-term trials. Adverse event frequencies were similar in both the tolvaptan and placebo groups.

For the long-term trial, the dual primary end points did not significantly differ between groups: death occurred in 25.9% in the tolvaptan group and 26.3% in the placebo group, and composite cardiovascular death or HF hospitalization occurred in 42.0% in the tolvaptan group and 40.2% in the placebo group (Figure 10.6). There was no subgroup, including severe HF, severely depressed LVEF, or hyponatremia, that appeared to benefit from tolvaptan over placebo. Cardiovascular mortality, cardiovascular hospitalization, and worsening HF also did not differ between treatment groups. Mean body weight was significantly reduced at day 1 with tolvaptan, compared to placebo—an effect that was observed at day 7 or discharge, and during the long-term follow-up

Figure 10.6. Long-term end points in 4133 patients hospitalized for worsening HF and reduced ejection fraction randomized to tolvaptan or placebo. Konstam MA, Gheorghiade M, Burnett JC, Jr., et al. Effects of oral tolvaptan in patients hospitalized for worsening heart failure: the EVEREST Outcome Trial. *JAMA.* 2007;297(12):1319–1331. Copyright © 2007 American Medical Association. All rights reserved.

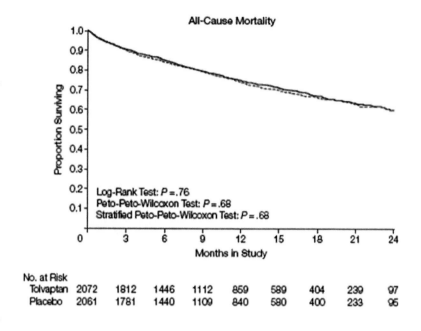

No. at Risk

Tolvaptan	2072	1812	1446	1112	859	589	404	239	97
Placebo	2061	1781	1440	1109	840	580	400	233	95

period. A similar trend was noted for improvement in hyponatremia (Figure 10.7). Dyspnea significantly improved at day 1 in patients receiving tolvaptan, with 74.3% in the tolvaptan group and 68.0% in the placebo group demonstrating improvement. Similarly, edema significantly improved at day 7 in patients receiving tolvaptan, with 73.8% in the tolvaptan group and 70.5% in the placebo group manifesting improvement in edema by at least 2 grades. There was no significant change observed in the KCCQ at outpatient week 1 in the 2 groups. Adverse events resulting in study drug discontinuation occurred in 6.5% of tolvaptan patients and 5.5% of placebo patients. Of all adverse events, only thirst differed significantly between treatment groups.

Tolvaptan has also been studied in other disease processes where correction of hyponatremia may be beneficial, such as cirrhosis or the syndrome of inappropriate antidiuretic hormone secretion. The Study of Ascending Levels of Tolvaptan in Hyponatremia 1 and 2 (SALT-1 and -2) studies

enrolled 448 patients with euvolemic or hypervolemic hyponatremia (serum sodium < 135 mEq/L), of which approximately 30% had hyponatremia due to HF, into 1 of 2 identical prospective, multicenter, randomized, double-blind, placebo-controlled trials to test the efficacy of tolvaptan in correcting hyponatremia after 30 days of treatment.[38] Patients were randomized to tolvaptan, 15 mg daily, with escalation to 30 mg daily and then 60 mg daily if necessary, based on serum sodium. Primary end points were change in the average AUC for serum sodium levels from baseline to day 4 and from baseline to day 30. Secondary end points included changes in the AUC in patients with marked hyponatremia (serum sodium < 130 mEq/L) and the percentage of patients with severe hyponatremia and normalized sodium after treatment. There was a significant increase in the AUC for serum sodium levels from baseline to 4 days and baseline to 30 days with tolvaptan compared to placebo, an effect observed in patients with marked and mild hyponatremia (serum sodium 130–134 mEq/L).

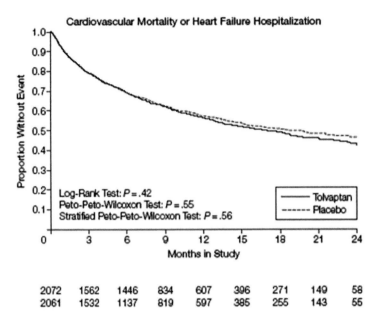

Figure 10.6.
(Continued)

Tolvaptan's effects on hyponatremia were observed as early as 8 hours after administration (Figure 10.8). In addition, significantly more patients had normal serum sodium and fewer patients had severe hyponatremia at days 4 and 30 with tolvaptan compared to placebo. However, hyponatremia recurred 1 week after discontinuation of tolvaptan at day 30. Side effects with tolvaptan were thirst, dry mouth, and urinary frequency.

Based on available evidence, tolvaptan was approved by the US Food and Drug Administration (FDA) for the treatment of hyponatremia but not for acute HF, in June 2008, making it the only available oral vasopressin antagonist.

Lixivaptan (VPA 459)

Similar to tolvaptan, lixivaptan is an orally active V2 receptor antagonist, with a even greater selectivity for the V2 receptor compared to tolvaptan.[39] A phase 2 randomized, double-blind, placebo-controlled trial in 42 patients with NYHA class II or III HF and LVEF ≤ 35% on standard medical ther-apy, including diuretics, randomized to 1 of 6 doses of lixivaptan (10, 30, 75, 150, 250, and 400 mg) or placebo administered as a single dose, was performed to determine the renal effects of this drug.[40] Doses of lixivaptan were escalated only after blinded safety data were evaluated by the principal investigator and study sponsor. End points observed were mostly related to short-term renal, electrolyte, and urinary parameters. Dose-dependent increases in urine volume were observed over 4 hours with all doses except for the 10-mg dose, compared to placebo, with 24-hour urine volume ranging from 1.8 L with placebo to 3.9 L with 400 mg lixivaptan. These increases were accompanied by significant increases in solute-free water excretion as well as increases in serum sodium with lixivaptan doses > 75 mg. The most frequent adverse events were diarrhea, headache, dizziness, orthostatic tachycardia, dry mouth, and flatulence.

Based on the favorable short-term efficacy and safety of lixivaptan, the phase 3 Treatment of Hyponatremia Based on Lixivaptan

Figure 10.7. Long-term effects of tolvaptan on body weight, sodium, and renal function in 4133 patients hospitalized for worsening HF and reduced ejection fraction randomized to tolvaptan or placebo. Data for serum sodium are for patients with serum sodium levels < 134 mEq/L at baseline. Konstam MA, Gheorghiade M, Burnett JC, Jr., et al. Effects of oral tolvaptan in patients hospitalized for worsening heart failure: the EVEREST Outcome Trial. *JAMA.* 2007;297(12):1319–1331. Copyright © 2007 American Medical Association. All rights reserved.

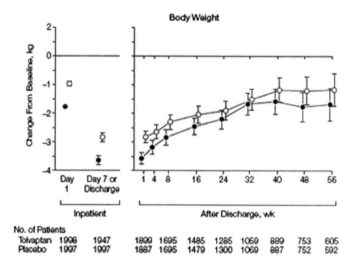

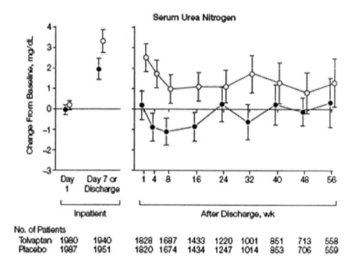

in NYHA Class III/IV Cardiac Patient Evaluation (BALANCE) trial is currently in the recruitment phase (clinicaltrials.gov identifier: NCT00578695). The study will randomize approximately 650 patients hospitalized with worsened HF with hyponatremia to lixivaptan versus placebo, administered over 60 days. The primary end point will be an increase in serum sodium levels from baseline. Secondary end points will be all-cause mortality, cardiovascular hospitalization, HF hospitalization, and changes in body weight.

Other investigations currently underway are studying the effects of lixivaptan in patients with euvolemic hyponatremia.

SR 121463

SR 121463 is also an oral V2 antagonist with high affinity for animal and human V2 receptors similar to lixivaptan.[41] The drug was under development for HF with the initiation of the phase 2 Safety Study of Vasopressin V2 Receptor Antagonist on Patients with Severe Chronic Heart Failure (AQUAVIT) study, ini-

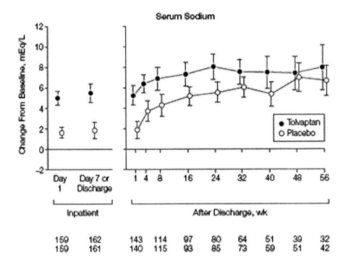

Figure 10.7.
(Continued)

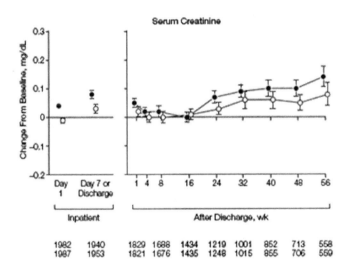

tiated in August 2001, and completed in February 2003. It was a multicenter, randomized, double-blind, placebo-controlled study of 338 patients with severe chronic HF on standard medical therapy, including diuretics, randomized to SR 121463 in a forced up-titration dosing strategy versus placebo for a period of 120 days (clinicaltrials.gov identifier: NCT00032747). The primary end point was clinical status at day 120. Although the trial is complete, there is no published data from this trial to date.

Combined V1a/V2 Antagonist (Conivaptan)

Conivaptan (YM087, Astellas Pharma) is a nonapeptide intravenous agent that antagonizes both the V1a and V2 receptors at a 10:1 ratio,[42] approved for the treatment of euvolemic hyponatremia by the FDA in December 2005. The first larger-sized study of conivaptan in HF was a phase 2 randomized, multicenter, double-blind, placebo-

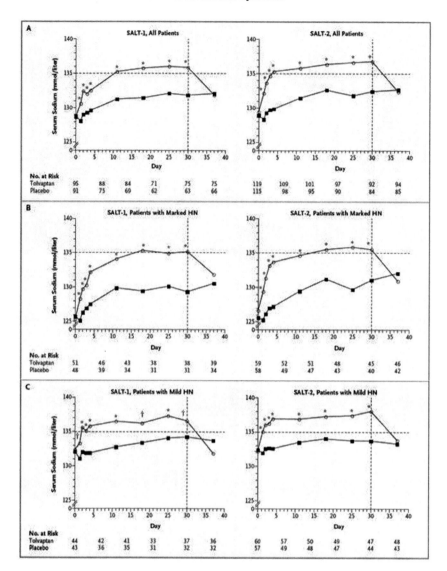

Figure 10.8. Serum sodium concentration in 448 patients with euvolemic or hypervolemic hyponatremia (serum sodium < 135 mEq/L) treated with escalating doses of tolvaptan or placebo. (A) All randomized patients, (B) patients with marked baseline hyponatremia (serum sodium < 130 mEq/L), and (C) patients with mild baseline hyponatremia (serum sodium 130–134 mEq/L). Schrier RW, Gross P, Gheorghiade M, Berl T, Verbalis JG, Czerwiec FS, Orlandi C. Tolvaptan, a selective oral vasopressin V2-receptor antagonist, for hyponatremia. *N Engl J Med.* 2006;355(20):2099–2112. With permission of the Massachusetts Medical Society.

controlled invasive hemodynamic trial of 140 patients with severe chronic HF (NYHA class III or IV), regardless of LVEF, on standard medical therapy including diuretics.[25] Patients were randomized in a 1:1:1:1 manner to a 30-minute intravenous infusion of conivaptan (10, 20, or 40 mg) or placebo if the PCWP was ≥ 16 mm Hg and cardiac index ≤ 2.8 L/min/m² on 2 consecutive recordings at least 30 minutes apart after a 6- to 16-hour stabilization period. Hemodynamic and renal parameters were then measured at multiple time points over a 12-hour assessment period, during which time background diuretics and other cardiac medications were held, and fluid was restricted to no more than 1.5 L over 12 hours. Primary end points were peak change from baseline in PCWP within 3 to 6 hours after infusion, and change from baseline PCWP as measured by AUC over the 12-hour evaluation period. Secondary end points included peak change at 3 to 6 hours in other pulmonary artery catheter measurements, as well as renal and electrolyte parameters. Conivaptan at 20- and 40-mg doses had a significant reduction in PCWP and AUC for PCWP over 12 hours compared to placebo, an effect sustained until approximately 8 hours after drug infusion, and remained below baseline at 12 hours. A similar trend was noted for right atrial pressure, but not mean arterial pressure, heart rate, cardiac index, or systemic or pulmonary vascular resistance. Similar to the acute effects of tolvaptan, conivaptan demonstrated a dose-dependent increase in urine output and reduction in urine osmolality compared to placebo.

In another phase 2 multicenter, randomized, double-blind, placebo-controlled trial, 162 patients hospitalized for worsening HF, irrespective of LVEF, were randomized in a 1:1:1:1 manner to intravenous conivaptan (two 24-hour infusions of 40, 80, or 120 mg, after 20-mg loading dose) or placebo,

and followed for 72 hours.[43] Primary end points were the AUC change from baseline to 48 hours in patient-assessed respiratory symptoms and global status, total 72-hour urine output, and daily urine output. There were no differences in respiratory symptoms or global status between the conivaptan and placebo groups, although the total and daily urine outputs were significantly greater in the conivaptan groups. The 72-hour total urine output appeared to be dose-dependent. There was no difference in blood pressure change in all 3 conivaptan groups compared to placebo. Conivaptan was well-tolerated, with no significant adverse reactions compared to placebo, with the exception of infusion-site reactions.

The ADVANCE (A Dose Evaluation of a Vasopressin Antagonist in CHF Patients Undergoing Exercise) trial was a double-blind, placebo-controlled study of 345 patients with chronic (NYHA class II–IV) HF, regardless of ventricular function, randomized in a 1:1:1:1 manner to 12 weeks of 1 of 3 doses of oral conivaptan (10, 20, or 40 mg daily) versus placebo, designed to study the effects of conivaptan on exercise tolerance.[44] The primary end point was time to reach 70% peak oxygen consumption during an incremental exercise test, while secondary end points included Minnesota Living with Heart Failure score and NYHA class. To date, results of ADVANCE have not been published, however, it has been reported that there was no improvement in overall functional capacity, exercise tolerance, or quality of life when conivaptan was compared with placebo.[45]

V1a Antagonists

Infusion of an intravenous peptide V1a antagonist resulted in a fall in systemic vascular resistance and increase in CO in patients with HF and elevated AVP levels.[46] There are no V1a antagonists under development for use in HF, although relcovaptan (SR 49059, Sanofi-Aventis), when initially tested for treatment of hypertension, demonstrated only a transient vasodilatory effect, which was not associated with sustained blood pressure reduction.[46]

Vasopressin Antagonists Summarized

Vasopressin plays an important pathophysiologic role in HF, with elevated levels predictive of poor prognosis in acute and chronic HF. Vasopressin exerts its effects on the V1a receptor, which causes smooth muscle vasoconstriction, and the cortical collecting duct V2 receptor, which leads to aquaporin channel insertion in the basolateral membrane resulting in free water absorption. Despite the promising hypothesis of blocking V1a and V2 receptors, studies to date have not led to improved morbidity and mortality in HF. Nevertheless, vasopressin antagonists, namely tolvaptan, have a favorable safety profile. When combined with normalization of serum sodium, reduction in body weight, along with improvement in signs and symptoms, suggests that with further study, vasopressin antagonists still hold promise in the treatment of HF. Currently, both tolvaptan and conivaptan are approved by the FDA for the treatment of hyponatremia and not HF.

Adenosine Receptor Antagonists

Pathophysiology of Adenosine in Heart Failure

Adenosine is a purine nucleoside produced from hydrolysis of adenosine triphosphate (ATP).[47] Found in all body cells, it is involved in multiple physiologic and pathophysiologic processes.[48] There are 4 distinct adenosine

receptor (AR) subtypes: A1R, A2aR, A2bR, and A3R (Table 10.2).[49] All are membrane-bound G-protein–coupled receptors of the P1 class sensitive to adenosine analogues. By contrast, receptors of the P2 class are sensitive to ATP. A1R and A3R are coupled to the pertussis toxin–sensitive Gi proteins and inhibit adenylyl cyclase and cAMP, while A2aR and A2bR activate Gs proteins and stimulate adenylyl cyclase.[49]

The physiological effects resulting from activation of these receptors are diverse and are outlined in Table 10.2. However, this discussion focuses on the A1R in the kidney, as this is the primary mechanism of interest currently studied in HF. The A1Rs are found in the renal afferent arteriole and proximal tubules. Their stimulation leads to reduced glomerular filtration rate (GFR) via afferent arteriolar vasoconstriction and increased proximal sodium absorption via stimulation of proximal sodium/bicarbonate transporters, along with suppression of renin release.[50,51]

The regulation of fluid and sodium delivery to the distal nephron is tightly regulated within narrow limits to ensure homeostasis. A negative feedback loop called tubuloglomerular feedback (TGF) is part of the homeostatic mechanism that regulates sodium delivery.[52,53] In the distal convoluted tubule, specialized cells called the macula densa are in close contact with the afferent arteriole, and they release adenosine in response to increases in solute delivery. This in turn leads to the stimulation of the A1R, afferent arteriolar vasoconstriction, and reduced GFR, which leads to enhanced proximal sodium absorption and reduced distal sodium delivery[54,55] (Figure 10.9). It has been suggested that IV non-potassium–sparing loop diuretics further activate adenosine release via TGF as a result of increasing sodium delivery because of their mechanism of action.

Table 10.2 Actions of Adenosine

Receptor	Signaling Pathway	Location	Actions
A1	Gi protein, IP3	Brain (cortex, hippocampus, cerebellum, thalamus), spinal cord, testes, adipose tissue, heart, kidney	Decreases CNS electrical excitability, reduces heart rate, decreases atrial contraction, renal vasoconstriction, antidiuresis, antinatriuresis
A2a	Gs protein	Brain (striatum, nucleus accumbens, tuberculum olfactorium), heart, lungs, thymus, spleen, adipose tissue	Increases cerebral blood flow, takes part in wound healing, coronary vasodilation, increases renal medullary blood flow
A2b	Gs protein	Lung, large intestine, bladder	Bronchoconstriction
A3	Gi protein, IP3	Lung, liver, placenta >> brain, aorta, kidney > testes > heart	Cardioprotective, allergic responses

Adapted from Slawsky MT, Givertz MM. Rolofylline: a selective adenosine 1 receptor antagonist for the treatment of heart failure. *Expert Opin Pharmacother.* 2009;10(2):311-322; and Poulsen SA, Quinn RJ. Adenosine receptors: new opportunities for future drugs. *Bioorg Med Chem.* 1998;6(6):619–641.

In HF, reduction of GFR may be detrimental. Available evidence strongly suggests that baseline renal dysfunction,[56] as well as worsening renal function (WRF) during hospitalization,[57,58] is a poor prognostic marker in acute HF syndrome. Although the mechanism by which WRF develops during hospitalization is debated, adenosine is thought to be a potential mediator, given adenosine serum levels are more elevated with higher classes of chronic HF (Figure 10.10)[59] As adenosine has adverse effects on GFR, the A1R has emerged as a potential target for treating acute HF syndrome in an attempt to preserve GFR.

Adenosine-1 Receptor Antagonists and Heart Failure

There are no A1R antagonists currently available for clinical use. The following compounds have been studied in humans.

BG 9719 and BG 9928 (Biogen)

The first human study of an A1R antagonist was a single-center, randomized, double-blind trial in 12 patients with stable NYHA class III to IV HF on stable medical therapy excluding loop diuretics, given either intravenous BG 9719 (1 mg/kg over 60 min) or placebo as a single dose, followed by a cross-

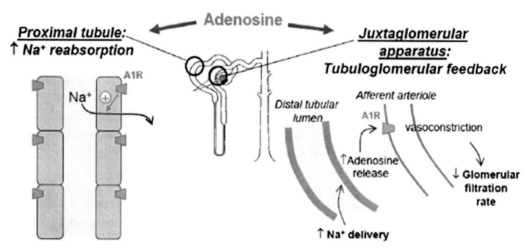

Figure 10.9. Mechanism of adenosine in the kidneys through TGF. Reduced sodium (Na) delivery to the distal tubule leads to adenosine release, which in turn stimulates the A1R, leading to afferent arteriolar vasoconstriction, reduced GFR, and enhanced proximal Na reabsorption. De Luca L, Mebazaa A, Filippatos G, et al. Overview of emerging pharmacologic agents for acute heart failure syndromes. *Eur J Heart Fail.* 2008;10(2):201–213. With permission from the European Society of Cardiology.

over, then intravenous furosemide, over several days.[60] Renal hemodynamics and GFR were measured using radionuclide imaging. It was demonstrated that renal blood flow and sodium excretion increased with both furosemide and BG 9719, however, furosemide, but not BG 9719 or placebo, was associated with reduction in GFR. This study was followed by a larger randomized, double-blind, placebo-controlled crossover study in 63 patients with chronic HF (NYHA class II–IV), and LVEF ≤ 40%, randomized to 1 of 3 different intravenous doses of BG 9719 (to yield serum concentrations of 0.1, 0.75, and 2.5 µg/mL) infused over 7 hours in an ascending dosing scheme.[61] The infusions were given over 3 days, with furosemide or placebo administered and crossed over on days 2 and 3. Study end points were urine volume, creatinine clearance, and electrolyte excretion as measured by urine collection. Compared to placebo, BG 9719 administration resulted in modest but significant increases in urine volume, which was greatly

increased with coadministration with furosemide. In addition, there was an increase in creatinine clearance over placebo with the lower 2 doses of BG 9719, an effect that was maintained after coadministration with furosemide (Figure 10.11).

Another A1R antagonist, BG 9928, was tested in 50 patients with chronic HF (NYHA class II–IV) and LVEF ≤ 40%. This was a multicenter, randomized, double-blind, placebo-controlled, dose-escalation study that randomized patients to 1 of 4 oral doses of BG 9928 or placebo.[62] Primary end points were changes in urinary sodium excretion and urine volume, while secondary end points were symptom and body weight assessments. Compared with placebo, BG 9928 increased sodium excretion and urine volume over 10 days without causing kaliuresis or renal dysfunction. There was a nonsignificant reduction in body weight, and nonsignificant trends toward improvement in edema, physician-assessed global status, and NYHA class.

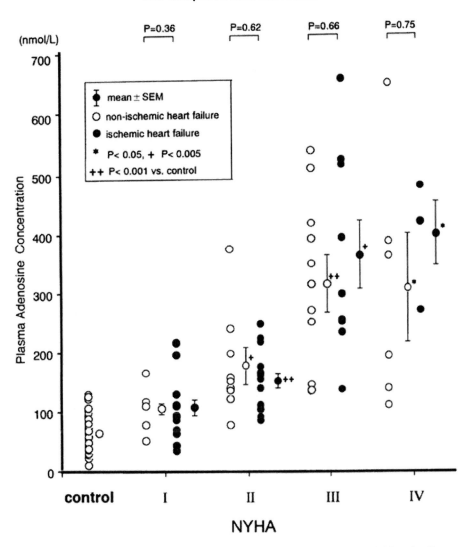

Figure 10.10. Plasma adenosine levels in patients with HF. Funaya H, Kitakaze M, Node K, Minamino T, Komamura K, Hori M. Plasma adenosine levels increase in patients with chronic heart failure. *Circulation*. 1997; 95(6):1363–1365. With permission.

SLV 320 (Solvay Pharmaceuticals)

Another A1R antagonist, SLV 320, was studied in a multicenter, randomized, double-blind, placebo-controlled invasive hemodynamic study in 111 patients with worsening chronic HF (NYHA class II–IV), LVEF < 35%, requiring diuretic therapy.[63] All patients had a pulmonary artery catheter placed and were randomized to 1 of 3 intravenous doses of SLV 320, placebo, or furosemide after CO

and heart rate measurements, determined at 10-minute intervals, had < 10% variability at 2 consecutive measurements, and followed for 24 hours. End point measurements were urinary parameters, renal function, and hemodynamic improvement. Compared to the placebo group, patients treated with SLV 320 had a small, nonsignificant decrease from baseline in cystatin C, whereas there was an increase from baseline in furosemide, which

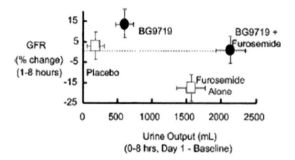

Figure 10.11. Relationship between urine output and GFR with BG 9719, alone or with furosemide in 15 patients with chronic systolic HF. Data is from the middle of the 3 doses tested. Gottlieb SS, Brater DC, Thomas I, et al. BG9719 (CVT-124), an A1 adenosine receptor antagonist, protects against the decline in renal function observed with diuretic therapy. *Circulation.* 2002;105(11):1348–1353. With permission.

was significant when compared with the SLV 320 groups. In addition, a nonsignificant trend toward reduced PCWP with SLV 320 was noted but no change in blood pressure or heart rate compared to placebo.

Rolofylline (KW 3902, Merck)

The most extensively studied A1R antagonist to date is rolofylline (KW 3902). Originally developed as an adjunct to cisplatin chemotherapy, its utility in preventing renal dysfunction in HF was later tested. Phase 1 studies testing different intravenous doses (1–60 mg) of rolofylline in a double-blind, randomized, placebo–controlled trial of 36 patients with HF demonstrated a dose-dependent natriuresis with a peak effect at the 30-mg dose, occurring 3 hours after drug administration.[64] This led to phase 2 studies, the first of which was a randomized, double-blind, placebo–controlled study designed to determine the optimal dose range of intravenous rolofylline as monotherapy and in combination with intravenous furosemide in 2 clinically challenging populations: acute

decompensated heart failure (ADHF) and diuretic resistance.[65] The ADHF population involved 159 patients hospitalized with HF (NYHA class II–IV), regardless of LVEF and renal impairment (creatinine clearance [CrCl] 20–80 mL/min using the Cockroft-Gault equation), who were administered 40 mg intravenous furosemide. If no additional furosemide was needed after 12 hours of the initial dose, as determined by the treating physician or site coordinator, then patients were randomized to 1 of 4 rolofylline doses (2.5, 15.0, 30.0, or 60.0 mg). Loop diuretics were not permitted until 6 hours after study drug infusion, and on days 2 and 3, the study drug was again administered with intravenous furosemide at any time at the investigator's discretion. The diuretic–resistant protocol involved 35 patients hospitalized with HF (NYHA class III–IV), regardless of LVEF, determined by the investigator to have reached a point where further increases in diuretic therapy were unlikely to be effective. Patients were randomized to receive a single intravenous dose of rolofylline (10, 20, 30, or 60 mg) or placebo, with diuretics held at least 5 hours prior to infusion. For the ADHF protocol, mean baseline serum creatinine was 1.8 mg/dL, and CrCl was 48 mL/min. In all groups, rolofylline monotherapy resulted in higher urine output during the first 6 hours compared to placebo, but achieved statistical significance only in the 30-mg group. By 24 hours, cumulative urine volumes were similar between groups. Mean serum creatinine had decreased compared to baseline in all rolofylline groups at day 2, whereas it increased in the placebo group. This trend was similar at day 4, with the exception of an increase in mean serum creatinine in the 60-mg rolofylline group. Cumulative intravenous furosemide was significantly less in the 30-mg rolofylline group compared to placebo. There were no significant differences in systolic blood pressure or heart rate from baseline to 6 hours between groups, and there were no significant adverse effects compared to placebo. For the diuretic-resistant group, there was a modest increase in urine output observed in all rolofylline groups compared to placebo, which was not statistically significant after 6 hours. Mean CrCl significantly increased from baseline in the 30-mg rolofylline group at all time points compared to placebo. Again, adverse events were not different in the rolofylline groups compared to placebo. It appeared that in these 2 clinically challenging groups, the greatest clinical effect was achieved with the 30-mg rolofylline dosing, with no further urine output with 60 mg, and possible WRF at this dose.

Another phase 2 study of 32 patients with chronic HF (NYHA class II–IV) and CrCl 30 to 80 mL/min, on oral doses of loop diuretic equivalent to at least 80 mg of furosemide, was designed to test the effects of outpatient infusion of rolofylline on urine volume and renal function. This was a randomized, double-blind, placebo-controlled, 2-way crossover study in which patients were randomized to either 30 mg intravenous rolofylline or placebo, followed by administration of 80 mg intravenous furosemide 30 minutes later, and repetition of the process after crossover on day 5. Urine volume, electrolytes, and renal function were measured over 8 days. GFR and renal plasma flow (RPF) were measured using established protocols that administered and measured iothalamate and para–amino-hippurate. Compared to placebo plus furosemide, rolofylline plus furosemide resulted in a slightly higher 8-hour urine volume (3.0 vs 2.5 L). This was associated with a significant increase from baseline in GFR (32% vs 8% at 8 hours) with rolofylline versus placebo. This effect was redemonstrated after washout of drug and crossover (Figure 10.12).

Promising results from phase 1 and 2 studies led to the design of the phase 3 multicenter, randomized, double-blind, placebo-controlled PROTECT studies (PROTECT-1 and -2). These 2 studies were identical in design and initiated during the same time period. The prespecified intention was to combine data from the first 300 patients in both trials with 60-day follow-up as the pilot phase of PROTECT to determine study end points and

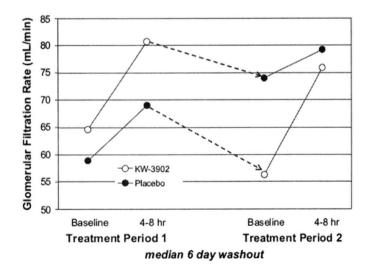

Figure 10.12. Effects of rolofylline (KW 3902) on GFR in patients with chronic HF and mild to moderate renal impairment. Baseline GFR between groups is not significantly different. Dittrich HC, Gupta DK, Hack TC, Dowling T, Callahan J, Thomson S. The effect of KW-3902, an adenosine A1 receptor antagonist, on renal function and renal plasma flow in ambulatory patients with heart failure and renal impairment. *J Card Fail.* 2007;13(8):609–617. With permission from Elsevier.

optimal dose and sample size required for an adequately powered pivotal study. The pilot data were not to be combined with the subsequent main study.

The PROTECT pilot study randomized 301 patients hospitalized with acute HF, irrespective of LVEF, CrCl 20 to 80 mL/min, and brain natriuretic peptide (BNP) > 250 pg/mL or N-terminal pro-BNP > 1000 pg/mL to 1 of 3 intravenous doses of rolofylline (10, 20, or 30 mg) or placebo for 3 days or until discharge, with telephone follow-up at 60 days.[66] Due to prior data that adenosine antagonists lower seizure threshold, patients at high risk for seizures were excluded,[67] and those at moderate risk were pretreated with 1 mg oral lorazepam 30 minutes before the study drug. A new trichotomous end point was developed for the study that was further modified after study completion and made more stringent: treatment success, failure, or unchanged. Success was defined as improvement in patient-reported dyspnea (moderately or markedly better than at randomization on a 7-point Likert scale); failure defined as death, early HF readmission (within 7 days of randomization, worsening HF defined by physician assessment by day 7), or persistent renal impairment (serum creatinine increase ≥ 0.3 mg/dL from randomization to day 7, confirmed at day 14, or initiation of hemofiltration or dialysis through day 7); or unchanged if neither criteria for success nor failure were met. It is important to note that this study was not powered to achieve a statistically significant end point.

Patients treated with rolofylline were more likely to achieve treatment success (53% vs 37%) and less likely to experience failure (16% vs 28%) compared to placebo (Figure 10.13). Other findings included a trend toward reduction in body weight and initial improvement in dyspnea, and a significantly lesser increase in creatinine in patients treated with rolofoylline compared to placebo, which appeared to be dose-related. There was a nonsignificant trend toward reduced 60-day mortality (5% vs 10%), and combined mortality, cardiovascular readmission, or renal readmission (16% vs 29%) at 60 days in the rolofylline versus placebo groups. There was no significant difference in adverse events in the treatment groups, and no seizures were reported, although 27% required seizure prophylaxis.

The favorable trends from the PROTECT pilot led to continuation with the main PROTECT trial.[68] There were 2033 patients randomized in a 2:1 ratio to either 30 mg rolofylline or placebo for up to 3 days. There was no difference in patients achieving treatment success (40.6% vs 36.0%) or failure (21.8% vs 19.8%) in the rolofylline or placebo groups, as defined in the PROTECT pilot study. In addition, there were no differences between rolofylline or placebo in any of the prespecified secondary end points of death from any cause or rehospitalization for cardiovascular or renal causes through day 60, and proportion of patients with persistent renal impairment. A trend toward more seizures and strokes in patients treated with rolofylline versus placebo occurred. Importantly, only a small percentage of the population experienced persistent renal impairment in both the placebo and rolofylline arms, 12.7% and 11.1%, respectively. Given the mechanism of action of rolofylline, it has been suggested that the hypothesis for which rolofylline was intended, protection or prevention of the kidneys, was not sufficiently tested given the low number of patients with persistent renal impairment.

Adenosine-1 Receptor Antagonists Summarized

A1R antagonists cause a modest natriuresis without kaliuresis or changes in blood pressure that is augmented with furosemide.

Figure 10.13. Primary trichotomous end point in 301 patients hospitalized for acute HF and mild to moderately impaired renal function showing the distribution of patients by classification as improved, unchanged, or worse at 7 days. Cotter G, Dittrich HC, Weatherley BD, Bloomfield DM, O'Connor CM, Metra M, Massie BM. The PROTECT pilot study: a randomized, placebo-controlled, dose-finding study of the adenosine A1 receptor antagonist rolofylline in patients with acute heart failure and renal impairment. *J Card Fail.* 2008;14(8):631–640. With permission from Elsevier.

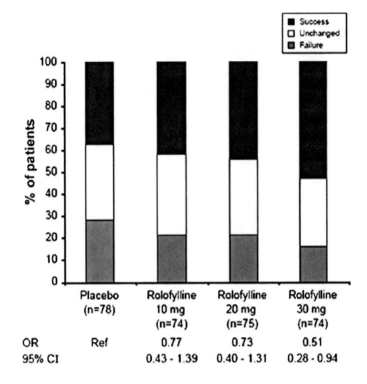

Symptoms also improve modestly with these agents. In patients with mild or moderate renal impairment, it does not appear to worsen renal function as measured by both serum and urine indicators. Given the disappointing results of the PROTECT study, further development of intravenous A1R blockers for acute HF has been halted at the time of this writing. What remains striking were the significant trends noted during earlier development phases and the absence of any positive findings as defined by primary or secondary end points during the pivotal trial. In addition, the prevalence of persistent renal impairment was substantially less than predicted. What future role adenosine antagonists have in acute HF syndrome remains to be determined.

Conclusion

Fluid management in acute HF syndrome remains challenging despite initial promise from the development of vasopressin and adenosine receptor antagonists. In the case of vasopressin antagonists, the modest clinical effects combined with the overall safe clinical profile may prove to be useful on a case–by–case basis, for example, in patients with acute HF syndrome and symptomatic hyponatremia. In the case of adenosine antagonists, further long–term efficacy and safety data will be needed to justify its use, given the unfavorable short–term effects on the central nervous system.

References

1. Gheorghiade M, Filippatos G, De Luca L, Burnett J. Congestion in acute heart failure syndromes: an essential target of evaluation and treatment. *Am J Med.* 2006;119(12 suppl 1):S3-S10.

2. Gheorghiade M, Pang PS. Acute heart failure syndromes. *J Am Coll Cardiol.* 2009;53(7):557-573.

3. Dickstein K, Cohen-Solal A, Filippatos G, et al. ESC guidelines for the diagnosis and treatment of acute and chronic heart failure 2008: the Task Force for the Diagnosis and Treatment of Acute and Chronic Heart Failure 2008 of the European Society of Cardiology. Developed in collaboration with the Heart Failure Association of the ESC (HFA) and endorsed by the European Society of Intensive Care Medicine (ESICM). *Eur Heart J.* 2008;29(19): 2388-2442.

4. Weber KT. Furosemide in the long-term management of heart failure: the good, the bad, and the uncertain. *J Am Coll Cardiol.* 2004;44(6):1308-1310.

5. Hasselblad V, Gattis Stough W, Shah MR, et al. Relation between dose of loop diuretics and outcomes in a heart failure population: results of the ESCAPE trial. *Eur J Heart Fail.* 2007;9(10):1064-1069.

6. Francis GS, Siegel RM, Goldsmith SR, Olivari MT, Levine TB, Cohn JN. Acute vasoconstrictor response to intravenous furosemide in patients with chronic congestive heart failure. Activation of the neurohumoral axis. *Ann Intern Med.* 1985;103(1):1-6.

7. McCurley JM, Hanlon SU, Wei SK, Wedam EF, Michalski M, Haigney MC. Furosemide and the progression of left ventricular dysfunction in experimental heart failure. *J Am Coll Cardiol.* 2004;44(6):1301-1307.

8. Domanski M, Norman J, Pitt B, Haigney M, Hanlon S, Peyster E. Diuretic use, progressive heart failure, and death in patients in the Studies Of Left Ventricular Dysfunction (SOLVD). *J Am Coll Cardiol.* 2003;42(4):705-708.

9. Manning M, Sawyer WH. Discovery, development, and some uses of vasopressin and oxytocin antagonists. *J Lab Clin Med.* 1989;114(6):617-632.

10. Goldsmith SR, Gheorghiade M. Vasopressin antagonism in heart failure. *J Am Coll Cardiol.* 2005;46(10):1785-1791.

11. Oghlakian G, Klapholz M. Vasopressin and vasopressin receptor antagonists in heart failure. *Cardiol Rev.* 2009;17(1):10-15.

12. Jard S. Mechanisms of action of vasopressin and vasopressin antagonists. *Kidney Int Suppl.* 1988;26:S38-42.

13. Nabika T, Velletri PA, Lovenberg W, Beaven MA. Increase in cytosolic calcium and phosphoinositide metabolism induced by angiotensin II and [Arg]vasopressin in vascular smooth muscle cells. *J Biol Chem.* 1985;260(8):4661-4670.

14. Tahara A, Tomura Y, Wada K, et al. Effect of YM087, a potent nonpeptide vasopressin antagonist, on vasopressin-induced hyperplasia and hypertrophy of cultured vascular smooth-muscle cells. *J Cardiovasc Pharmacol.* 1997;30(6):759-766.

15. Tahara A, Saito M, Tsukada J, et al. Vasopressin increases vascular endothelial growth factor secretion from human vascular smooth muscle cells. *Eur J Pharmacol.* 1999;368(1):89-94.

16. Nakamura Y, Haneda T, Osaki J, Miyata S, Kikuchi K. Hypertrophic growth of cultured neonatal rat heart cells mediated by vasopressin V(1A) receptor. *Eur J Pharmacol.* 2000;391(1-2):39-48.

17. Hirsch AT, Dzau VJ, Majzoub JA, Creager MA. Vasopressin-mediated forearm

vasodilation in normal humans. Evidence for a vascular vasopressin V2 receptor. *J Clin Invest.* 1989;84(2):418–426.

18. Verbalis JG. Vasopressin V2 receptor antagonists. *J Mol Endocrinol.* 2002;29(1): 1–9.

19. Antoni FA, Holmes MC, Makara GB, Karteszi M, Laszlo FA. Evidence that the effects of arginine-8-vasopressin (AVP) on pituitary corticotropin (ACTH) release are mediated by a novel type of receptor. *Peptides.* 1984;5(3):519–522.

20. Szatalowicz VL, Arnold PE, Chaimovitz C, Bichet D, Berl T, Schrier RW. Radioimmunoassay of plasma arginine vasopressin in hyponatremic patients with congestive heart failure. *N Engl J Med.* 1981;305(5):263–266.

21. Goldsmith SR, Francis GS, Cowley AW Jr, Levine TB, Cohn JN. Increased plasma arginine vasopressin levels in patients with congestive heart failure. *J Am Coll Cardiol.* 1983;1(6):1385–1390.

22. Preibisz JJ, Sealey JE, Laragh JH, Cody RJ, Weksler BB. Plasma and platelet vasopressin in essential hypertension and congestive heart failure. *Hypertension* 1983;5(2 pt 2):I129–138.

23. Riegger GA, Liebau G, Kochsiek K. Antidiuretic hormone in congestive heart failure. *Am J Med.* 1982;72(1):49–52.

24. Blair JE, Zannad F, Konstam MA, et al. Continental differences in clinical characteristics, management, and outcomes in patients hospitalized with worsening heart failure results from the EVEREST (Efficacy of Vasopressin Antagonism in Heart Failure: Outcome Study with Tolvaptan) program. *J Am Coll Cardiol.* 2008;52(20):1640–1648.

25. Udelson JE, Smith WB, Hendrix GH, et al. Acute hemodynamic effects of conivaptan, a dual V(1A) and V(2) vasopressin receptor antagonist, in

patients with advanced heart failure. *Circulation.* 2001;104(20):2417–2423.

26. Schrier RW, Berl T, Anderson RJ. Osmotic and nonosmotic control of vasopressin release. *Am J Physiol.* 1979;236(4):F321–332.

27. Schrier RW, Abraham WT. Hormones and hemodynamics in heart failure. *N Engl J Med.* 1999;341(8):577–585.

28. Goldsmith SR, Francis GS, Cowley AW Jr, Goldenberg IF, Cohn JN. Hemodynamic effects of infused arginine vasopressin in congestive heart failure. *J Am Coll Cardiol.* 1986;8(4):779–783.

29. Yamamura Y, Nakamura S, Itoh S, et al. OPC-41061, a highly potent human vasopressin V2-receptor antagonist: pharmacological profile and aquaretic effect by single and multiple oral dosing in rats. *J Pharmacol Exp Ther.* 1998;287(3):860–867.

30. Hirano T, Yamamura Y, Nakamura S, Onogawa T, Mori T. Effects of the V(2)-receptor antagonist OPC-41061 and the loop diuretic furosemide alone and in combination in rats. *J Pharmacol Exp Ther.* 2000;292(1):288–294.

31. Gheorghiade M, Niazi I, Ouyang J, et al. Vasopressin V2-receptor blockade with tolvaptan in patients with chronic heart failure: results from a double-blind, randomized trial. *Circulation.* 2003;107(21):2690–2696.

32. Gheorghiade M, Gattis WA, O'Connor CM, et al. Effects of tolvaptan, a vasopressin antagonist, in patients hospitalized with worsening heart failure: a randomized controlled trial. *JAMA.* 2004;291(16):1963–1971.

33. Udelson JE, Orlandi C, Ouyang J, et al. Acute hemodynamic effects of tolvaptan, a vasopressin V2 receptor blocker, in patients with symptomatic heart failure and systolic dysfunction: an international, multicenter, randomized,

placebo-controlled trial. *J Am Coll Cardiol.* 2008;52(19):1540–1545.

34. Udelson JE, McGrew FA, Flores E, et al. Multicenter, randomized, double-blind, placebo-controlled study on the effect of oral tolvaptan on left ventricular dilation and function in patients with heart failure and systolic dysfunction. *J Am Coll Cardiol.* 2007;49(22):2151–2159.

35. Gheorghiade M, Konstam MA, Burnett JC Jr, et al. Short-term clinical effects of tolvaptan, an oral vasopressin antagonist, in patients hospitalized for heart failure: the EVEREST Clinical Status Trials. *JAMA.* 2007;297(12): 1332–1343.

36. Konstam MA, Gheorghiade M, Burnett JC Jr, et al. Effects of oral tolvaptan in patients hospitalized for worsening heart failure: the EVEREST Outcome Trial. *JAMA.* 2007;297(12):1319–1331.

37. Gheorghiade M, Orlandi C, Burnett JC, et al. Rationale and design of the multicenter, randomized, double-blind, placebo-controlled study to evaluate the Efficacy of Vasopressin antagonism in Heart Failure: Outcome Study with Tolvaptan (EVEREST). *J Card Fail.* 2005;11(4):260–269.

38. Schrier RW, Gross P, Gheorghiade M, et al. Tolvaptan, a selective oral vasopressin V2-receptor antagonist, for hyponatremia. *N Engl J Med.* 2006;355(20):2099–2112.

39. Chan PS, Coupet J, Park HC, et al. VPA-985, a nonpeptide orally active and selective vasopressin V2 receptor antagonist. *Adv Exp Med Biol.* 1998;449:439–443.

40. Abraham WT, Shamshirsaz AA, McFann K, Oren RM, Schrier RW. Aquaretic effect of lixivaptan, an oral, non-peptide, selective V2 receptor vasopressin antagonist, in New York Heart Association functional class II and

III chronic heart failure patients. *J Am Coll Cardiol.* 2006;47(8):1615–1621.

41. Serradeil-Le Gal C. An overview of SR121463, a selective non-peptide vasopressin V(2) receptor antagonist. *Cardiovasc Drug Rev.* 2001;19(3):201–214.

42. Lee CR, Watkins ML, Patterson JH, et al. Vasopressin: a new target for the treatment of heart failure. *Am Heart J.* 2003;146(1):9–18.

43. Goldsmith SR, Elkayam U, Haught WH, Barve A, He W. Efficacy and safety of the vasopressin V1A/V2-receptor antagonist conivaptan in acute decompensated heart failure: a dose-ranging pilot study. *J Card Fail.* 2008;14(8):641–647.

44. Russell SD, Selaru P, Pyne DA, et al. Rationale for use of an exercise end point and design for the ADVANCE (A Dose evaluation of a Vasopressin ANtagonist in CHF patients undergoing Exercise) trial. *Am Heart J.* 2003;145(1): 179–186.

45. Hoque MZ, Arumugham P, Huda N, Verma N, Afiniwala M, Karia DH. Conivaptan: promise of treatment in heart failure. *Expert Opin Pharmacother.* 2009;10(13):2161–2169.

46. Thibonnier M, Kilani A, Rahman M, et al. Effects of the nonpeptide V(1) vasopressin receptor antagonist SR49059 in hypertensive patients. *Hypertension.* 1999;34(6):1293–1300.

47. Shah RH, Frishman WH. Adenosine1 receptor antagonism: a new therapeutic approach for the treatment of decompensated heart failure. *Cardiol Rev.* 2009;17(3):125–131.

48. Slawsky MT, Givertz MM. Rolofylline: a selective adenosine 1 receptor antagonist for the treatment of heart failure. *Expert Opin Pharmacother.* 2009;10(2):311–322.

49. Poulsen SA, Quinn RJ. Adenosine receptors: new opportunities for future drugs. *Bioorg Med Chem.* 1998;6(6):619–641.

50. Modlinger PS, Welch WJ. Adenosine A1 receptor antagonists and the kidney. *Curr Opin Nephrol Hypertens.* 2003;12(5):497–502.

51. Takeda M, Yoshitomi K, Imai M. Regulation of Na(+)-3HCO3- cotransport in rabbit proximal convoluted tubule via adenosine A1 receptor. *Am J Physiol.* 1993;265(4 pt 2):F511–519.

52. Singh P, Thomson SC. Renal homeostasis and tubuloglomerular feedback. *Curr Opin Nephrol Hypertens.* 2010;19(1):59–64.

53. Braam B, Mitchell KD, Koomans HA, Navar LG. Relevance of the tubuloglomerular feedback mechanism in pathophysiology. *J Am Soc Nephrol.* 1993;4(6):1257–1274.

54. Vallon V, Miracle C, Thomson S. Adenosine and kidney function: potential implications in patients with heart failure. *Eur J Heart Fail.* 2008;10(2):176–187.

55. Vallon V, Muhlbauer B, Osswald H. Adenosine and kidney function. *Physiol Rev.* 2006;86(3):901–940.

56. Heywood JT, Fonarow GC, Costanzo MR, Mathur VS, Wigneswaran JR, Wynne J. High prevalence of renal dysfunction and its impact on outcome in 118,465 patients hospitalized with acute decompensated heart failure: a report from the ADHERE database. *J Card Fail.* 2007;13(6):422–430.

57. Butler J, Forman DE, Abraham WT, et al. Relationship between heart failure treatment and development of worsening renal function among hospitalized patients. *Am Heart J.* 2004;147(2):331–338.

58. Forman DE, Butler J, Wang Y, et al. Incidence, predictors at admission, and impact of worsening renal function among patients hospitalized with heart failure. *J Am Coll Cardiol.* 2004;43(1):61–67.

59. Funaya H, Kitakaze M, Node K, Minamino T, Komamura K, Hori M. Plasma adenosine levels increase in patients with chronic heart failure. *Circulation.* 1997;95(6):1363–1365.

60. Gottlieb SS, Skettino SL, Wolff A, et al. Effects of BG9719 (CVT-124), an A1-adenosine receptor antagonist, and furosemide on glomerular filtration rate and natriuresis in patients with congestive heart failure. *J Am Coll Cardiol.* 2000;35(1):56–59.

61. Gottlieb SS, Brater DC, Thomas I, et al. BG9719 (CVT-124), an A1 adenosine receptor antagonist, protects against the decline in renal function observed with diuretic therapy. *Circulation.* 2002;105(11):1348–1353.

62. Greenberg B, Thomas I, Banish D, et al. Effects of multiple oral doses of an A1 adenosine antagonist, BG9928, in patients with heart failure: results of a placebo-controlled, dose-escalation study. *J Am Coll Cardiol.* 2007;50(7): 600–606.

63. Mitrovic V, Seferovic P, Dodic S, et al. Cardio-renal effects of the A1 adenosine receptor antagonist SLV320 in patients with heart failure. *Circ Heart Fail.* 2009;2(6):523–531.

64. Chaparro S, Dittrich HC, Tang WW. Rolofylline (KW-3902): a new adenosine A1-receptor antagonist for acute congestive heart failure. *Future Cardiol.* 2008;4(2):117–123.

65. Givertz MM, Massie BM, Fields TK, Pearson LL, Dittrich HC. The effects of KW-3902, an adenosine A1-receptor antagonist,on diuresis and renal function in patients with acute decompensated heart failure and renal impairment or diuretic resistance. *J Am Coll Cardiol.* 2007;50(16):1551–1560.

66. Cotter G, Dittrich HC, Weatherley BD, et al. The PROTECT pilot study: a randomized, placebo-controlled, dose-finding study of the adenosine

A1 receptor antagonist rolofylline in patients with acute heart failure and renal impairment. *J Card Fail.* 2008;14(8):631-640.

67. Dunwiddie TV, Worth T. Sedative and anticonvulsant effects of adenosine analogs in mouse and rat. *J Pharmacol Exp Ther.* 1982;220(1):70-76.

68. Massie BM, O'Connor CM, Metra M, et al. Rolofylline, an adenosine A1-receptor antagonist, in acute heart failure. *N Engl J Med.* 363(15):1419-1428.

69. De Luca L, Mebazaa A, Filippatos G, et al. Overview of emerging pharmacologic agents for acute heart failure syndromes. *Eur J Heart Fail.* 2008;10(2):201-213.

70. Dittrich HC, Gupta DK, Hack TC, Dowling T, Callahan J, Thomson S. The effect of KW-3902, an adenosine A1 receptor antagonist, on renal function and renal plasma flow in ambulatory patients with heart failure and renal impairment. *J Card Fail.* 2007;13(8):609-617.

Ultrafiltration for the Treatment of Heart Failure

11

Piergiuseppe Agostoni
Giancarlo Marenzi

An increasing awareness exists that renal dysfunction represents an important epidemiological, clinical, and prognostic problem in both acute and chronic cardiovascular conditions, in particular in the settings of heart failure (HF).[1,2]

As the prevalence of HF is dramatically growing, hospitalization for acute destabilization of chronic patients has markedly increased. Considerable efforts have been made to improve both quality of life and clinical outcome of patients with HF, as well as to reduce hospitalizations.

Ultrafiltration, as supportive care in patients with coexisting cardiac and renal dysfunction (cardiorenal syndrome), has been a matter of intense investigative interest in recent years, and it is clearly emerging as a useful therapeutic strategy in both elective and emergency situations.[3-6] Nevertheless, no official guidelines for the use of ultrafiltration or other renal replacement therapies in patients with cardiac disease have been defined. Information about clinical indications, therapeutic protocols, and impact of these adjunctive treatments on hard clinical end points is still lacking. This is likely due to the limited number of randomized, controlled studies published in selected HF populations. Thus, most of the existing knowledge on the use of ultrafiltration has been indirectly acquired from noncardiologic clinical backgrounds, such as nephrology and intensive care settings.

In this chapter, we discuss the potential applications of ultrafiltration in patients with

The Cardiorenal Syndrome: A Clinician's Guide to Pathophysiology and Management, 1st ed. © 2012 J. Thomas Heywood and John C. Burnett Jr., eds. Cardiotext Publishing, ISBN: 978-0-9790164-7-9.

HF and fluid overload on the basis of clinical and investigational experience. A brief updated overview on the objective impact of this condition is provided to better define the clinical scenarios in which ultrafiltration therapy may be used. Finally, the pathophysiology insights from this mechanical therapy for the HF syndrome and its possible future applications are briefly highlighted.

The Clinical Impact of Heart Failure and Associated Renal Dysfunction

Current estimates of the prevalence of HF vary widely, but it is reported to be ≥ 5% in the general population over 65 years of age. Patients with advanced HF have a very high 1-year mortality rate, reaching about 50% for patients in New York Heart Association (NYHA) class IV.[7,8] In addition to cardiac mortality, all-cause mortality has been shown to be increased 3-fold in HF patients when compared to the general population. Renal dysfunction is clearly recognized as the most important independent predictor of mortality in both chronic and acute HF.[2,9] Increases in serum creatinine during hospitalization for HF occurs in almost 30% of patients. Notably, even a > 0.3 mg/dL increase in serum creatinine concentration has a prognostic relevance, with a 7-fold higher in-hospital mortality rate.[10]

Although patients with severe HF (NYHA class IV) represent only 13% of the whole HF patient population, they are responsible for almost 50% of the cost of HF hospitalizations.[7] The exact triggers of acute destabilization and congestion are not known. However, excessive salt intake, renal dysfunction, neurohormonal activation, and medications may contribute to fluid retention and edema.

Ultrafiltration for Management of Fluid Overload in Heart Failure

The primary therapeutic goals for acute HF exacerbation include removal of excess fluid, reduction in ventricular filling pressures and increase in cardiac output, myocardial protection, neurohormonal modulation, and renal function preservation. Although intensive intravenous treatment with loop diuretics may initially facilitate fluid loss and improve symptoms, their use is associated with increased neurohormonal activation, intravascular volume depletion, hemodynamic impairment, and renal function decline. Moreover, a worse outcome has been associated with the use of diuretics, and a dose–dependent inverse relation between loop diuretics dose and survival has been demonstrated in advanced HF.[8,11] However, because fluid overload heavily impacts on the quality of life of these patients, alternative therapeutic strategies are needed to counteract the development of diuretic refractoriness, particularly in those cases in which progressively increasing diuretic doses are required.

Ultrafiltration was first utilized for the treatment of fluid overload in HF more than 55 years ago,[12] and in the last 25 years several studies have confirmed its clinical efficacy, as well as its safety profile.[3,4,12,13] When applied to HF patients, ultrafiltration, in the short term, may reverse the vicious circle responsible for the progression of the disease – in which cardiac output reduction, neurohormonal activation, and renal dysfunction negatively impact each other.[14] The peculiar feature of ultrafiltration is its capability of removing excessive fluid from the extravascular space, without affecting circulating volume. Most of the observed clinical, hemodynamic, and respiratory effects are the result of this property.[3,4,13,14] Reduction of extravascular lung water with ultrafiltration allows the rapid improvement of respiratory symptoms (dyspnea and orthopnea), pulmonary gas exchanges, lung mechanics and radiological signs of pulmonary vascular congestion, and alveolar and interstitial edema. Removal of systemic extravascular water allows resolution of peripheral edema and, when present, ascites and pleural effusions.[3] The subtraction of extravascular pulmonary water, by reducing the intrathoracic pressure and, thus, the diastolic burden on the heart, exerts a positive influence on cardiac dynamics.[15] The hemodynamic improvement following ultrafiltration is the result of both the reduction of the extracardiac constraint and the optimization of circulating volume. Even withdrawal of several liters of fluid,

over a period of a few hours, can be safely performed without detrimental hemodynamic consequences, and clinical improvement is usually maintained for a long time following a single session.[3,4] During ultrafiltration, circulating volume – the true cardiac preload – is preserved, or even optimized, by fluid refilling from the extravascular space. The decrease in the ventricular filling pressures reflects the reduction of intrathoracic pressure and of pulmonary stiffness due to reabsorption of the excessive extravascular lung water that burdens the heart (Figure 11.1). Improvement in pulmonary mechanics favorably affects the heart with a reduction in size and in Doppler–derived restrictive filling, as well as with the improvement of circulatory hemodynamics.[5,15,16]

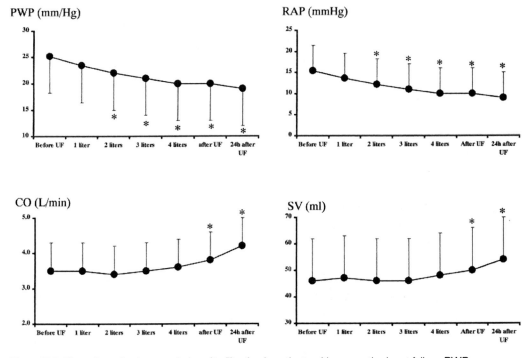

Figure 11.1. Hemodynamic changes during ultrafiltration in patients with congestive heart failure. PWP = pulmonary wedge pressure; RAP = right atrial pressure; CO = cardiac output; SV = stroke volume; UF = ultrafiltration. Marenzi G, Lauri G, Grazi M, Assanelli E, Campodonico J, Agostoni P. Circulatory response to fluid overload removal by extracorporeal ultrafiltration in refractory congestive heart failure. *J Am Coll Cardiol.* 2001;38:963–968. With permission from Elsevier.

In addition to edema removal, ultrafiltration allows for other effects that are particularly useful in patients with advanced HF and associated renal insufficiency: correction of hyponatremia, restoration of urine output and diuretic responsiveness, reduction of circulating levels of neurohormones, and, possibly, removal of other cardiac-depressant mediators.[3,6,14,17] The mechanism by which ultrafiltration may improve renal function is still unclear, but it can be possibly explained by the interaction of multiple factors, such as reduction in venous congestion and improvement of cardiac output and intravascular volume. All these factors allow the recovery of an effective transrenal arterial-venous pressure gradient, and they increase the glomerular filtration rate.[18] Recovery of diuretic responsiveness is a major clinical effect, because it allows for maintenance, and even improvement in the following days and months, of the clinical benefits achieved at the end of a single session of ultrafiltration. Moreover, it permits the use of lower dosages of diuretics, with potentially fewer side effects.

It should be pointed out that the favorable effects of ultrafiltration are not reproducible when equivalent fluid volume is removed by high-dose diuretic infusion.[19] When the 2 strategies—mechanical and pharmacological—for fluid withdrawal are compared, divergent effects on sodium removal capacity, on intravascular volume, and on renin-angiotensin-aldosterone (RAAS) system activity are usually achieved. Indeed, the fluids removed with the 2 treatments have a different tonicity (isotonic with ultrafiltration and hypotonic with furosemide), and intravascular volume is preserved with ultrafiltration and reduced with furosemide. These differences, regarding the amount of sodium removed and the intravascular volume, in spite of a similar fluid volume withdrawn, are thought to be responsible for the diverse

neurohormonal reaction, with consequent achievement of a more favorable water and salt balance after ultrafiltration (less input of water without recovery in body weight). This hypothesis emphasizes the clinical relevance of a "physiologic" dehydration in HF.

Hyponatremia, hypokalemia, and RAAS activation associated with chronic diuretic treatment are recognized to be negative prognostic indicators in HF. Presumably, long-term treatment with periodic sessions of ultrafiltration, which typically does not impact on sodium and potassium serum concentrations and does not activate the RAAS axis, could have a positive impact on the progression of the disease, on the formation of edema, and, finally, on mortality. To date, the ability of ultrafiltration to prolong survival in patients with HF has not been fully established. The UNLOAD trial (ultrafiltration vs intravenous diuretics for patients hospitalized for acute decompensated congestive heart failure) has demonstrated that early treatment with ultrafiltration in patients with acute HF safely produces greater weight and fluid loss than intravenous diuretics, and that is associated with a 44% reduction of rehospitalizations for HF in the following 3 months (Figure 11.2).[20] Randomized trials designed to evaluate the long-term effectiveness of ultrafiltration in acute and chronic HF are ongoing. The results of these studies should definitely establish their clinical impact in HF, in terms of morbidity (rate and duration of hospitalizations), mortality, and overall cost of care. The Continuous Ultrafiltration for cOngestive heaRt failurE (CUORE) trial is one of the ongoing studies.[21] The CUORE trial is a randomized, case-control study on conventional HF treatment versus conventional treatment plus ultrafiltration with, in both groups, aggressive patient follow-up. Preliminary results from the CUORE trial suggest that time to hospital discharge after decompensated HF is re-

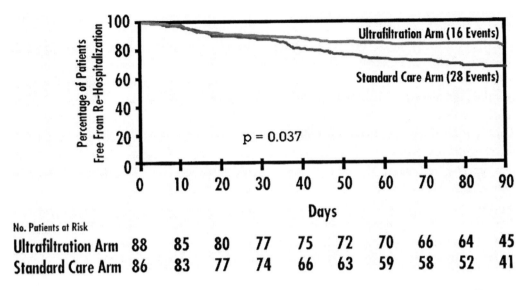

Figure 11.2. Percent of patients freer from rehospitalization in the UNLOAD trial. Costanzo MR, Guglin ME, Saltzberg MT, et al. UNLOAD Trial Investigators. Ultrafiltration versus intravenous diuretics for patients hospitalized for acute decompensated heart failure. *J Am Coll Cardiol.* 2007;49:675–683. With permission from Elsevier.

duced in ultrafiltration-treated patients, as well as the rehospitalization rate in the following year.[21] Because HF imposes a heavy burden on individuals, in terms of low tolerance of physical exertion, lengthy hospital admissions, and reduced survival improvement in quality of life, reduction in hospitalization episodes and hospitalization length via ultrafiltration are clearly attractive.

Ultrafiltration as a Window on Cardiac Physiology in Heart Failure

Besides the clinical results reported here, one of the major impacts of ultrafiltration on HF medicine has been a significant advance in our understanding of pathophysiology of fluid overload and, most importantly, of lung fluid excess. Moreover, studies of ultrafiltration have increased our capability to

properly treat HF patients, even using other therapeutic tools. It is well known that respiratory abnormalities have a major role in reducing exercise capacity in HF patients. Specifically, exercise of HF patients is characterized by (1) lower total ventilation and tidal volume (VT) at peak exercise; (2) higher ventilation for a given workload and/or oxygen consumption (VO_2) due to higher respiratory rate, albeit lower VT; and (3) higher dead space/tidal volume ratio (VD/VT) during exercise and, consequently, higher waste ventilation and higher inefficiency of ventilation during exercise, as inferable from the higher ventilation to carbon dioxide (VE/VCO_2) relationship slope.[22,23] Ultrafiltration may improve exercise capacity in HF patients through several mechanisms, including increase of VT during exercise and, through it, of total ventilation.[5] These effects are due to a reduced lung stiffness mediated by a lower extravascular lung fluid content,[14] which has been demonstrated by extravascular fluid measurement done indirectly through a chest x-ray score, and directly through a single breath constant expiratory flow technique.[5,24] Physiologically important consequences of extravascular lung fluid reduction by ultrafiltration are the improvement of lung mechanics at rest, as shown by improvement of alveolar volume, forced expiratory volume in 1 second (FEV₁), vital capacity, and maximal voluntary ventilation, and during exercise, as shown by improvement of VT and dynamic lung compliance.[5,16,19,24] Furthermore, ultrafiltration-induced upward and leftward shifts of the Frank-Starling relationship (ventricular filling pressure–cardiac output) during exercise have been demonstrated in both the right and left ventricle (Figure 11.3).[16] This shift is hypothesized to be due to an improved heart–lung interaction mediated by a less stiff "cardiac fossa," which reduces the external constraint on the heart.[25] Consequently, ultrafiltration facilitates diastolic filling and reduces the external work of the heart in systole.[15] Indeed, it should be remembered that cardiac volume changes during systole and diastole are paralleled by opposite changes in lung volume. In other words, ultrafiltration facilitates the "push and pull" action generated by the heart on the lung during the cardiac cycle.[25]

The most unexpected and probably important lesson of ultrafiltration studies has been on the pathophysiology of the alveolar-capillary membrane in HF syndrome. Indeed, gas diffusion through the alveolar–capillary membrane is impeded in patients with chronic HF and, notably, lung diffusion capacity is associated with their prognosis, exercise capacity, and adaptation to

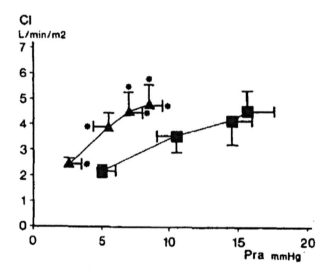

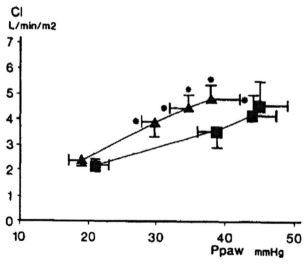

Figure 11.3. Cardiac index (CI) vs right atrial pressure (Pra; upper panel) and vs pulmonary artery wedge pressure (Ppaw) during exercise before (■) and after (▲) ultrafiltration. Modified from Agostoni PG, Marenzi GC, Sganzerla P, et al. Lung-heart interaction as a substrate for the improvement in exercise capacity after body fluid volume depletion in moderate congestive heart failure. *Am J Cardiol.* 1995;76:793–798. With permission from Elsevier.

high altitude.[26,27] Reduction of lung fluid by ultrafiltration, however, does not increase alveolar capillary diffusion (Table 11.1).[24] This observation was, at the beginning, surprising, but it well matches with the observation that even cardiac transplant is not associated with lung diffusion improvement.[28,29] So, we can postulate that in chronic HF, during stable resting condition, alveolar gas exchange reduction is due to membrane fibrosis, connective tissue derangement, and deposition of cells, but not to fluid accumulation. The opposite happens in acute HF and in chronic HF during exercise, where extra fluid accumulates along the alveolar capillary membrane, thus reducing alveolar gas exchange.[30] The fact that ultrafiltration reduces lung water content but does not affect lung diffusion is consistent with the observation that drugs, such as ACE inhibitors and antialdosteronic compounds, improve lung diffusion without affecting pulmonary hemodynamics.[31-33]

Future Directions

Although ultrafiltration has been used for treatment of HF for many years, several issues still need to be clarified. First, we do not

Table 11.1: Lung Diffusing Capacity for Carbon Monoxide (DLco), Alveolar-Capillary Membrane Diffusing Capacity for Carbon Monoxide (Dm), Capillary Volume (Vc), Alveolar Volume (Va) and Lung Tissue (Lt) in Controls (n = 18) and in Chronic Congestive Heart Failure Patients Undergoing Ultrafiltration (n = 28)

	CONTROLS	CONGESTIVE HEART FAILURE PATIENTS	
		Before UF	4 Days After UF
DLco (mL/min/mm Hg)	29.0 ± 5.0	17.1 ± 4.0*	17.0 ± 5.0*
Dm (mL/min/mm Hg)	47.0 ± 11.0	24.1 ± 6.5*	24.8 ± 7.9*
Vc (mL)	102 ± 20	113 ± 38	100 ± 39
Lt (mL)	420 ± 130	620 ± 180*	550 ± 170*§

DLco = total lung diffusion for carbon monoxide; Dm = specific membrane diffusing capacity; Lt = lung tissue; UF = ultrafiltration; Vc = capillary volume

* = $p < 0.01$ vs. controls, § = $p < 0.02$ vs. before ultrafiltration

Agostoni PG, Guazzi M, Bussotti M, Grazi M, Palermo P, Marenzi G. Lack of improvement of lung diffusing capacity following fluid withdrawal by ultrafiltration in chronic heart failure. *J Am Coll Cardiol.* 2000;36: 1600–1604. With permission from Elsevier.

know whether repeated sessions of ultrafiltration may provide the same benefit of the first treatment and, eventually, which clinical criteria should be considered for the best timing of ultrafiltration repetition. Indeed, several clinical criteria, or even a composite score, could be applied including symptoms worsening, body weight increase, diuretic dosage requirement, BNP level increase, renal function deterioration, and fixed time intervals.

Second, the more appropriate time to initiate ultrafiltration for treatment of congestive HF, in order to obtain the maximal clinical advantage and minimize kidney damage, is still uncertain.

Third, it is at present unknown which renal replacement therapy (ultrafiltration, hemofiltration, hemodiafiltration, peritoneal dialysis, other) is the preferred treatment modality for management of fluid overload in congestive HF. This is a compelling question because renal replacement therapy has been successfully used in refractory HF for clinical stabilization and/or prevention of hospitalization for acute decompensated HF. Future randomized studies are needed to compare the efficacy of these treatment modalities in HF, with particular emphasis on their possible different sodium removal capacity. Another point of investigative interest is the possible advantage of combining techniques in different phases of the clinical course of HF patients, that is, ultrafiltration or hemofiltration for removal of fluid overload and rapid clinical stabilization, and long-term treatment with peritoneal dialysis for prevention of water and salt retention, and of hospitalization recurrence.[34]

Finally, because renal insufficiency is a frequent comorbidity of HF, and vice versa, there is likely a cutoff area of kidney dysfunction, unidentified yet, where hemofiltration or hemodiafiltration should be preferred to ultrafiltration.

Conclusion

The application of ultrafiltration in HF patients allows improvement of clinical and hemodynamic conditions. Moreover, it reestablishes neurohormonal imbalances, and restores diuresis and diuretic responsiveness. Further investigation is needed to confirm the positive clinical impact of ultrafiltration, to better define protocols and more appropriate renal replacement modalities, to identify patients and clinical settings in which the greatest benefit can be obtained, and, finally, to definitively establish the effect of ultrafiltration on hard clinical end points.

Acknowledgment

The authors are indebted to Elisabetta Salvioni, PhD, for the revision of the manuscript and the technical help.

References

1. Heywood JT, Fonarow GC, Costanzo MR, Mathur VS, Wigneswaran JR, Wynne J; ADHERE Scientific Advisory Committee and Investigators. High prevalence of renal dysfunction and its impact on outcome in 118,465 patients hospitalized with acute decompensated heart failure: a report from the ADHERE database. *J Card Fail.* 2007;13:422–430.
2. Marenzi G, Lauri G, Guazzi M, et al. Cardiac and renal dysfunction in chronic heart failure: Relation to neurohumoral activation and prognosis. *Am J Med Sci.* 2001;321:359–366.
3. Rimondini A, Cipolla CM, Della Bella P, et al. Hemofiltration as short-term treatment for refractory congestive heart failure. *Am J Med.* 1987;83:43–48.
4. Marenzi G, Lauri G, Grazi M, Assanelli E, Campodonico J, Agostoni P. Circulatory response to fluid overload removal

by extracorporeal ultrafiltration in refractory congestive heart failure. *J Am Coll Cardiol.* 2001;38:963–968.

5. Agostoni PG, Marenzi GC, Pepi M, et al. Isolated ultrafiltration in moderate congestive heart failure. *J Am Coll Cardiol.* 1993;21:424–431.

6. Costanzo MR, Saltzberg M, O'Sullivan J, Sobotka P. Early ultrafiltration in patients with decompensated heart failure and diuretic resistance. *J Am Coll Cardiol.* 2005;46:2047–2051.

7. Muntwyler J, Abetel G, Gruner C, Follath F. One-year mortality among unselected outpatients with heart failure. *Eur Heart J.* 2002;23:1861–1866.

8. Emerman CL DMT, Costanzo MR, Peacock WF; for the ADHERE Scientific Advisory Committee. Impact of intravenous diuretics on the outcomes of patients hospitalized with acute decompensated heart failure: insights from the ADHERE registry. *J Card Fail.* 2004;10:S116.

9. Fornarow GC, Adams KF Jr, Abraham WT, Yancy CW, Boscardin WJ; for the ADHERE Scientific Advisory Committee, Study Group, and Investigators. Risk stratification for the hospital mortality in acutely decompensated heart failure: classification and regression tree analysis. *JAMA.* 2005;293:572–580.

10. Krumholz HM, Chen YT, Vaccarino V, et al. Correlates and impact on outcomes of worsening renal function in patients > or = 65 years of age with heart failure. *Am J Cardiol.* 2000;85:1110–1113.

11. Eshaghian S, Horwich TB, Fonarow GC. Relation of loop diuretic dose to mortality in advanced heart failure. *Am J Cardiol.* 2006;97:1759–1764.

12. Kolff WJ, Leonards JR. Reduction of otherwise intractable edema by dialysis or filtration. *Cleve Clin Q.* 1954;21:61–71.

13. Lauer A, Saccaggi A, Ronco C, Belledonne M, Glabman S, Bosch JP. Continuous arteriovenous hemofiltration in the critically ill patient. Clinical use and operational characteristics. *Ann Intern Med.* 1983;99:455–460.

14. Marenzi G, Grazi S, Giraldi F, et al. Interrelation of humoral factors, hemodynamics, and fluid and salt metabolism in congestive heart failure: effects of extracorporeal ultrafiltration. *Am J Med.* 1993;94:49–56.

15. Pepi M, Marenzi GC, Agostoni PG, et al. Sustained cardiac diastolic changes elicited by ultrafiltration in patients with moderate congestive heart failure: pathophysiological correlates. *Br Heart J.* 1993;70:135–140.

16. Agostoni PG, Marenzi GC, Sganzerla P, et al. Lung–heart interaction as a substrate for the improvement in exercise capacity after body fluid volume depletion in moderate congestive heart failure. *Am J Cardiol.* 1995;76:793–798.

17. Cipolla CM, Grazi S, Rimondini A, et al. Changes in circulating norepinephrine with hemofiltration in advanced congestive heart failure. *Am J Cardiol.* 1990;66:987–994.

18. Mullens W, Abrahams Z, Francis GS, et al. Importance of venous congestion for worsening of renal function in advanced decompensated heart failure. *J Am Coll Cardiol.* 2009;53:589–596.

19. Agostoni P, Marenzi G, Lauri G, et al. Sustained improvement in functional capacity after removal of body fluid with isolated ultrafiltration in chronic cardiac insufficiency: failure of furosemide to provide the same result. *Am J Med.* 1994;96:191–199.

20. Costanzo MR, Guglin ME, Saltzberg MT, et al; UNLOAD Trial Investigators.

Ultrafiltration versus intravenous diuretics for patients hospitalized for acute decompensated heart failure. *J Am Coll Cardiol.* 2007;49:675–683.

21. Muratori M, Marenzi G, Casentino E, et al. Preliminary report on the effects of ultrafiltration in severe heart failure: the Continuous Ultrafiltration for cOngestive heaRt failurE (CUORE) trial. *Eur J Heart Fail.* 2008;7(suppl 1):72.

22. Wasserman K, Zhang YY, Gitt A, et al. Lung function and exercise gas exchange in chronic heart failure. *Circulation.* 1997;96:2221–2227.

23. Agostoni P, Pellegrino R, Conca C, Rodarte JR, Brusasco V. Exercise hyperpnea in chronic heart failure: relationships to lung stiffness and expiratory flow limitation. *J Appl Physiol.* 2002;92:1409–1416.

24. Agostoni PG, Guazzi M, Bussotti M, Grazi M, Palermo P, Marenzi G. Lack of improvement of lung diffusing capacity following fluid withdrawal by ultrafiltration in chronic heart failure. *J Am Coll Cardiol.* 2000;36:1600–1604.

25. Agostoni P, Butler J. Cardio-pulmonary interrelations on exercise. In: Wasserman K, Whipp BJ, eds. *Exercise: Physiology and Pathophysiology.* New York: Marcel Dekker; 1992:221–252.

26. Agostoni PG, Bussotti M, Palermo P, Guazzi M. Does lung diffusion impairment affect exercise capacity in patients with heart failure? *Heart.* 2002;88:453–459.

27. Agostoni P, Bussotti M, Cattadori G, et al. Gas diffusion and alveolar-capillary unit in chronic heart failure. *Eur Heart J.* 2006;27:2538–2543.

28. Ohar J, Osterloh J, Ahmed N, Miller L. Diffusing capacity decreases after heart transplantation. *Chest.* 1993;103:857–861.

29. Bussieres LM, Pflugfelder PW, Ahmad D, Taylor AW, Kostuk WJ. Evolution of resting lung function in the first year after cardiac transplantation. *Eur Respir J.* 1995;8:959–962.

30. Cattadori G, Wasserman K, Meloni C, et al. Alveolar membrane conductance decreases as BNP increases during exercise in heart failure. Rationale for BNP in the evaluation of dyspnea. *J Card Fail.* 2009;15:136–144.

31. Guazzi M, Marenzi G, Alimento M, Contini M, Agostoni P. Improvement of alveolar-capillary membrane diffusing capacity with enalapril in chronic heart failure and counteracting effect of aspirin. *Circulation.* 1997;95:1930–1936.

32. Guazzi M, Agostoni P, Guazzi MD. Modulation of alveolar-capillary sodium handling as a mechanism of protection of gas transfer by enalapril, and not by losartan, in chronic heart failure. *J Am Coll Cardiol.* 2001;37:398–406.

33. Agostoni P, Magini A, Andreini D, et al. Spironolactone improves lung diffusion in chronic heart failure. *Eur Heart J.* 2005;26:159–164.

34. Mehrotra R, Khanna R. Peritoneal ultrafiltration for chronic congestive heart failure: rationale, evidence and future. *Cardiology.* 2001;96:177–182.

Renal Cell Therapy

A Novel Approach to the Treatment of Cardiorenal Syndrome

12

GRETCHEN HAGEMAN

H. DAVID HUMES

The pathophysiology of cardiorenal syndrome is complex due to the multifaceted interaction of cardiac and renal failure. Current treatment approaches have not shown consistent benefits and in some cases are associated with increased risk of mortality.[1] As cardiac function declines, diuretics required for treatment of fluid overload can have acute and chronic effects on the kidney. Eventually this clinical state with associated renal insufficiency results in the inability of the kidney to respond to diuretics to relieve congestive heart failure. In cardiorenal syndrome, the intricate neurohormonal feedback system that modulates euvolemia malfunctions within 2 organ systems, creating conflicting physiologic signals. The addition of more renal cells could have the potential to reset this vascular feedback system and replace some intrinsic mechanisms to improve both cardiac and renal function.

The kidney may function as the primary mode of homeostatic regulation during acute or chronic heart failure (HF). As low blood flow and pharmacologic intervention injure the kidneys, the operating healthy cell mass is depleted, which is clinically reflected in decreasing glomerular filtration rate (GFR) or creatinine clearance. Replacement of metabolic and hormonal functions using renal progenitor cell therapy could help to restore native kidney cell function in this disorder. The healthy cells have the potential to provide a rebalancing of the cardiorenal axis and ultimately a positive systemic cardiac effect.

Clinical Indicators

Healthy kidneys play a critical role in cardiovascular homeostasis, with sympathetic

The Cardiorenal Syndrome: A Clinician's Guide to Pathophysiology and Management, 1st ed. © 2012 J. Thomas Heywood and John C. Burnett Jr., eds. Cardiotext Publishing, ISBN: 978-0-9790164-7-9.

nervous system (SNS) signaling mechanisms precisely controlling vascular response and blood pressure. The kidney's role in fluid homeostasis is best understood through the renin-angiotensin-aldosterone system (RAAS). As blood volume or vascular efficiency decreases, the kidney increases the concentration of renin, which in turn up-regulates angiotensin production by converting liver-produced angiotensinogen. This elevation of both angiotensin and renin causes blood pressure to increase, and aldersterone is then up-regulated as well, causing fluid reabsorption by the kidney and increasing blood volume and water retention. Improper activation of the RAAS cycle in cardiorenal syndrome further exacerbates this concurrent SNS response. RAAS alterations in other hormones produced by the kidney play a critical role in vascular integrity and modulation beyond fluid volume.

Data suggest that the metabolism of catecholamines by monoamine oxidases, specifically renalase, significantly contributes to the regulation of vascular tone and hypervolemia in cardiorenal syndrome.[2-6] Renalase also has been shown to metabolize dopamine, lowering the concentration of this circulating neurotransmitter and modulating natriuresis.[7] The kidney is the major producer of renalase, and decreases in the production of both renalase and pro-renalase (inactive form) following kidney injury, and without compensation by other sources, have been documented. This suggests that systemic concentrations of renalase and pro-renalase could be used as early identifiers of kidney injury and progression of cardiorenal syndrome. Moreover they may play a critical role in the progression of hypertension, cardiovascular disease, oxidative stress, inflammation, and atherosclerosis.[2,3,5,6]

Systemic inflammation plays a significant role in the progression of cardiorenal syndrome. Acute or chronic kidney or heart injury affects the overall inflammatory state of the body and its long-term response. This chronic systemic inflammatory condition is thought to be caused by an elevated state of oxidative stress, a state that is due to the production of reactive oxygen species, which are chemically reactive molecules containing oxygen such as hydrogen peroxide and superoxide, and nitric oxide imbalance. It has been suggested that leptin levels also correlate with oxidative stress and cardiovascular incidents, due to decreased kidney clearance.[8] This elevated oxidative status in conjunction with the pathways noted interacts with and causes incorrect oxidation of compounds, resulting in further inflammatory signaling.[9] This counterproductive state of oxidative stress results in an up-regulation of inflammatory markers within systemic vasculature and improper signaling through the SNS.

Plasma concentrations of proinflammatory cytokines such as interleukin 6 (IL-6) and tumor necrosis factor-alpha (TNF-α) increase appreciably as disease processes such as cardiorenal syndrome and chronic HF advance. Their detrimental role is not well understood, but numerous studies show statistically significant correlations between increases in IL-6 and TNF-α and increased mortality.[10-12] Additionally, there are suggestions that IL-6-like cytokines can cause increases in angiotensinogen, directly affecting the efficacy of the RAAS to control volume homeostasis. This overproduction is also thought to cause cardiac myocyte hypertrophy.[12] Elevated oxidative stress and chronic systemic inflammation cause systemic desensitization by reducing nitric oxide, elevating secretion of inflammatory markers, and inhibiting production of anti-inflammatory markers.[9,13] Additional inflammatory markers used to document this occurrence are myeloperoxidase, IL-1, and C-reactive protein (CRP). The chronically inflamed state also impairs the body's ability to fight infections appropriately, further compounding systemic dysregulation. Data collected from our group with preclinical animal studies and phase 2 human clinical trials mimicking these states of systemic proinflammation suggest that renal cell therapy devices may be an innovative approach to the treatment of cardiorenal syndrome and may impact clinical indicators associated with this multifarious disease process.

Cell Source and Usage

An extracorporeal cell therapy device utilizing a standard hemofiltration cartridge has been successfully fabricated with human cells.[14] The device contains approximately 10^8 renal tubule cells grown from adult stem/progenitor cells as confluent monolayers along the inner surface of the fibers. The initial cell therapy device was large (12- × 4-in cylinder) and required an additional extracorporeal pump circuit to deliver blood and plasma ultrafiltrate to the cells. These elements were designed as an add-on to current dialysis treatment in patients with acute renal failure. This device is commonly known as the renal assist device (RAD). For preclinical application, the RAD was seeded with primary porcine renal epithelial cells expanded from kidneys harvested from Hampshire breed pigs and used in a large-animal porcine model of septic shock.[13] *In vitro* experiments with the RAD utilized porcine or human proximal tubule progenitor cells and showed differentiated transport and metabolic functions.[14-16] The *ex vivo* circuit design requires placement of hemofilters prior to and following the cell device for creation of ultrafiltrate. These hemofilter membranes serve the additional purpose of immunoprotection of the cells; this is achieved due to the impenetrability of immunoglobulins and immunocompetent cells across the hollow fibers. Therefore, opportunity for rejection of nonautologous cells is reduced.

Therapeutic Application

Preclinical Studies

Preclinical studies were conducted to demonstrate the effects of a renal tubule cell–seeded device in a pig with multiorgan failure (MOF) and systemic inflammatory response syndrome caused by the induction of sepsis by an intraperitoneal infusion of *E. coli*. While these conditions are not identical to those of cardiorenal syndrome, the presence of MOF and systemically activated inflammation mimics the multiorgan effects and inflammatory conditions seen in cardiorenal syndrome.[17] All animals developed acute tubular necrosis with oliguria/anuria within 2 to 4 hours following administration, and renal cell treatment resulted in systemic physiologic improvements. Overall, the cell-treated group lived 40% longer than the sham-treated group, as shown in Figure 12.1.

Renal blood flow was significantly improved in RAD–treated animals compared to the sham control group. This indicates a critical role of the renal cell device in improving renal perfusion in the presence of hypotension. The cell therapy effect on renal blood flow becomes apparent after 2 hours and continues until the study termination (Figure 12.2).

Heart function also demonstrated direct improvement with the use of the RAD. Cardiac output improved by almost 30% compared to the sham-treated group, with an average difference of 1.2 L/min (Figure 12.3).

These results indicate a significant role of the renal cells in improving cardiac vascular

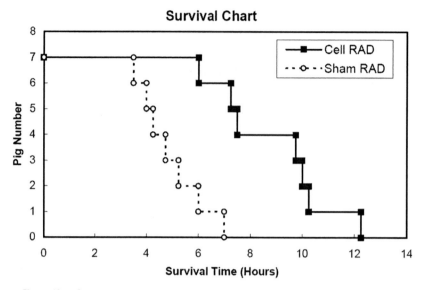

Figure 12.1. Survival curves comparing cell RAD therapy and the sham control therapy in a porcine model of sepsis. Humes HD, Buffington DA, Lou L, Abrishami S, Wang M, Xia J, Fissell WH. Cell therapy with a tissue-engineered kidney reduces the multiple-organ consequences of septic shock. *Crit Care Med.* 2003;31:2421–2428. With permission.

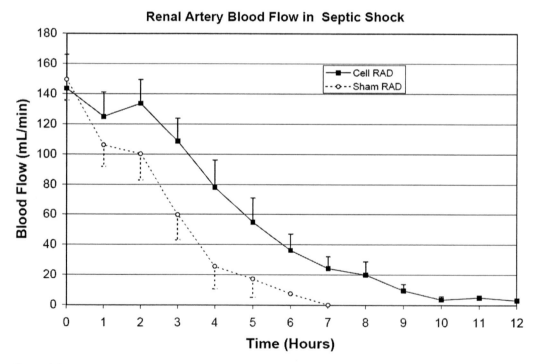

Figure 12.2. Maintenance of renal blood flow in RAD-treated vs sham control animals in a porcine model of septic shock. Humes HD, Buffington DA, Lou L, Abrishami S, Wang M, Xia J, Fissell WH. Cell therapy with a tissue-engineered kidney reduces the multiple-organ consequences of septic shock. *Crit Care Med.* 2003;31:2421–2428. With permission.

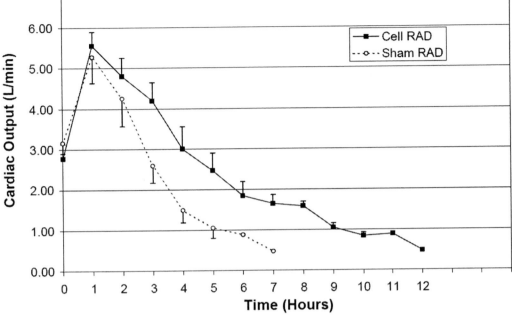

Figure 12.3. Maintenance of cardiac output in RAD-treated vs sham control animals in a porcine model of septic shock. Humes HD, Buffington DA, Lou L, Abrishami S, Wang M, Xia J, Fissell WH. Cell therapy with a tissue-engineered kidney reduces the multiple-organ consequences of septic shock. *Crit Care Med.* 2003;31:2421–2428. With permission.

performance during multiorgan dysfunction and a systemically inflamed state such as sepsis or cardiorenal syndrome. In additional studies (data not shown), the average mean arterial pressure showed improvement during renal cell treatment, further supporting the role the cell device plays in vascular modulation.

Lower levels of proinflammatory cytokines were seen in the plasma of the cell-treated group in the porcine sepsis study. Specifically, IL-6 modulation was demonstrated in the cell-treated group over the sham, as shown in Figure 12.4. In comparison to the sham–treated group, IL-6 was controlled to nearly half of the systemic elevation.

These findings further exhibit the possible role of the kidney in immunomodulation during a systemic immune response.

Additional preclinical studies in acutely uremic dogs have demonstrated that the bioartificial kidney successfully replaced filtration, transport, metabolic, and endocrinologic functions of the kidney.[16] Further preclinical experiments in acutely uremic dogs evaluated the influence of the RAD under stress states. Acutely nephrectomized animals were challenged with infusions of endotoxin (lipopolysaccharide) intravenously or with intraperitoneal administration of doses of viable *E. coli* before treatment with either cell or sham control RADs in a bioartificial kidney.[18–20] In these experiments, cell RADs provided metabolic renal replacement and resulted in higher anti–inflammatory plasma levels, better hemodynamic stability, and, in the *E. coli* sepsis model, longer survival times compared to sham controls.

Plasma IL-6 in Septic Shock

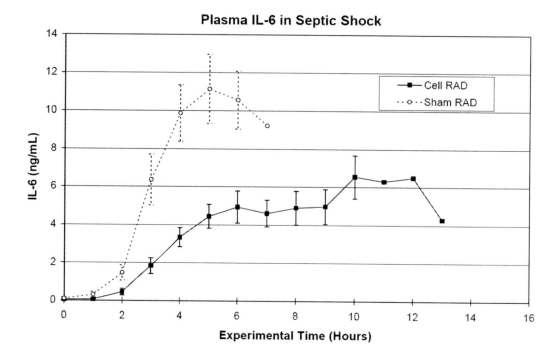

Figure 12.4. Plasma concentrations of IL-6 in septic animals treated with the cell RAD compared to a group receiving noncell, sham treatment. The increase in IL-6 concentrations was considerably less in the cell-RAD group compared to the control group. Humes HD, Buffington DA, Lou L, Abrishami S, Wang M, Xia J, Fissell WH. Cell therapy with a tissue-engineered kidney reduces the multiple-organ consequences of septic shock. *Crit Care Med*. 2003;31:2421–2428. With permission.

Clinical Studies

These supportive preclinical experiments were the basis for testing human cell RADs in phase 1/2 and phase 2 clinical trials in intensive care unit patients with acute renal failure and MOF. A favorable phase 1/2 safety trial[16] led to an FDA-approved, randomized, controlled open-label phase 2 investigation at 12 clinical sites to determine whether this cell therapy approach alters patient mortality. This phase 2 study involved 58 patients, of whom 40 were randomized to RAD therapy and 18 made up a control group with comparable demographics and severity of illness. Renal cell therapy improved the 28-day mortality rate from 61% in the conventional hemofiltration–treated control group

to 34% in the RAD–treated group.[21,22] This survival impact continued through the 90- and 180–day follow-up periods ($P < 0.04$), with the Cox proportional hazard ratio indicating that the risk of death was 50% of that observed in the conventional continuous renal replacement therapy group. This survival advantage with renal cell therapy was observed for various etiologies of acute renal failure and regardless of organ failure number (1–5+) or the presence of sepsis. Subset analysis of patients with concomitant severe sepsis or septic shock demonstrated incidences of sepsis of 73% and 67% in the cell therapy and conventional therapy groups, respectively. RAD therapy was associated with a mortality rate of 34% in patients with sepsis, compared with 67% in the conventional treatment group. Thus, these clinical results suggest an effect of renal cell therapy on survival rates in these desperately ill patients, although in a very small group of patients. Overall, these data suggest a possible role of renal cell therapy in immunomodulation, as was seen during sepsis in the preclinical large-animal trials. Important cardiovascular effects were also seen.

As demonstrated in Figure 12.5, the course of renal cell treatment in an individual patient in these studies highlights the effect of renal cells on improved cardiovascular parameters in this patient with MOF secondary to toxic shock syndrome.[23] This patient required high levels of 3 different vasopressors to stabilize blood pressure prior to therapy. After just a half day of treatment with the RAD, dopamine was reduced significantly and levarterenol was discontinued as blood pressure steadied.

Upon removal of the RAD, pressors were immediately required for restabilization, as shown in Figure 12.5.

In acute kidney injury (AKI), the presence of oliguria and anuria is common. The urine output response over the course of RAD treatment in an individual patient with AKI is shown in Figure 12.6.[23] In another study (data not shown), 72-hour cell therapy resulted in an overall 50% increase in urine output, maintained during the posttherapy period, compared to patients receiving standard continuous venovenous hemofiltration.

Potential Mechanism of Action

Renal cell therapy might impact systemic inflammation and hormonal abnormalities when incorporated into cardiorenal syndrome clinical treatment approaches. These

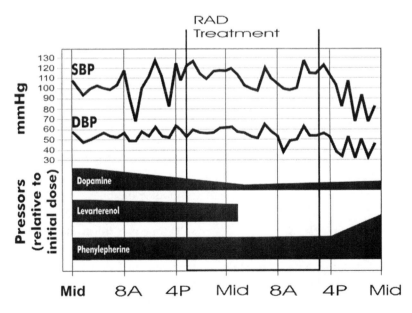

Figure 12.5. Correlation of RAD therapy session with decrease in patient vasopressor requirement. Humes HD, Weitzell WF, Bartlett RH, Swaniker FC, Paganini EP. Renal cell therapy is associated with dynamic and individualized responses in patients with acute renal failure. *Blood Purif.* 2003;21:64–71. With permission from S. Karger AG, Basel.

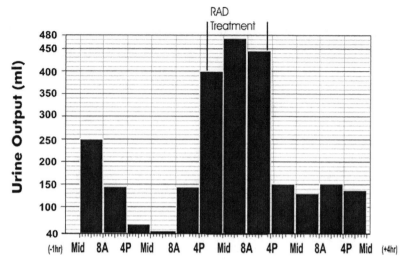

Figure 12.6. Correlation of RAD therapy session with patient urine output. Humes HD, Buffington DA, Lou L, Abrishami S, Wang M, Xia J, Fissell WH. Cell therapy with a tissue-engineered kidney reduces the multiple-organ consequences of septic shock. *Crit Care Med.* 2003;31:2421–2428. With permission.

two aspects, regulation of the systemic inflammatory state and appropriate hormonal signaling, are critically interconnected and interdependent. Further, hormonal effects impact beyond inflammation to improve RAAS pathway signaling, prorenalase and renalase production, and dopamine metabolism. This intervention could improve blood pressure, vascular response, and fluid homeostasis. Figure 12.7 diagrams the hypothetical involvement of tubule cell therapy in the complicated cascade of events resulting from acute tubular necrosis, sepsis, or cardiorenal syndrome.

Future Studies

Future studies are planned for a small-scale RAD system, called the bioartificial renal epithelial cell system (BRECS), in a canine model of chronic HF.[24-28] Additionally, *in vitro* studies are being conducted to determine the effects of preconditioned renal cell media on isolated cardiac myocytes. These

studies are expected to provide significant insight into the role that renal epithelial cell hormonal production may play in cardiac events and CHF.

Conclusion

The complexity of the development and pharmacological management of cardiorenal syndrome demands an innovative and multifaceted therapy approach. Renal cell therapy demonstrates the potential to ameliorate this complex disease process and restabilize the body, reset SNS dysfunction, and support systemic homeostasis. The results from preclinical and clinical studies are promising, suggesting a potential improvement in renal perfusion and urine formation. In turn, a reduction in pharmacological intervention provides the ideal opportunity for native physiologic modulation. There are many components to renal cell therapy to be evaluated to further understand the homeostatic role that has been suggested by

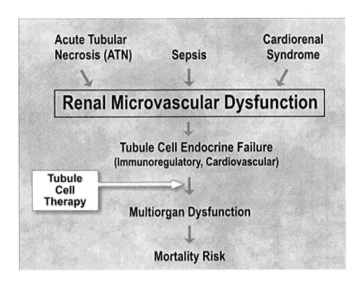

Figure 12.7. Schematic showing the integrated role tubule cell therapy devices may play in diseases that have a systemic effect on overall homeostasis.

the preclinical studies and phase 1/2 clinical trials discussed in this chapter. With the growing population of people with HF a new therapeutic method is required to reduce symptoms and improve quality of life. The future preclinical chronic HF and *in vitro* myocyte studies are expected to shed light on many of these areas and evaluate the role renal cell therapy may play in improving cardiac function by enhancing myocyte contractility, vascular regulation, and immunoregulation. Advancement in the physiologic understanding of native heart and kidney function interactions will improve our understanding of cardiorenal syndrome and possibly result in new treatment options to improve the lives of patients.

Disclosures

H. David Humes is a shareholder of Innovative BioTherapies, Inc., and Nephrion, Inc., biotechnology spinout companies of the University of Michigan.

References

1. Aaronson KD, Sackner-Bernstein J. Risk of death associated with nesiritide in patients with acutely decompensated heart failure. *JAMA*. 2006;296: 1465–1466.

2. Schlaich MP, Socratous F, Hennebry S, et al. Sympathetic activation in chronic renal failure. *J Am Soc Nephrol*. 2009;20:933–939.

3. Desir GV. Renalase deficiency in chronic kidney disease, and its contribution to hypertension and cardiovascular disease. *Curr Opin Nephrol Hypertens*. 2008;17:181–185.

4. Seno Di Marco G, Vio CP, Pavão dos Santos OF, Casarini DE. Catecholamine production along the nephron. *Cell Physiol Biochem*. 2007;20:919–924.

5. Xu J, Desir GV. Renalase, a new renal hormone: its role in health and disease. *Curr Opin Nephrol Hypertens*. 2007;16: 373–378.

6. Xu J, Li G, Wang P, et al. Renalase is a novel soluble monoamine oxidase that regulates cardiac function and blood pressure. *J Clin Invest*. 2005;115:1275–1280.

7. Ibarra FR, Armando I, Nowicki S, et al. Dopamine is metabolised by different enzymes along the rat nephron. *Pfluger Arch- Eur J Physiol*. 2005;450:185–191.

8. Horoz M, Aslan M, Koylu AO, et al.

The relationship between leptin level and oxidative status parameters in hemodialysis patients. *Artif Organs.* 2009;33:81–85.

9. Tsagalis G, Zerefos S, Zerefos N. Cardiorenal syndrome at different stages of chronic kidney disease. *Artif Organs.* 2007;30:564–576.

10. Deswal A, Petersen NJ, Feldman AM, Young JB, White BG, Mann DL. Cytokines and cytokine receptors in advanced heart failure: an analysis of the cytokine database from the vesnarinone trial (VEST). *Circulation.* 2001;103:2055–2059.

11. Rauchhaus M, Doehner W, Francis DP, et al. Plasma cytokine parameters and mortality in patients with chronic heart failure. *Circulation.* 2000;102:3060–3067.

12. Wollert KC, Drexler H. The role of interleukin-6 in the failing heart. *Heart Fail Rev.* 2001;6:95–103.

13. Rodrigo R, Prat H, Passalacqua W, Araya J, Guichard C, Bächler JP. Relationship between oxidative stress and essential hypertension. *Hypertens Res.* 2007;30: 1159–1167.

14. Humes HD, Fissell WH, Weitzel WF, et al. Metabolic replacement of renal function in uremic animals with a bioartificial kidney containing human cells. *Am J Kidney Dis.* 2002;39:1078–1087.

15. Humes HD, Weitzel WF, Bartlett RH, et al. Initial clinical results of the bioartificial kidney containing human cells in ICU patients with acute renal failure. *Kidney Int.* 2004;66:1578–1588.

16. Humes HD, Buffington DA, MacKay SM, Funke AJ, Weitzel WF. Replacement of renal function in uremic animals with a tissue-engineered kidney. *Nat Biotechnol.* 1999;17:451–455.

17. Ronco C, Haapio M, House AA, Anavekar N, Bellomo R. Cardiorenal syndrome. *J Am Coll Cardiol.* 2008;52:1527–1539.

18. Humes HD, Buffington DA, Lou L, et al. Cell therapy with a tissue-engineered kidney reduces the multiple-organ consequences of septic shock. *Crit Care Med.* 2003;31:2421–2428.

19. Fissell WH, Dyke DB, Weitzel WF, et al. Bioartificial kidney alters cytokine response and hemodynamic in endotoxin challenged dogs. *Blood Purif.* 2002;20:55–60.

20. Fissell WH, Lou L, Abrishami S, Buffington DA, Humes HD. Bioartificial kidney ameliorates gram-negative bacteria-induced septic shock in uremic animals. *J Am Soc Nephrol.* 2003;14: 454–461.

21. Tumlin J, Wali R, Brennan HD, Humes HD. Effect of the renal assist device (RAD) on mortality of dialysis-dependent acute renal failure: a randomized, open-labeled, multicenter, Phase II trial [Abstract]. *J Am Soc Nephrol.* 2005;16:46A.

22. Williams W, Tumlin J, Murray P, Tolwani A; RAD-002 Study Investigators. Renal bioreplacement therapy (RBT) reduces mortality in ICU patients with acute renal failure (ARF). *J Am Soc Nephrol.* 2006;17:49A.

23. Humes HD, Weitzell WF, Bartlett RH, Swaniker FC, Paganini EP. Renal cell therapy is associated with dynamic and individualized responses in patients with acute renal failure. *Blood Purif.* 2003;21:64–71.

24. Sabbah HN, Stein PD, Kono T, et al. A canine model of chronic heart failure produced by multiple coronary microembolizations. *Am J Physiol.* 1991;260:H1379–H1384.

25. Hasenfuss G. Animal models of human cardiovascular disease, heart failure and hypertrophy. *Cardiovasc Res.* 1998;39:60–76.

26. Baartscheer A, Schumacher CA, Belterman CN, Coronel R, Fiolet JW. SR

calcium handling and calcium after transients in a rabbit model of heart failure. *Cardiovasc Res.* 2003;58:99–108.

27. Maurice JP, Shah AS, Kypson AP, et al. Molecular beta-adrenergic signaling abnormalities in failing rabbit hearts after infarction. *Am J Physiol Heart Circ Physiol.* 1999;276:H1853–H1860.

28. Thakar CV, Worley S, Arrigain S, Yared JP, Paganini EP. Influence of renal dysfunction on mortality after cardiac surgery: modifying effect of preoperative renal function. *Kidney Int.* 2005;67:1112–1119.

The Role of Renal Replacement Therapy and Transplantation in Patients with Cardiorenal Syndrome

13

JIGAR PATEL

LOUIS R. ALVAREZ-CONTRERAS

ANDREW J. KING

With an aging population and rising incidence of diabetes mellitus and hypertension, there has been a commensurate increase in the incidence of chronic kidney disease (CKD). People with CKD are at increased risk of cardiovascular disease and congestive heart failure (CHF). A significant portion of patients with CHF develop progressive loss of kidney function, with or without overt renal parenchymal disease.[1] This disorder, termed *cardiorenal syndrome*, portends a poor overall prognosis.[2] In fact, there is some evidence that glomerular filtration rate (GFR) may be one of the most important predictors of mortality in patients with HF, perhaps more important than left ventricular ejection fraction (LVEF).[3] CHF and CKD frequently coexist, and it is difficult for the clinician to determine the relative contribution of low GFR to the heightened mortality. This raises the important question about the role of renal replacement therapy and kidney transplantation in the management of combined CKD and CHF.

Epidemiology and Morbidity of Chronic Kidney Disease with Cardiovascular Disease

CKD is associated with cardiovascular morbidity, as shown by the analysis of Weiner et al[4] of ARIC and Cardiovascular Health Study (CHS) cohorts. That report observed a 9.8% rate of cardiac events over 5 years in

The Cardiorenal Syndrome: A Clinician's Guide to Pathophysiology and Management, 1st ed. © 2012 J. Thomas Heywood and John C. Burnett Jr., eds. Cardiotext Publishing, ISBN: 978–0–9790164–7–9.

stage 3 to 4 CKD, compared with 3.7% in a more general population (the original Framingham cohort). In a longitudinal study of the large Kaiser Permanente renal registry, Go et al[5] followed a group of patients for a median of 2.8 years. The researchers found a correlation between estimated GFR and rate of cardiovascular events, with a 2.1% rate of events in the group with GFR ≥ 60 mL/min/1.73 m^2, 3.65% in the group with GFR 45 to 59, 11.3% in the group with GFR 30 to 44, 21.8% in the group with GFR 15 to 29, and 36% in the group with GFR < 15.

The greatest morbidity and mortality resulting from CKD and end-stage renal disease (ESRD) is that related to cardiovascular disease. The US Renal Data System (USRDS) provides a comprehensive report on the US End-stage Renal Disease Program, which in 2006 covered 506,256 patients.[6] The most recent data reveal that, among this population, hospitalizations for cardiovascular disease are 44 to 62 per 100 patient years at risk; the number has increased steadily from 1993 to 2005. In comparison, the American Heart Association Heart Disease and Stroke Statistics[7] showed that the incidence of HF has also risen over time, and currently the rate of hospital discharges for HF stands at 0.46 per 100 patients per year, indicating a near 100-fold difference compared to the USRDS population. During the first year of ESRD, cardiovascular deaths account for 100 deaths per 1000 patient years.[6] Indeed, 45% of all deaths relate to cardiovascular disease, making cardiovascular disease the single most common cause of death. One reason for this grim statistic may be the poor prognosis of dialysis patients after myocardial infarction. In a study of 34,189 dialysis patients with acute myocardial infarction, 59% were dead after the first year, and 73% were dead by 2 years.[8] Even in the reperfusion era, 1990–1995, 61% were dead by the first year and 74% by the second year.

Linkage of Chronic Kidney Disease and Heart Failure

Heart failure is a significant source of morbidity and mortality among patients with renal disease (Figure 13.1). According to the USRDS, the mortality at 1 year in Medicare patients with CKD was 20%, whereas the combination of CKD and HF increased the mortality to 32% at 1 year.[6] In a separate study of CKD patients, the median survival of patients with CKD and HF was 36 months, whereas in the absence of HF survival was 62 months.[9] This trend was also seen in the USRDS Dialysis Morbidity and Mortality Study, Wave 2.[10] In this observational study of 3925 patients starting dialysis therapy in 1996 and 1997, the prevalence of HF was noted to be related to gender (women 37%, men 34%) and diabetes (diabetics 45%, nondiabetics 28%). Multivariate analysis of this data set also revealed coronary artery disease, pericarditis, and LV hypertrophy as independent risk factors for HF. The authors postulate that the association of pericarditis with HF raises the likelihood that uremia per se plays a role in myocardial dysfunction.

A relationship between uremia and LV function was investigated by a German group in 1988.[11] An animal model for uremia was created by performing sequential nephrectomy of Sprague-Dawley rats. On microscopic examination, the hearts of the uremic rats showed marked activation of interstitial cells, with increased cytoplasmic volume compared to control animals. In the cardiomyocytes, there was swelling of mitochondria. These changes were the early indicators of myocardial fibrosis in response to uremia. Similar changes were seen in human dialysis patients from Zurich, Switzerland.[12] In this study, 200 patients, who had died while on chronic dialysis, were studied by histologic analysis of the myocardium. In

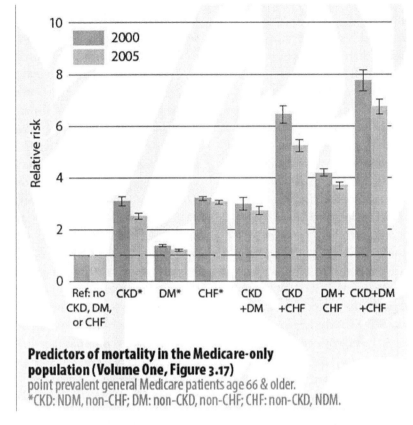

Predictors of mortality in the Medicare-only population (Volume One, Figure 3.17)
point prevalent general Medicare patients age 66 & older.
*CKD: NDM, non-CHF; DM: non-CKD, non-CHF; CHF: non-CKD, NDM.

Figure 13.1 Effect of comorbidities such as heart failure on mortality in patients with CKD. From US Renal Data System, USRDS 2008 Annual Data Report: Atlas of Chronic Kidney Disease and End-Stage Renal Disease in the United States, National Institutes of Health, National Institute of Diabetes and Digestive and Kidney Diseases, Bethesda, MD, 2008. (*Notice: The data reported here have been supplied by the US Renal Data System (USRDS). The interpretation and reporting of these data are the responsibility of the authors, and in no way should be seen as an official policy or interpretation of the US government.*)

those with chronic uremia but not on dialysis, the degree of diffuse fibrosis was 6%. Whereas 20% of those on chronic dialysis for at least 6 months had diffuse fibrosis, by contrast diffuse fibrosis was 0% in controls.

Role of Standard Therapeutic Measures for Heart Failure

The morbidity and mortality figures for cardiovascular disease in the background of CKD, and particularly ESRD, are grim. Unfortunately, this risk does not seem to be mitigated by therapeutic maneuvers proven efficacious in the general population. For example, in the 4D study, Wanner et al[13] investigated the effect of atorvastatin on the long-term outcomes of diabetic patients on hemodialysis. This study enrolled 1255 diabetic patients on hemodialysis, with a mean age of 65. Subjects were randomized to atorvastatin 20 mg versus placebo, for a median follow-up of 4 years. After 4 years of therapy, there was no statistical difference between the groups in the primary composite outcome of death from cardiac causes, nonfatal myocardial infarction, and stroke. The primary composite outcome occurred in 38% of the placebo group, and 37% of the atorvastatin group. Similarly, there were nonsignificant differences in the rate of death from cardiac causes, nonfatal myocardial infarction, and all-cause death. In a trend that runs counter to prevailing thought, the rate of fatal stroke was significantly higher in the atorvastatin group (2% placebo vs 4% atorvastatin, 95% CI, 1.05–3.93), with the increased risk being primarily from fatal ischemic stroke. This result should be considered cautiously, as it is not the primary end point, the number of stroke event was small (40 total strokes), and the confidence interval is wide.

More recently, the AURORA study group[14] looked at the effect of the newer agent rosuvastatin in dialysis patients, 28% of whom had diabetes, with an average time on dialysis of 3.5 years. There were a total of 2776 patients randomized to receive rosuvastatin 10 mg daily or placebo. The mean follow-up was 3 years, after which the rosuvastatin group had mean LDL of 60, compared to LDL of 100 in the placebo group. Despite this, there was no significant difference in the occurrence of major cardiovascular events—9.2% in the rosuvastatin group and 9.5% in the placebo group (HR 0.96, CI 0.84–1.11). There was no relationship between cardiovascular events with either baseline LDL cholesterol or LDL cholesterol after 3 months of treatment.

The poor outcomes in patients with renal disease and HF also do not seem to improve with revascularization. For example, an analysis of the USRDS data from 1995 to 1998 looked at patients on dialysis for at least 60 days prior to revascularization.[15] There were 15,784 dialysis patients who had coronary revascularization—6668 had coronary artery bypass grafting (CABG), 4836 had percutaneous transluminal coronary angioplasty (PTCA) only, and 4280 had coronary stent placement. These patients were followed for a mean of 13 to 18 months. The all-cause survival after coronary stent placement was 67% at 1 year, 48% at 2 years, and 29% at 3.5 years. After CABG, the survival was 71% at 1 year, 56% at 2 years, and 37% at 3.5 years, a statistically significant difference when compared to the stent group. The difference in survival was driven by the diabetic group, with a 19% reduction in risk of death with CABG compared with PTCA (relative risk 0.81; 95% CI, 0.75–0.88). In contrast, stents had no statistically significant advantage over PTCA alone in diabetic patients (relative risk 0.99; 95% CI, 0.91–1.08). These data suggest a possible advantage of CABG over stents in this population, echoing the findings of people with diabetes and multivessel coronary artery disease without CKD.[16] Despite this small possible therapeutic advantage, the survival rate remains abysmal, and newer approaches are required.

Role of Dialysis

Patients with HF and CKD frequently experience diminishing effectiveness of diuretic therapy, leading to consideration of renal replacement therapy. The National Kidney Foundation guidelines indicate that dialysis should be considered when the GFR is below 15 mL/kg/1.73 m^2 body surface area.[17] The guidelines also state that dialysis may be considered when the patient presents with fluid overload refractory to diuretics, progressive uremic encephalopathy, persistent metabolic disturbances refractory to medical therapy, or pericarditis. Although there are very few absolute contraindications for dialysis, its use for the long-term care of HF patients must be tempered by several considerations. First, these patients have significant disability that markedly restricts their activity. Travel to and from an outpatient dialysis unit may be overwhelming for these individuals. Furthermore, intradialysis hypotension is frequent and can lead to emergent need for hospitalization.[18] Indeed, HF patients tend to have chronic low-normal blood pressures, both as a result of their poor LV systolic performance, and due to the multiple neurohormonal medications that are typically given. Other considerations include the need for establishing permanent vascular access, which creates a 0.5- to 1.0-L arteriovenous shunt. The volume load resulting from this shunt can further decompensate a heart that is already at the limits of its compensation. Alternative strategies for dialysis, including peritoneal dialysis, nocturnal dialysis, and short daily in-home dialysis, may avoid some of these problems and lead to better quality of life.[19] A strong social support system is imperative for any long-term success. Patients may decline dialysis therapy, which is perfectly reasonable, given the poor prognosis of HF complicated by renal failure (Figure 13.1).

Role of Kidney Transplantation

To make a significant impact on survival, attention has to turn to other therapies, such as renal transplantation or newer modalities of dialysis. Many studies show improved survival of dialysis patients who undergo renal transplantation.[20,21] Selection bias is always an issue when comparing therapies, particularly those that require a subjective evaluation of the patient for referral. However, an intriguing study addressed this limitation by comparing the survival of transplant recipients to those still on the transplant waiting list as well as the "non-referred" dialysis population.[22] This study used data from the USRDS from 1991 to 1996. After excluding patients older than 70, there were 228,552 total dialysis patients, of

whom 46,164 were on the transplant list for the first time. From this population, 23,275 patients received a renal transplant. The rate of death from initial placement on the transplant list was 6.3 per 100 patient years in the group that remained on the waiting list, 3.8 per 100 patient years in the group that received transplant, and 16.1 per 100 patient years in the entire dialysis group. This study indicated that patients referred for renal transplant are indeed selected for their health and predicted survival. However, renal transplant still was associated with a considerable 40% reduction in mortality in the first year, compared to patients on the waiting list, and a 66% reduction of mortality at 3 to 4 years of follow-up. Although impressive, the data are observational in nature and do not entirely remove selection bias. To date, there have been no prospective clinical trials, and, given the complexity of this disease, there likely never will be. However, there are data that suggest kidney transplant does affect cardiac structure and function, and hence may confer an independent survival advantage.

Renal transplantation was shown to improve cardiac structure in a small study from the renal transplant program at Universidade Federal, Brazil.[23] Patients were prospectively followed for 12 months posttransplant with 2-dimensional echocardiography. Consistent with numerous other studies, 75% of these patients had LV hypertrophy prior to transplant. The presence of LV dilatation (defined as LV end-diastolic diameter > 52 mm) decreased from 58% prior to transplant to 17% at 12 months after transplantation. LV mass decreased from an average of 164 g/m^2 prior to transplant, to 130 g/m^2 after transplantation ($P = 0.009$). This was associated with improvement in blood pressure.

In another investigation, the effect on LV hypertrophy was followed in 433 dialysis patients from eastern Canada from 1982 to

1991, 143 of whom received renal allografts.[24] Echocardiography was used to measure the dimensions, thickness, and mass of the left ventricle. However, only 113 of the patients with renal allografts had echocardiograms that were of sufficient quality to make those measurements, and only 70 of these had repeat echocardiograms enabling serial comparisons. From year 1 to year 2, LV mass, indexed to body surface area, decreased from 161 g/m^2 to 146 g/m^2. Also during this time period, LV cavity volume decreased from 81 to 75 mL/m^2. No further changes of significance were seen in LV mass or LV cavity volume in years 3 and 4. Echocardiography is currently recommended by the National Kidney Foundation for all patients initiating hemodialysis.

The best study of cardiac structure and function posttransplantation comes from Wali et al[25] from the University of Maryland. From 1998 to 2002, this group enrolled 138 patients with ESRD and a reduced LVEF (EF 30%–33% at baseline). Of these, 103 patients remained after exclusion of concomitant pancreas transplant recipients, repeat renal transplant, valvular heart disease, obstructive sleep apnea, amyloidosis, and early loss of graft within the first 3 months. The investigators screened for cardiovascular disease in all patients over the age of 50, or any patients with diabetes, using dobutamine stress echocardiogram or SPECT myocardial perfusion scans. Based on these tests, patients with suspected coronary artery disease had coronary angiograms and, if needed, percutaneous revascularization prior to listing for transplant. To measure cardiac function serially, the patients underwent radionuclide ventriculography gated–blood pool scans (MUGA) before transplant listing, 6 months after renal transplantation, and 12 months after transplantation. LVEF, which averaged 31% ± 6% prior to transplantation, improved to 47% ± 10% at 6 months after transplanta-

tion. Indeed, 70% of patients had normalized LVEF, and more than 86% had at least 5% improvement in their EF. An inverse association was noted between normalization of EF and the duration of dialysis prior to transplantation. On multivariate analysis, the strongest predictor for normalization of EF was the pretransplant time on dialysis. There was a significantly decreased mortality in the group that experienced normalization of EF after renal transplant (Figure 13.2).

Despite the impressive benefits in mortality and morbidity, consideration of renal transplantation in this high-risk population must always be tempered by the availability of resources. In 2006, there were over 18,000 kidney transplants in the United States, an increase of 3.5%.[6] To put this number in context, there were over 350,000 patients on dialysis that year, and 70,000 were on the waiting list for a kidney.[6] The expected median wait time for an organ is 4 years. Therefore, patient selection for renal transplant must include careful consideration for anticipated mortality of comorbid conditions, including HF. The expected survival of HF patients without kidney disease is 79% at 2 years and 59% at 5 years after diagnosis.[26] However, the USRDS suggested that the combination of HF and CKD was particularly lethal.[6] Some of the patients with HF and ESRD have the potential to improve or even normalize, as seen in the data from Wali et al[25] at the University of Maryland. Until these data are confirmed, or there are independent markers to identify people who will benefit most, it is a difficult ethical question whether patients with HF should receive such a scarce resource.

Included in the 18,000 transplants in 2006, approximately 3000 were from living related donors, and another 3000 were from living distantly related or unrelated donors. Living donors make up a significant portion of the supply of organs. However, there are

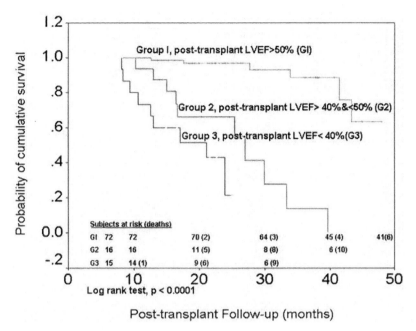

Figure 13.2 Cumulative probability of survival after renal transplant, according to improvement in LVEF. Wali RK, Wang GS, Gottlieb SS, et al. Effect of kidney transplantation on left ventricular systolic dysfunction and congestive heart failure in patients with end-stage renal disease. *J Am Coll Cardiol.* 2005;45:1051–1060. With permission from Elsevier.

special ethical considerations. Although the nephrectomy to harvest the organ is a relatively safe procedure for the donor, there is the risk of small–bowel obstruction, estimated to be about 2% over long–term follow-up.[27] There is also the risk of depression in the person after donating a kidney.[28] Because of these risks, certain ethical concerns exist about organ donation by living donors, particularly for recipients with comorbid conditions likely to shorten survival, such as HF.[29] One concern is that living related or emotionally related donors may feel coerced or even compelled to donate. Another concern is that directed donation, where a donor specifies a particular stranger or the characteristics of a stranger that will receive the organ, involves ethically thorny issues such as financial incentive or racial inequality.

Referral to Transplant Team

Many patients with cardiorenal syndrome are followed simultaneously by the cardiology and nephrology teams; hence the decision of whether to refer for transplant evaluation frequently lies with the nephrology consultant. Although there are general guidelines regarding the criteria for patient referral,[30] this is a decision that requires good clinical judgment under the best of circumstances, that is, even in the absence of cardiorenal syndrome. Eligibility in the general dialysis population relates to numerous factors including degree of disability, obesity, age, time on dialysis, and presence of comorbid conditions. People with cardiorenal syndrome by definition have at least one serious comorbid condition, are frequently older, and have severe disability. These factors alone account for the low number of patients who are actually referred. As discussed, confirmation of the strong beneficial effects of transplant on cardiac function observed in the University of Maryland data might alter future practice patterns, but organ shortages persist. In the absence of confirmatory data, we would recommend that referral be restricted to those with clinical features suggesting a reasonable prognosis from the underlying cardiac condition.

Conclusion

Heart failure and end-stage renal disease are both disorders that are associated with significant morbidity and mortality. When present in the same individual, the effect on mortality is magnified. The evidence-based therapies for cardiovascular disease and HF have been strikingly disappointing in the ESRD population. Relatively small studies suggest that renal transplant may improve cardiac function, and in some, even normalize the echocardiogram. Uremia may directly injure the cardiomyocyte, contributing to the development of HF, which may account for the inverse correlation between time on dialysis and improvement in cardiac function after renal transplant. It is an exciting prospect that a disease with such morbidity as HF can be addressed in such an effective way. However, our enthusiasm must be supported by further studies specifically investigating this link, the predictors of outcome after renal transplantation must be further explored, and we must thoroughly consider the ethical issues regarding the use of limited resources for a population with uncertain prognosis.

References

1. Patel J, Heywood JT. Management of the cardiorenal syndrome in heart failure. *Curr Cardiol Rep.* 2006;8:211–216.

2. Fonarow GC, Adams KF, Abraham WT; ADHERE Investigators. Risk stratification for in-hospital mortality in heart failure using classification and regression tree (CART) methodology: analysis of 33,046 patients in the ADHERE registry [abstract 290]. *J Card Fail.* 2003;9(suppl):S79.

3. Hillege HL, Girbes AR, de Kam PJ, et al. Renal function, neurohormonal activation, and survival in patients with chronic heart failure. *Circulation.* 2000;102:203–210.

4. Weiner DE, Tighiouart H, Elsayed EF, et al. The Framingham predictive instrument in chronic kidney disease. *J Am Coll Cardiol.* 2007;50:217–224.

5. Go AS, Chertow GM, Fan D, McCulloch CE, Hsu CY. Chronic kidney disease and the risks of death, cardiovascular events, and hospitalization. *N Engl J Med.* 2004;351:1296–1305.

6. U.S. Renal Data System, USRDS 2008 Annual Data Report: Atlas of Chronic Kidney Disease and End-Stage Renal Disease in the United States, National Institutes of Health, National Institute of Diabetes and Digestive and Kidney Diseases, Bethesda, MD, 2008. (*Notice: The data reported here have been supplied by the United States Renal Data System (USRDS). The interpretation and reporting of these data are the responsibility of the authors, and in no way should be seen as an official policy or interpretation of the U.S. government.*)

7. Thom T, Haase N, Rosamond W, et al; American Heart Association Statistics Committee and Stroke Statistics Subcommittee. Heart disease and stroke statistics—2006 update: a report

from the American Heart Association Statistics Committee and Stroke Statistics Subcommittee. *Circulation.* 2006;113: e85-151.

8. Herzog CA, Ma JZ, Collins AJ. Poor long-term survival after acute myocardial infarction among patients on long-term dialysis. *N Engl J Med.* 1998;339:799-805.

9. Harnett JD, Foley RN, Kent GM, Barre PE, Murray D, Parfrey PS. Congestive heart failure in dialysis patients: prevalence, incidence, prognosis, and risk factors. *Kidney Int.* 1995;47:884-890.

10. Stack AG, Bloembergen WE. A cross-sectional study of the prevalence and clinical correlates of congestive heart failure among incident US dialysis patients. *Am J Kidney Dis.* 2001;38: 992-1000.

11. Mall G, Rambausek M, Neumeister A, Kollmar S, Vetterlein F, Ritz E. Myocardial interstitial fibrosis in experimental ischemia—Implications for cardiac compliance. *Kidney Int.* 1988; 33:804-811.

12. Mall G, Huther W, Schneider J, Lundin P, Ritz E. Diffuse intermyocardiocytic fibrosis in uraemic patients. *Nephrol Dial Transplant.* 1990;5:39-44.

13. Wanner C, Krane V, März W, et al; German Diabetes and Dialysis Study Investigators. Atorvastatin in patients with type 2 diabetes mellitus undergoing hemodialysis. *N Engl J Med.* 2005;353:238-248.

14. Fellström BC, Jardine AG, Schmieder RE, et al; AURORA Study Group. Rosuvastatin and cardiovascular events in patients undergoing hemodialysis. *N Engl J Med.* 2009;360:1395-1407.

15. Herzog CA, Ma JZ, Collins AJ. Comparative survival of dialysis patients in the United States after coronary angioplasty, coronary artery stenting, and coronary artery bypass surgery and impact of diabetes. *Circulation.* 2002;106:2207-2211.

16. The BARI Investigators. The final 10-year follow-up results from the BARI randomized trial. *J Am Coll Cardiol.* 2007;49:1600-1606.

17. Hemodialysis Adequacy 2006 Work Group. Clinical practice guidelines for hemodialysis adequacy, update 2006. *Am J Kidney Dis.* 2006;48(suppl 1):S2-S90.

18. Zager PG, Nikolic J, Brown RH, et al. "U" curve association of blood pressure and mortality in hemodialysis patients. Medical Directors of Dialysis Clinic, Inc. *Kidney Int.* 1998;54:561-569.

19. Puñal Rioboó J, Sánchez-Iriso E, Ruano-Ravina A, et al. Short daily versus conventional hemodialysis quality of life: a cross-sectional multicentric study in Spain. *Blood Purif.* 2009;28:159-164.

20. Russell JD, Beecroft ML, Ludwin D, Churchill DN. The quality of life in renal transplantation—A prospective study. *Transplantation.* 1992;54:656-660.

21. Cosio FG, Alamir A, Yim S, et al. Patient survival after renal transplantation. I. The impact of dialysis pre-transplant. *Kidney Int.* 1998;53:767-772.

22. Wolfe RA, Ashby VB, Milford EL, et al. Comparison of mortality in all patients on dialysis, patients on dialysis awaiting transplantation, and recipients of a first cadaveric transplant. *N Engl J Med.* 1999;341:1725-1730.

23. Ferreira SR, Moisés VA, Tavares A, Pacheco-Silva A. Cardiovascular effects of successful renal transplantation: a 1-year sequential study of left ventricular morphology and function, and 24-hour blood pressure profile. *Transplantation.* 2002;74:1580-1587.

24. Rigatto C, Foley RN, Kent GM, Guttmann R, Parfrey PS. Long-term changes in

left ventricular hypertrophy after renal transplantation. *Transplantation.* 2000;70:570-575.

25. Wali RK, Wang GS, Gottlieb SS, et al. Effect of kidney transplantation on left ventricular systolic dysfunction and congestive heart failure in patients with end-stage renal disease. *J Am Coll Cardiol.* 2005;45:1051-1060.

26. Mosterd A, Cost B, Hoes AW, et al. The prognosis of heart failure in the general population: The Rotterdam Study. *Eur Heart J.* 2001;22:1318-1327.

27. Dunn JF, Nylander WA Jr, Richie RE, Johnson HK, MacDonell RC Jr, Sawyers JL. Living related kidney donors. A 14-year experience. *Ann Surg.* 1986; 203:637-643.

28. Kasiske BL, Ravenscraft M, Ramos EL, Gaston RS, Bia MJ, Danovitch GM. The evaluation of living renal transplant donors: clinical practice guidelines. Ad Hoc Clinical Practice Guidelines Subcommittee of the Patient Care and Education Committee of the American Society of Transplant Physicians. *J Am Soc Nephrol.* 1996;7:2288-2313.

29. Truog RD. The ethics of organ donation by living donors. *N Engl J Med.* 2005;353:444-446.

30. Knoll G, Cockfield S, Blydt-Hansen T, et al; Kidney Transplant Working Group of the Canadian Society of Transplantation. Canadian Society of Transplantation consensus guidelines on eligibility for kidney transplantation. *CMAJ.* 2005;173:1181-1184.

Selection of Heart Failure Patients with Renal Dysfunction for Cardiac Transplantation

14

Tong Liu

Mariell Jessup

Heart transplantation is currently the standard, definitive therapy for patients with end-stage heart failure (HF) for whom all medical or alternative therapies have been exhausted. Since the introduction of the calcineurin inhibitors as a critical part of an immunosuppressive regimen, survival after transplantation exceeds 83% at 1 year and 75% at 5 years after the operation.[1] Up to 85% of heart transplant recipients report improvement in quality of life, and approximately 50% return to work after the procedure. But advanced HF patients with renal dysfunction are generally excluded from heart transplantation because abnormal renal function increases morbidity post-transplantation.[2-5] Thus, it is important to clearly distinguish patients with potentially

reversible renal failure from those patients in whom renal dysfunction is associated with advanced, irreversible end-stage renal disease (ESRD). Accordingly, this chapter focuses on strategies to identify the causes of renal dysfunction in the patient with advanced HF under consideration for heart transplantation. Ideally, heart transplantation can be offered to those patients with reversible renal dysfunction, while those selected patients with intrinsic renal disease might require a combined heart–kidney transplant instead.

Renal Dysfunction in Heart Failure

The number of patients with advanced chronic HF is increasing secondary to better treatment modalities of acute ischemic heart disease, as well as advances in the treatment of chronic HF. Nevertheless, patients with

The Cardiorenal Syndrome: A Clinician's Guide to Pathophysiology and Management, 1st ed. © 2012 J. Thomas Heywood and John C. Burnett Jr., eds. Cardiotext Publishing, ISBN: 978-0-9790164-7-9.

advanced HF commonly have renal insufficiency[6]; HF and renal insufficiency frequently coexist in the same patients.[7-9] As a reference for this chapter, the National Kidney Foundation's classification of kidney disease ranges from stage 1 (GFR > 90 mL/min/m²), stage 2 (GFR 60–89 mL/min/m²), stage 3 (GFR 30–59 mL/min/m²), stage 4 (GFR 15–29 mL/min/m²), to stage 5 (GFR < 15 mL/min/m²).[10] Progressive renal dysfunction in the setting of treatment for HF has been defined by either an increase in creatinine of at least 0.3 g/dL or GFR < 59 mL/min/m², obtained after treatment.[11-13] Contributing factors to progressive renal dysfunction in this setting include poor cardiac output (CO), low effective circulatory volume, neurohormonal activation, and high prevalence of problems such as diabetes, atherosclerosis, and hypertension. Added to these factors is the increasingly long waiting time for many patients eligible for heart transplantation, so that more and more patients on the transplantation recipient list develop renal dysfunction while waiting. Attempts are necessary to understand the underlying etiology of the renal dysfunction in individual patients because some factors are potentially reversible, especially if diagnosed early. Appropriate treatment strategies could theoretically improve the prognosis of patients with HF and renal dysfunction, and more optimally guide the appropriate selection of transplant candidates.

Etiology of Comorbid Renal Dysfunction in Patients with Heart Failure

Data from several sources demonstrate that approximately 20% to 40% of patients admitted for acute decompensated heart failure (ADHF) have comorbid renal insufficiency (RI) based on their clinical history and serum creatinine levels.[11] In the ADHERE database,[14] over 60% of patients admitted for ADHF had at least moderate (stage 3) kidney disease, using the National Kidney Foundation classification.[10] Moreover, this comorbid RI is associated with significantly increased risk for morbidity and mortality.[15] Comorbid RI can result from hemodynamic abnormalities, intrinsic renal disease, or their combination, as outlined in Table 14.1.

The causes of HF-associated RI are diverse, but diminished renal perfusion is a common consequence of the hemodynamic changes associated with HF and its treatment. The primary causes of decreased renal perfusion are hypovolemia (inadequate preload), neurohormonally mediated vasoconstriction (increased afterload), and hypotension with preserved CO (vasodilatory shock) or low output syndrome. More recently, attention has focused on the role of abnormally high venous pressures as a critically important component of worsening renal dysfunction in the HF patient.[16,17] The role of certain drugs, such as nonsteroidal anti-inflammatory drugs (NSAIDs), in worsening renal function is especially problematic in the elderly patient with HF and arthritis. Renal dysfunction may also be caused by intrinsic renal disease, exacerbated by diabetes and hypertension.

Having outlined the list of potential causes, it is clear that, most often, renal dysfunction in HF patients is multifactorial in origin, necessitating an individual patient approach. Obviously, in the patient under consideration for heart transplantation, the role of diminished CO must be assessed. If CO and mean arterial pressure fall in the setting of myocardial failure, so too does renal blood flow, activating the renin-angiotensin-aldosterone system (RAAS), and the sympathetic nervous system (SNS), all of which, in a well-described circle, cause

Table 14.1 Etiologies of
Renal Dysfunction in Heart Failure

Hemodynamic Abnormalities
- Hypovolemia (inadequate preload)
- Neurohormonally mediated vasoconstriction (increased afterload)
- Hypotension: (1) with preserved CO (vasodilatory shock), (2) with low CO (severe pump failure, cardiogenic shock)
- Abnormally high central venous pressures
- Drug-induced (nonsteroidal anti-inflammatory drugs, angiotensin-converting enzyme inhibitors. angiotensin receptor blockers)

Intrinsic Renal Disease
- Vasculopathy of venal arteries and veins
- Nephron loss (diabetes and hypertension)

---

structural and functional damage to the kidney and heart. The fall in CO may be compounded by the concomitant hemodynamic abnormality of high cardiac filling pressure. This, in turn, increases renal interstitial pressure, as demonstrated years ago by Blake et al,[18] who showed that dogs with increased renal vein pressure were found to have increased renal interstitial pressure. Although experimentally demonstrated in animals, validation of this phenomenon in humans is lacking. Nonetheless, a growing body of evidence supports this hypothesis,[16,17] and it has been shown that lowering central venous pressure with ultrafiltration improves urine output.[19,20] Bertani et al[21] examined renal pathology in autopsy specimens from patients who died of end-stage HF and found that the HF patients had no arteriolar changes or glomerulosclerosis.

Thus, there may be clues to identifying the patient with primarily hemodynamically mediated renal failure who is without intrinsic kidney disease. These clues include an absence of proteinuria, normal kidney size at ultrasonography, and the absence of severe histopathology in renal biopsy specimens. As an extreme example, Bergler–Klein et al[22] reported that patients without native kidney disease but hemodynamically mediated dialysis–dependent renal failure of < 4 months were able to recover renal function after transplantation.

With the review of the potential causes of renal failure in mind, there are several steps to work through when a GFR of < 59 mL/min/m^2 or an increase in serum creatinine of 0.3 mg/dL is observed in HF patients during treatment[11]:

1. Volume status. Determination of fluid status is critical, because in some ways it is potentially the easiest abnormality to modify. The best clinical indicators of volume overload are the symptom of orthopnea and the sign of elevated jugular venous pressure.[23] Diuretics relieve both of these indicators, the foundation of therapy for advanced HF. However, overzealous use of diuretics can cause hypovolemia, reducing CO and, consequently, GFR.[24] Careful physical examination, noninvasive hemodynamic measurements (eg, limited echocardiographic evaluation of right atrial and left atrial pressures), and invasive hemodynamic monitoring are usually sufficient to diagnose this very common cause of renal dysfunction.[25] Judicious treatment, by withholding diuretics and administration of fluids, often results in prompt normalization of the serum creatinine.

2. Cardiac output. Invasive hemodynamic monitoring is often required to assess the CO and systemic vascular resistance, especially if there is concomitant low blood pressure. Inotropic agents are useful to augment CO, although these drugs have not been shown to improve survival in the long term. Renal function may actually improve as CO and, hence, renal perfusion are increased.[26] This specific result would tend to indicate that the underlying renal dysfunction was more likely cardiac in origin rather than intrinsic renal disease.

3. Intrinsic renal function. Parenchymal renal disease should be suspected if RI persists after abnormalities in volume status, CO, and systemic vascular resistance are corrected. Typically, this is due to nephron loss secondary to diabetes, hypertension, or renal vascular disease. If needed, a renal biopsy could be done to identify the histopathologic correlates. The presence of proteinuria usually indicates intrinsic renal disease and is associated with an increased risk for the development of chronic, progressive renal insufficiency.[27]

Irreversible renal dysfunction with serum creatinine > 2 mg/dL or creatinine clearance (CrCl) < 50 mL/min was considered at the Bethesda Conference as a secondary exclusion criterion for heart transplantation.[2] More recently, guidelines from the International Society for Heart and Lung Transplantation listed a serum creatinine level of > 3 mg/dL as a relative contraindication to transplantation.[5] However, creatinine blood level is not the most sensitive marker of kidney function. Creatinine depends on muscle mass, which varies with gender, ethnicity, and age. As a result, serum creatinine concentration alone may not accurately reflect renal function.[28,29] Although serum creatinine is used commonly, preferably eGFR, based on predictive equations that take into account not only serum creatinine level but also other factors, such as age, sex, and race,[29] should be evaluated.[5]

Heart Transplantation and Renal Dysfunction

Renal insufficiency after heart transplantation portends a poor prognosis.[30,31] Previous published reports indicate that 3% to 7% of patients who survive the initial month after transplantation become dialysis dependent within 5 to 10 years.[32,33] Several studies have reported that the risk of developing chronic RI after orthotopic heart transplantation is predicted by pretransplant renal function. Sehgal et al[34] followed 80 adult patients who had undergone heart transplantation over a mean period of 4.7 years. These patients were divided into 2 groups according to the last follow-up serum creatinine. The renal insufficiency group was defined as a serum creatinine $\geq$ 2.4 mg/dL while the remaining patients were defined by a serum creatinine $\leq$ 1.7 mg/dL. They found that the patients with posttransplant progressive RI tended to be older and had a lower mean GFR at initial evaluation. Ostermann et al[35] analyzed data on 1180 recipients of cardiac allografts from the United Kingdom Adult Transplant Audit Database in the years 1996 to 2002. Recipients with a CrCl < 51 mL/min at transplantation (using the Cockroft–Gault formula) had twice the mortality (19.7%) of those patients with a CrCl > 51 mL/min (9.5%) (P < 0.001). Vossler et al[36] conducted a retrospective analysis on 160 patients who survived more than 1 year after heart transplantation. They reported that those patients with preoperative serum creatinine concentration > 1.5 mg/dL were at the highest risk of chronic RI after transplantation. In that cohort, 55.3% of patients with pre–heart transplant creatinine > 1.5 mg/dL had chronic RI after surgery, and for this subgroup, 28.5% became dialysis dependent. This study also demonstrated that the significance of the pretransplant correlation was robust even when other potential confounding variables were considered.

These earlier studies have been more recently confirmed by an analysis of 622 patients by Odim et al.[37] In this study, the recipients were divided into either normal or impaired preoperative renal function. Impaired renal function was defined as a CrCl of < 40 mL/min (Cockroft-Gault formula). In the impaired preoperative renal function group, the incidence of early mortality was 17%. It was significantly higher than in those patients with normal renal function. The patients in the impaired renal function group had a 2.6 fold (95% CI, 1.4–4.9) higher incidence of early mortality than those with normal preop renal function (Figure 14.1). Moreover, patients with preoperative RI re-

quired dialysis in the early postoperative period more frequently than did the patients with normal preoperative renal function (32% vs 9%, respectively; $P < 0.0001$). Therefore, CrCl < 40 mL/min is a useful marker for increased postoperative renal failure and mortality. Ojo et al[31] conducted a population-based cohort analysis to evaluate the risk factors for chronic renal failure in recipients of nonrenal transplants. They found that a decrement in GFR of 10 mL/min/1.73 m^2 in the pretransplant time period was associated with an increase of 9% for the risk of chronic renal failure (relative risk, 1.09; 95% CI, 1.07–1.10). Greater reductions in the pretransplant GFR were also associated with progressive increases in the risk of chronic renal failure. These findings are in accordance with the study by Al Aly et al,[38] who showed that pretransplant GFR is an important risk factor for any decrement in renal function after the procedure. In addition, Rubel et al[39] studied 370 patients who received heart transplants, with up to 10 years of follow-up. They found low preoperative GFR to be a significant predictor of subsequent ESRD. The significance of poor preoperative GFR as a predictor of subsequent ESRD was maintained on multivariate analysis as well, with an associated hazard ratio of 3.69.

Figure 14.1. Actuarial survival following heart transplant for patients with CrCl above or below 40 mL/min, illustrating the superior outcomes for the patients with preserved renal function following transplant. Odim J, Wheat J, Laks H, et al. Peri-operative renal function and outcome after orthotopic heart transplantation. *J Heart Lung Transplant.* 2006;25:162–166. With permission from Elsevier.

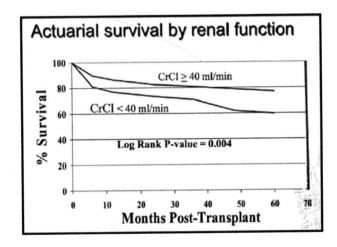

In contrast to these studies, other investigations have reported that there are no significant correlations between the preoperative GFR and postoperative renal function. In a case-controlled study, van Gelder et al[40] reported some patients with pretransplant CrCl above 70 mL/min who developed renal failure. Another study of 187 patients with variable duration of follow-up (1–60 months) suggested that pretransplant serum creatinine was not predictive of long-term renal function.[41] Lindelow et al[42] also demonstrated that no relationship could be found between the preoperative GFR and postoperative renal function. Nevertheless, these authors did indicate that patients with preoperative depressed renal function who improved on inotropic treatment seemed to have a poor outcome; 40% of such patients needed early dialysis and 20% needed late dialysis. Vossler et al[36] also found that despite the strong correlation between preoperative serum creatinine and development of chronic RI, 19% of patients with normal preoperative creatinine experienced chronic renal failure, suggesting that the pathophysiology of this process could result from multiple interacting factors. Taken together, the results of these studies do not support the strategy of applying even more stringent renal function criteria in the selection of transplant candidates, as there does not appear to be overwhelming evidence that posttransplant renal failure can be avoided entirely. Conflicting evidence exists regarding the relationship between preoperative renal function and the development of chronic RI after heart transplantation. We suggest that renal functional reserve before transplantation is a key factor in determining whether an individual will tolerate the transplant operation itself, with associated cardiopulmonary bypass, and long-term treatment with immunosuppressive agents, most notably the calcineurin antagonists. It

is likely that all patients treated with calcineurin antagonists have some renal damage but that the degree of functional impairment is highly dependent on the degree of pretransplant renal disease.[30,31,34,42]

We would propose, in summary, the following approach for the possible cardiac transplant candidate with a preoperative GFR value < 40 mL/min/1.73 m² or a serum creatinine > 1.7 mg/dL. Attempts should be made to optimize the renal function through improved hemodynamics by using pharmacologic interventions such as inotropes, vasodilators, and diuretics (or withholding diuretics as the case may be) according to the hemodynamic parameters. Once the lowest serum creatinine value is achieved, GFR can be determined. If GFR is > 40 mL/min/1.73 m², the patient can be accepted for heart transplantation. This reversibility test of renal dysfunction might be an adequate method of identifying a renal reserve before heart transplantation.

Combined Simultaneous Heart-Kidney Transplantation

Current surgical skills and immunosuppressive strategies now permit simultaneous heart and kidney transplantation,[43] and this approach is increasingly being considered for the patient with advanced renal disease who needs heart transplantation. The first successful heart and kidney transplant with long-term survival was performed in 1986.[44] Since then, the number of simultaneous heart-kidney transplantations has increased every year. The Registry of the International Society for Heart and Lung Transplantation (ISHLT) has recorded more than 350 such procedures.[45] Narula et al[46] published a collective review of 84 combined cardiorenal transplants performed in 82 patients in the United States between October 1987 and May 1995. The mean duration of post-transplant follow-up was 780 ± 744 days. The patient survival at 1, 6, 12, and 24 months posttransplant was 92%, 79%, 76%, and 67%, respectively. The actuarial survival rates in the heart-kidney recipients were statistically similar to those observed in 14,340 isolated heart recipients (United Network for Organ Sharing [UNOS] Scientific Registry) during the same period (92%, 86%, 83%, and 79%, respectively). In 2001, Leeser et al[47] presented the results of their single-center series of 13 patients undergoing simultaneous heart and kidney transplantation. The mortality at 1 year was 25%, comparable to the published 24% mortality of the UNOS series.[46] A Kaplan-Meier analysis revealed a 1-year survival of 77% for heart-kidney recipients and 80% for heart alone at their institution.[47] Smith et al[48] reported on a 25-year experience with heart retransplantation at a single institution. They noted that in 28 patients undergoing heart retransplantation after cyclosporine therapy, the preoperative serum creatinine level seemed to have prognostic

importance. If the creatinine level was lower than 2 mg/dL, the incidence of postoperative dialysis was 6% (1/17), and 1-year patient survival was 100% (17/17). Conversely, if creatinine level was > 2 mg/dL, the incidence of dialysis was 7% (6/11), and the 1-year patient survival rate of those needing dialysis was 33% (2/16). Three patients with significant cyclosporine-induced renal dysfunction (a creatinine level of > 2 mg/dL) underwent simultaneous kidney transplantation and heart retransplantation; all were alive with excellent cardiac and renal function. The ISHLT's twenty-second official adult heart transplant report (2005) illustrated the survival curves for recipients undergoing simultaneous heart and kidney transplant, compared to the cohort receiving heart transplantation alone during the same period (Figure 14.2).[45] The actuarial survival rates in the heart-kidney recipients were similar to those isolated heart recipients. Compared to isolated heart transplantation, combined heart-kidney transplantation did not adversely affect intermediate survival.

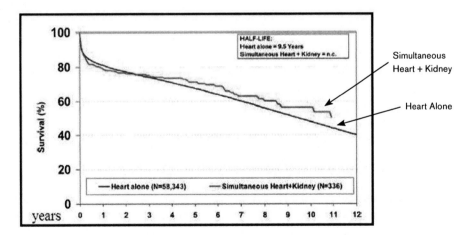

Figure 14.2. Kaplan-Meier survival for heart transplant recipients undergoing simultaneous kidney transplantation compared with heart transplant alone between January 1982 and June 2003, showing no significant difference in survival. Taylor DO, Edwards LB, Boucek MM, et al. Registry of the International Society for Heart and Lung Transplantation: Twenty-second official adult heart transplant report—2005. *J Heart Lung Transplant.* 2005;24:945–955. With permission from Elsevier.

However, survival for patients receiving a kidney transplant after a heart transplantation was significantly lower than for isolated heart recipients at the same time points after the index surgery.[45]

Thus, heart-kidney transplant as a single procedure can be performed successfully. It has been shown to not only reduce morbidity and cost associated with RI but also offers immunological benefits, as there appears to be a lower incidence of rejection.[43,46-53] Recipients of simultaneous heart and kidney transplant, by necessity coming from a single donor, have less acute rejection of the heart and the kidney allograft compared to isolated heart or kidney transplant recipients alone.[45,46-50] Simultaneous rejection of both organs is very uncommon.[46,47]

What, then, are the indications for combined heart-kidney transplantation for heart transplantation candidates with concurrent renal dysfunction? It is reasonable to include end-stage HF patients with dialysis-dependent renal failure or pathological kidney disease (such as polycystic kidney) for simultaneous heart and kidney procedures. But, it is more difficult to make the decision for patients not yet on dialysis. Jeyarajah et al[54] showed, in comparison, that in combined liver-kidney transplants with marginal renal function due to a reversible cause (eg, hepatorenal syndrome), patients can be managed effectively without a concomitant renal graft and have the same long-term outcomes. The same may be true in heart-kidney transplants. The preferred strategy may only be elucidated by a multicenter, randomized trial, using a clearly defined set of criteria for the renal dysfunction.

If fixed renal disease occurs in patients with end-stage HF, at what cutoff GFR value should they be considered for heart-kidney transplantation? Trachiotis et al[55] suggest that optimally managed patients with severe HF who have a serum creatinine > 1.8 mg/dL

and a GFR < 40 mL/min are potentially more suitable candidates for a simultaneous heart and kidney transplant, because they are at high risk of becoming dialysis-dependent heart transplant patients. In the National Taiwan University Hospital, Wang et al[56] reported that end-stage HF patients with a serum creatinine > 3.0 mg/dL or CrCl < 20 mL/min should undergo simultaneous heart and kidney transplantations. Savdie et al[50] and Leeser et al[47] suggest a GFR of < 30 mL/min. Finally, one study suggested that a GFR (as calculated by Cockroft-Gault formula) of < 60 mL/min might be a threshold predicting future need of heart-kidney transplantation; there is no consensus on this issue.[57] Further, studies are needed to establish guidelines of what preoperative GFR warrants heart and kidney transplantations.

Conclusion

Worsening renal function in most patients with advanced HF awaiting transplantation usually indicates severe end-organ compromise. However, the sole presence of renal dysfunction does not preclude, necessarily, a patient with HF from heart transplantation. If the cause of renal dysfunction is shown to be reversible prior to transplant, renal function should improve after heart transplantation alone, providing excellent outcomes for the majority of patients. For patients on chronic dialysis with end-stage heart disease, and candidates for heart transplantation with coexisting progressive irreversible renal disease, combined heart-kidney transplant may be an acceptable option in potential heart transplantation recipients.

References

1. Christie JD, Edwards LB, Aurora P, et al. Registry of the international society for heart and lung transplantation: twenty-

fifth official adult heart transplant report-2008. *J Heart Lung Transplant.* 2008;27:957–969.

2. Mudge GH, Goldstein S, Addonizio LJ, et al. 24th Bethesda conference: cardiac transplantation. Task force 3: recipient guidelines/prioritization. *J Am Coll Cardiol.* 1993;22:21–31.

3. Costanzo MR, Augustine S, Bourge R, et al. Selection and treatment of candidates for heart transplantation: a statement for health professionals from the Committee on Heart Failure and Cardiac Transplantation of the Council on Clinical Cardiology, American Heart Association. *Circulation.* 1995;92:3593–3612.

4. Miller LW. Listing criteria for cardiac transplantation: results of an American Society of Transplant Physicians-National Institutes of Health conference. *Transplantation.* 1998;66:947–951.

5. Mehra MR, Kobashigawa J, Starling R, et al. Listing criteria for heart transplantation: International Society for Heart and Lung Transplantation guidelines for the care of cardiac transplant candidates—2006. *J Heart Lung Transplant.* 2006;25:1024-1042.

6. D'Amico CL. Cardiac transplantation: patient selection in the current era. *J Cardiovasc Nurs.* 2005;20(5 suppl):S4–S13.

7. Hunt SA, Abraham WT, Chin MH, et al; American College of Cardiology; American Heart Association Task Force on Practice Guidelines; American College of Chest Physicians; International Society for Heart and Lung Transplantation; Heart Rhythm Society. ACC/AHA 2005 Guideline Update for the Diagnosis and Management of Chronic Heart Failure in the Adult: a report of the American College of Cardiology/American Heart Association Task Force on Practice Guidelines (Writing Committee to Update the 2001 Guidelines for the Evaluation and Management of Heart Failure): developed in collaboration with the American College of Chest Physicians and the International Society for Heart and Lung Transplantation: endorsed by the Heart Rhythm Society. *Circulation.* 2005;112:e154–e235.

8. Nieminen MS, Böhm M, Cowie MR, et al; ESC Committee for Practice Guideline (CPG). Executive summary of the guidelines on the diagnosis and treatment of acute heart failure: the Task Force on Acute Heart Failure of the European Society of Cardiology. *Eur Heart J.* 2005;26:384–416.

9. Swedberg K, Cleland J, Dargie H, et al; Task Force for the Diagnosis and Treatment of Chronic Heart Failure of the European Society of Cardiology. guidelines for the diagnosis and treatment of chronic heart failure: executive summary (update 2005): the Task Force for the Diagnosis and Treatment of Chronic Heart Failure of the European Society of Cardiology. *Eur Heart J.* 2005;26:1115-1140.

10. K/DOQI clinical practice guidelines for chronic kidney disease: evaluation, classification, and stratification. *Am J Kidney Dis.* 2002;39(2 suppl 1):S1–S266.

11. Krumholz HM, Chen YT, Vaccarino V, Wang Y, et al. Correlates and impact on outcomes of worsening renal function in patients > or =65 years of age with heart failure. *Am J Cardiol.* 2000;85:1110-1113.

12. Smith GL, Vaccarino V, Kosiborod M, et al. Worsening renal function: what is a clinically meaning change in creatinine during hospitalization with heart failure? *J Card Fail.* 2003;9:13-25.

13. Gottlieb SS, Abraham W, Butler J, et al. The prognostic importance of different definitions of worsening renal function

in congestive heart failure. *J Card Fail.* 2002;8:136-141.

14. Adams KF Jr, Fonarow GC, Emerman CL, et al; ADHERE Scientific Advisory Committee and Investigators. Characteristics and outcomes of patients hospitalized for heart failure in the United States: rationale, design, and preliminary observations from the first 100,000 cases in the Acute Decompensated Failure National Registry (ADHERE). *Am Heart J.* 2005;149:209-216.

15. Dries DL, Exner DV, Domanski MJ, Greenberg B, Stevenson LW. The prognostic implications of renal insufficiency in asymptomatic and symptomatic patients with left ventricular systolic dysfunction. *J Am Coll Cardiol.* 2000;35:681-689.

16. Damman K, van Deursen VM, Navis G, Voors AA, van Veldhuisen DJ, Hillege HL. Increased central venous pressure is associated with impaired renal function and mortality in a broad spectrum of patients with cardiovascular disease. *J Am Coll Cardiol.* 2009;53:582-588.

17. Mullens W, Abrahams Z, Francis GS, et al. Importance of venous congestion for worsening of renal function in advanced decompensated heart failure. *J Am Coll Cardiol.* 2009;53:589-596.

18. Blake WD, Wegria R, Keating RP, Ward HP. Effect of increased renal venous pressure on renal function. *Am J Physiol.* 1949;157:1-13.

19. Costanzo MR, Saltzberg M, O'Sullivan J, Sobotka P. Early ultrafiltration in patients with decompensated heart failure and diuretic resistance. *J Am Coll Cardiol.* 2005;46:2047-2051.

20. Rimondini A, Cipolla CM, Della Bella P, et al. Hemofiltration as short-term treatment for refractory congestive heart failure. *Am J Med.* 1987;83:43-48.

21. Bertani T, Ferrazzi P, Schieppati A, et al. Nature and extent of glomerular injury induced by cyclosporine in heart transplant patients. *Kidney Int.* 1991;40:243-250.

22. Bergler-Klein J, Pirich C, Laufer G, et al. The long-term effect of simultaneous heart and kidney transplantation on native renal function. *Transplantation.* 2001;71:1597-1600.

23. Butman SM, Ewy GA, Standen JR, Kern KB, Hahn E. Bedside cardiovascular examination in patients with severe chronic heart failure: importance of rest or inducible jugular venous distension. *J Am Coll Cardiol.* 1993;22:968-974.

24. Ikram H, Chan W, Espiner EA, Nicholls MG. Haemodynamic and hormone responses to acute and chronic furosemide therapy in congestive heart failure. *Clin Sci.* 1980;59:443-449.

25. Mullens W, Abrahams Z, Skouri HN, et al. Prognostic evaluation of ambulatory patients with advanced heart failure. *Am J Cardiol.* 2008;101: 1297-1302.

26. Stevenson LW. Clinical use of inotropic therapy for heart failure: looking backward or forward? Part I: inotropic infusions during hospitalization. *Circulation.* 2003;108: 367-372.

27. Keane WF. Proteinuria: its clinical importance and role in progressive renal disease. *Am J Kidney Dis.* 2000;35: S97-S105.

28. Heywood JT. The cardiorenal syndrome: lessons from the ADHERE database and treatment options. *Heart Fail Rev.* 2004;9:195-201.

29. Levey AS, Coresh J, Balk E, et al; National Kidney Foundation. National Kidney Foundation practice guidelines for chronic kidney disease: evaluation, classification, and stratification. *Ann Intern Med.* 2003;139:137-147.

30. Goldstein DJ, Zuech N, Sehgal V, Weinberg AD, Drusin R, Cohen D. Cyclosporine-associated end-stage nephropathy after cardiac transplantation: incidence and progression. *Transplantation.* 1997;63:664–668.

31. Ojo AO, Held PJ, Port FK, et al. Chronic renal failure after transplantation of a nonrenal organ. *N Engl J Med.* 2003;349:931–940.

32. Goldstein DJ, Zuech N, Sehgal V, Weinberg AD, Drusin R, Cohen D. cyclosporine-associated end-stage nephropathy after cardiac transplantation. *Transplantation.* 1997;63:644–668.

33. Greenberg A, Thompson ME, Griffith BJ, et al. Cyclosporine nephrotoxicity in cardiac allograft patients: a seven-year follow-up. *Transplantation.* 1990;50:589–593.

34. Sehgal V, Radhakrishnan J, Appel GB, Valeri A, Cohen DJ. Progressive renal insufficiency following cardiac transplantation: cyclosporine, lipids, and hypertension. *Am J Kidney Dis.* 1995;26:193–201.

35. Ostermann ME, Rogers CA, Saeed I, Nelson SR, Murday AJ; Steering Group of the UK Cardiothoracic Transplant Audit. Pre-existing renal failure doubles 30–day mortality after cardiac transplantation. *J Heart Lung Transplant.* 2003;22:S209.

36. Vossler MR, Ni H, Toy W, Hershberger RE. Pre-operative renal function predicts development of chronic renal insufficiency after orthotopic heart transplantation. *J Heart Lung Transplant.* 2002;21:874–881.

37. Odim J, Wheat J, Laks H, et al. Peri-operative renal function and outcome after orthotopic heart transplantation. *J Heart Lung Transplant.* 2006;25:162–166.

38. Al Aly Z, Abbas S, Moore E, Diallo O, Hauptman PJ, Bastani B. The natural history of renal function following orthotopic heart transplant. *Clin Transplant.* 2005;19:683–689.

39. Rubel JR, Milford EL, McKay DB, Jarcho JA. Renal insufficiency and end-stage renal disease in the heart transplant population. *J Heart Lung Transplant.* 2004;23:289–300.

40. van Gelder T, Balk AH, Zietse R, Hesse C, Mochtar B, Weimar W. Renal insufficiency after heart transplantation: a case-control study. *Nephrol Dial Transplant.* 1998;13:2322–2326.

41. Zietse R, Balk AH, vd Dorpel MA, Meeter K, Bos E, Weimar W. Time course of the decline in renal function in cyclosporine-treated heart transplant recipients. *Am J Nephrol.* 1994;14:1–5.

42. Lindelow B, Bergh CH, Herlitz H, Waagstein F. Predictors and evolution of renal function during 9 years following heart transplantation. *J Am Soc Nephrol.* 2000;11:951–957.

43. Blanche C, Valenza M, Czer LS, et al. Combined heart and kidney transplantation with allografts from the same donor. *Ann Thorac Surg.* 1994;58:1135–1138.

44. Faggian G, Bortolotti U, Stellin G, et al. Combined heart and kidney transplantation: a case report. *J Heart Transplant.* 1986;5:480–483.

45. Taylor DO, Edwards LB, Boucek MM, et al. Registry of the International Society for Heart and Lung Transplantation: twenty-second official adult heart transplant report—2005. *J Heart Lung Transplant.* 2005;24:945–955.

46. Narula J, Bennett LE, DiSalvo T, Hosenpud JD, Semigran MJ, Dec GW. Outcomes in recipients of combined heart-kidney transplantation: multiorgan, same-donor transplant

study of the International Society of Heart and Lung Transplantation/United Network for Organ Sharing Scientific Registry. *Transplantation.* 1997;63:861–867.

47. Leeser DB, Jeevanandam V, Furukawa S, et al. Simultaneous heart and kidney transplantation in patients with end-stage heart and renal failure. *Am J Transplant.* 2001;1:89–92.

48. Smith JA, Ribakove GH, Hunt SA, et al. Heart retransplantation: 25-year experience at a single institution. *J Heart Lung Transplant.* 1995;14:832–839.

49. Blanche C, Valenza M, Czer LS, et al. Combined heart and kidney transplantation with allografts from the same donor. *Ann Thorac Surg.* 1994;58:1135–1138.

50. Savdie E, Keogh AM, Macdonald PS, et al. Simultaneous transplantation of the heart and kidney. *Aust N Z J Med.* 1994;24:554–560.

51. Mistry BM, Memon MA, Jepson B, et al. Combined cardio-renal transplantation (CCRT) from the same donor: report of two cases and review of the literature. *Ann R Surg Engl.* 2001;83:339–342.

52. Bruschi G, Busnach G, Colombo T, et al. Long-term follow-up of simultaneous heart and kidney transplantation with single donor allografts: report of nine cases. *Ann Thorac Surg.* 2007; 84:522–527.

53. Hermsen JL, Nath DS, del Rio AM, et al. Combined heart-kidney transplantation: the University of Wisconsin experience. *J Heart Lung Transplant.* 2007;26:1119–1126.

54. Jeyarajah DR, McBride M, Klintmalm GB, Gonwa TA. Combined liver-kidney transplantation: what are the indications? *Transplantation.* 1997; 64:1091–1096.

55. Trachiotis GD, Vega JD, Johnston TS, et al. Ten-year follow-up in patients with combined heart and kidney transplantation. *J Thorac Cardiovasc Surg.* 2003;126:2065–2071.

56. Wang SS, Chou NK, Chi NH, et al. Simultaneous heart and kidney transplantation for combined cardiac and renal failure. *Transplant Proc.* 2006;38:2135–2137.

57. Lubitz SA, Pinney S, Wisnivesky JP, Gass A, Baran DA. Statin therapy associated with a reduced risk of chronic renal failure after cardiac transplantation. *J Heart Lung Transplant.* 2007;26:264–272.

Mechanical Circulatory Support and Cardiorenal Syndrome

15

Brian E. Jaski
Mrunalini A. Joshi

In patients with heart failure (HF), impaired renal function is independently associated with heightened risks for death, cardiovascular death, and hospitalization.[1,2] When HF leads to hospital admission, associated renal dysfunction predicts subsequent mechanical ventilation, cardiopulmonary resuscitation, and mortality.[3,4] When renal dysfunction deteriorates despite hospital admission, patient consequences are even further compromised.[5,6] Thus, in these individuals, application of advanced therapies, including mechanical circulatory support, may be necessary to abrogate these dismal outcomes.

General Considerations

Initiation of mechanical support should be considered when patients with progressive impairment in circulatory function do not achieve adequate compensation despite appropriate pharmacologic, percutaneous, electrical, and surgical therapies. There is a growing list of devices and surgical interventions to consider. Nuances of these therapies can be complex, requiring multidisciplinary teams and an assessment of the appropriate timing of initiation.

If the rate of patient deterioration is rapid—over minutes to days—augmentation of cardiac pump function for acute HF may be initiated by percutaneous devices designed to temporarily reverse progressive cardiogenic shock (intra-aortic balloon pump, transseptal or transaortic valvular left ventricular assist devices, or extracorporeal cardiopulmonary bypass; Table 15.1). In these situations, including acute myocardial

The Cardiorenal Syndrome: A Clinician's Guide to Pathophysiology and Management, 1st ed. © 2012 J. Thomas Heywood and John C. Burnett Jr., eds. Cardiotext Publishing, ISBN: 978-0-9790164-7-9.

Table 15.1: Devices Approved
for Temporary Mechanical Circulatory Support

Device	Brief Description	Degree of Circulatory Support	Cost
Intra-aortic balloon pump	Counterpulsation in the descending thoracic and abdominal aorta	+	$
Impella 2.5 (Abiomed, Danvers, MA)	Continuous flow from the left ventricle to the ascending aorta with an axial pump placed across the aortic valve	++	$$$
TandemHeart (CardiacAssist, Inc., Pittsburgh, PA)	Continuous flow from the left atria to iliac artery with external centrifugal pump	+++	$$$
Cardiopulmonary support	Continuous flow from central systemic veins/right artery to iliac artery with external centrifugal pump and oxygenator	+++	$$

infarction or fulminant myocarditis, etiologies of acute HF are potentially reversible.[7-9] If marked cardiac dysfunction persists despite temporary support, long-term mechanical support and/or cardiac transplant versus withdrawal of support and palliative care become important options. Although surgical implantation of a left ventricular assist device (LVAD) is the most common mechanical support for chronic HF intervention,[10] biventricular or total artificial heart support may be required.[11,12]

Whereas the presence of acute decompensated heart failure (ADHF) is often apparent, the gradual progression of chronic HF from American College of Cardiology (ACC)/American Heart Association (AHA) stage C to stage D[13] may be more subtle. This progression may require regular reassessment of patient clinical parameters, including renal function to gauge when mechanical support is indicated,[14] but before a patient has be-

come too sick to benefit. In this regard, the decision for therapy may overlap and parallel that for evaluation for cardiac transplant.

Similar to cardiac transplant, multidisciplinary teams are required with close collaboration between cardiologists, cardiac surgeons, and other clinicians. Postoperative adverse outcomes are associated with the severity of preoperative noncardiac end-organ dysfunction.[15,16] Both interventions are resource and time intensive and commit a patient to lifelong association with a specialized center. Many institutions with expertise in mechanical support are also centers of cardiac transplant.

Conversely, there are important differences between mechanical support and cardiac transplant. Evaluation of valvular (aortic, mitral, and tricuspid) and right ventricular (RV) function is important prior to placement of a LV assist device. Mechanical support does not consume a limited community resource of a donor organ. Immunosuppression is not needed. Compared to successful cardiac transplant, maximum exercise capacity is less[17,18] and patient daily concerns are greater (battery exchange/recharge, driveline maintenance).

In an individual patient, circulatory support should be identified as a bridge (to transplant, myocardial recovery, or decision after resuscitation) versus a definitive destination therapy. For example, if a patient with myocardial infarction and cardiorenal syndrome experiences a cardiac arrest that requires a prolonged resuscitation, percutaneous mechanical support could precede a potential need for an LVAD until neurologic status is determined to be adequate for recovery. If an LVAD is subsequently placed, candidacy for heart transplant could be considered versus discharge and long-term maintenance on LVAD support alone.

In general, a clinician should perform a thorough inventory of patients' risks of continued HF therapy compared to their reserve to tolerate surgery. Long-term prognosis of HF should be assessed based on symptoms, clinical events, physical exam, and laboratory and hemodynamic data, including exercise testing with oxygen consumption measurements.[19] Risk factors for LVAD placement include hemodynamic, hematologic, hepatorenal, nutritional, and neuropsychiatric function.[16] Patient priorities as related to quality of life and survival as well as the strength of family or other personal support should be considered.

Pulsatile Left Ventricular Assist Devices

In the 1960s, investigators and clinicians recognized the potential need for sustained circulatory support when patients developed postcardiotomy cardiogenic shock. In 1962,

in an animal model, Dennis et al[20] demonstrated that placement of an LVAD from the left atrium to the systemic arterial system decreased myocardial oxygen consumption while maintaining or increasing systemic perfusion and coronary blood flow. In 1971, DeBakey[21] reported the success of an extracorporeal pneumatic LVAD in postcardiotomy weaning, while Norman et al,[22] in 1978, reported the first clinical use of an implantable LVAD as a "bridge-to-transplantation." The US Food and Drug Administration (FDA) approved the HeartMate implantable pneumatic LVAD (Thoratec Corporation) in 1994, followed by the electrically powered LVAD in 1998 (Figure 15.1), both for supporting patients with end-stage HF as a bridge-to-cardiac transplantation.[23] Nevertheless, from the outset it was hoped that the experience with "bridge-to-transplant" could also serve as a model for "bridge-to-recovery" or as a permanent alternative to cardiac transplant ("destination therapy").

Following implantation, the LVAD acts as a series pump between the left ventricle and ascending aorta. Resting hemodynamics should return to normal. With exercise, parallel flow of blood through the native aortic valve may contribute to systemic circulation. The multicenter Experience with the left Ventricular Assist Device with Exercise (EVADE) trial reported patients achieving a peak oxygen consumption (VO2) of 14.6 mL/kg/min with exercise 1 to 3 months post-LVAD implantation, consistent with LVAD support permitting activities of daily life.[17,24] Dew et al[25] reported improved physical and emotional well-being of patients supported by an LVAD with increases in social function after leaving the hospital.

A variety of abnormalities seen in end-stage HF are reduced or reversed with implantation of an LVAD. Elevated plasma concentrations of several neurohormones, including aldosterone, renin, and norepi-

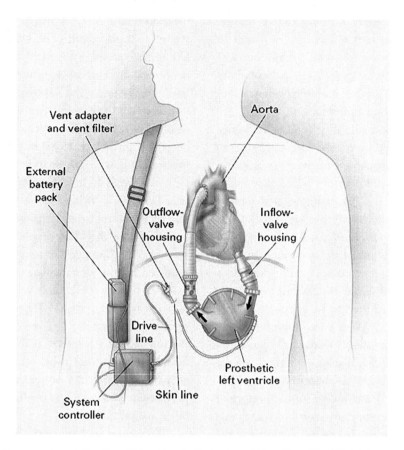

Figure 15.1. Components and direction of blood flow in the implanted HeartMate XVE LVAD. The pulsatile HeartMate XVE LVAD consists of an inflow conduit, inserted into the apex of the left ventricle, with an inflow valve that allows unidirectional flow of blood from the left ventricle into the device and prevents regurgitation during mechanical systole. The outflow conduit is anastomosed to the ascending aorta. A pusher plate forces a flexible diaphragm upward and pressurizes the blood chamber. The prosthetic pumping chamber actively propels blood through the outflow conduit, equipped with an outflow valve, into the ascending aorta, simulating the cyclic systole and diastole function of the heart, generating pulsatile blood flow. The pump is placed within the abdomen. The drive line is connected to a systemic controller and battery pack, worn on a belt or waist pack. A vent tube and filter aids in air exchange with the LVAD, avoiding a vacuum from forming with each ejection cycle. Adapted from Rose EA, Gelijns AC, Moskowitz AJ, et al. Randomized Evaluation of Mechanical Assistance for the Treatment of Congestive Heart Failure (REMATCH) Study Group. Long-term mechanical left ventricular assistance for end-stage heart failure. *N Engl J Med.* 2001;345:1435–1443.With permission from the Massachusetts Medical Society.

nephrine, are reduced by LVAD support.[26] Burnett et al[27] reported improved renal function with LVAD use, which included a decline in BUN and serum creatinine levels, and restoration of normal urine outputs. In addition, LVAD support was shown to normalize hepatic and pulmonary functions in patients with pre–LVAD hepatic dysfunction and mechanical ventilation.

Structural cardiac properties that regress toward normal with an LVAD include decreases in the cardiothoracic ratio, LV end-diastolic dimension and mass, posterior and septal wall thickness, and left atrial dimension.[26,28-33] Levin et al[26] found a leftward shift of the end–diastolic pressure–volume relationship (EDPVR) in hearts explanted in patients after LVAD support compared to medically treated patients, confirming lower volumes for any filling cardiac pressures and documenting the similarity of EDPVRs to those of normal hearts. In some LVAD–supported patients with nonischemic cardiomyopathy, left ventricular ejection fraction improved to > 45% with the LVAD temporarily turned off.[34] Abnormal cardiac cellular properties favorably affected by LVAD use include a 32% reduction in myocyte size, a reduction in the score of myocytolysis from 2.9 to 1.0, and improvement in the contractile properties of isolated myocytes.[29,33,35]

Overall, the long–term use of an intracorporeal pulsatile LVAD has been found to provide circulatory support and improve end-organ perfusion. Beyond these effects, LVAD implantation is associated with reduced neurohormonal activation and mechanical stress on the myocardium, reversal of some structural and geometric abnormalities in the heart, and salutary changes in myocyte size and function. Despite these findings, the clinical rate of myocardial recovery adequate to permit LVAD explant without heart transplant has been low.[36] A preliminary report with use of the novel beta-2 agonist clenbuterol described successful LVAD explant in 11/15 patients with nonischemic cardiomyopathy.[37] Currently, a multicenter trial with use of clenbuterol to promote LVAD bridge-to-recovery is in progress in the United States.

The success with LVAD implantation as a bridge-to-transplant provided a basis for the landmark Randomized Evaluation of Mechanical Assistance for the Treatment of Congestive Heart Failure (REMATCH) trial, which evaluated the pulsatile HeartMate XVE left ventricular assist device as a "destination therapy." One hundred twenty-nine patients with end-stage HF, who were ineligible for cardiac transplantation, received either an LVAD or optimal medical management. The primary end point of survival demonstrated a 48% reduction in the risk of death from any cause in the device group as compared with the medical therapy group, with an absolute reduction in the mortality rate of 27% at 1 year (Figure 15.2). Important limitations of the LVAD include mechanical failure of the device, sepsis, postoperative bleeding, and neurologic complications (Table 15.2). Although the frequency of adverse events in the device group was 2.35 times that in the medical therapy group, there was still a marked improvement in the quality of life at 1 year in the device group. The REMATCH trial led to the FDA approval in 2002 of the HeartMate XVE as an acceptable alternative therapy in selected patients with advanced HF contraindicated for cardiac transplantation.

Despite regulatory approval, clinical adoption of pulsatile LVADs has been modest in part due to their limited long-term mechanical durability. Specifically, pulsatile LVADs may develop tissue valvular failure or ball bearing wear requiring replacement within 2 years.[38] These degenerative modes of failure are usually gradual over days to weeks and replacement is associated with a low operative mortality. Although LVAD late deterioration is less important in a bridge-to-transplant patient, it is a major limitation in a destination therapy application.

Continuous Axial Flow Left Ventricular Assist Devices

The desire to improve long-term mechanical reliability and reduce device size spurred efforts to develop a continuous axial flow, rotary-pump intracorporeal LVAD.[39] Although trials with multiple axial flow devices are

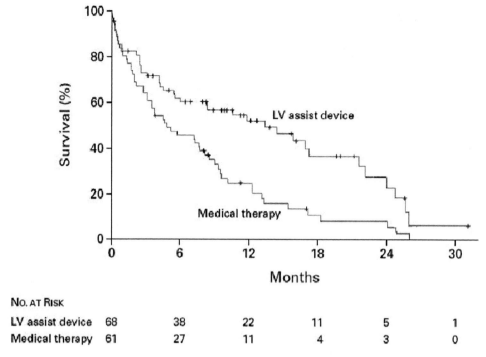

Figure 15.2. Kaplan-Meier analysis of survival, comparing the group of patients who received LVAD vs those who received optimal medical therapy. Survival rates in patients implanted with the HeartMate XVE LVAD were significantly improved compared with the medical therapy group (relative risk, 0.52; 95% CI, 0.34–0.78; $P = 0.001$). The survival at 1 year was 52% in the device group and 25% in the medical therapy group ($P = 0.002$) and at 2 years was 23% and 8%, respectively ($P = 0.09$). The median survival was 408 days in the device group and 150 days in the medical therapy group. Adapted from Rose EA, Gelijns AC, Moskowitz AJ, et al. Randomized Evaluation of Mechanical Assistance for the Treatment of Congestive Heart Failure (REMATCH) Study Group. Long-term mechanical left ventricular assistance for end-stage heart failure. *N Engl J Med.* 2001;345:1435–1443. With permission from the Massachusetts Medical Society.

in progress, the largest experience has been with the HeartMate II device (Figure 15.3, Thoratec Corporation). This new–generation LVAD is one-seventh the size and one-fourth the weight of the previous HeartMate XVE.[40] The first human implant occurred in July 2000. Although pump rotational speeds are constant, some pulsatile arterial pressure and flow is usually present via the contribution of native LV function through the pump and possibly the native aortic valve.

In a sheep model of long-term continuous flow circulatory support,[41] no functional or morphologic changes in major end organs were found. Radovancevic and coworkers[42] studied the effects of continuous flow pumps on end-organ perfusion in HF patients with prolonged circulatory support and similarly concluded that LVAD implantation was associated with adequate renal and hepatic perfusion comparable to that provided by pulsatile support up to 15 months after implant. BUN, creatinine, and creatinine clearance either improved or stayed within normal range at 6, 9, 12, and 15 months postoperatively.

Miller et al[39] reported outcomes with the HeartMate II LVAD in bridge-to-transplant patients. The results from this prospective multicenter study in 133 patients

Table 15.2: Causes of Death:
LVAD vs Optimal Medical Management

Cause of Death	Medical Therapy Group*	LVAD Group*	Total*
LV dysfunction	50	1	51
Sepsis	1	17	18
Failure of LVAD	0	7	7
Miscellaneous Noncardiovascular Causes			
Cerebrovascular disease	0	4	4
Miscellaneous cardiovascular causes	1	2	3
Pulmonary embolism	0	2	2
Acute myocardial infarction	1	0	1
Cardiac procedure	1	0	1
Perioperative bleeding	0	1	1
Unknown	0	2	2
Total	**54**	**41**	**95**

* Number of patients

Adapted from Rose EA, Gelijns AC, Moskowitz AJ, et al. Randomized Evaluation of Mechanical Assistance for the Treatment of Congestive Heart Failure (REMATCH) Study Group. Long-term mechanical left ventricular assistance for end-stage heart failure. *N Engl J Med*. 2001;345:1435–1443. With permission from the Massachusetts Medical Society.

showed that the overall rate of survival to transplantation, cardiac recovery, or ongoing support with no pump replacement in patients implanted with the continuous flow device was 75% at 6 months (Figure 15.4). Actuarial survival for patients was 89% at 1 month, 75% at 6 months, and 68% at 12 months post–LVAD implantation. Reductions in both serum creatinine (from 1.4 ± 0.5 to 1.1 ± 0.5 mg/dL, $P < 0.001$) and BUN (30.3 ± 16.9 to 18.6 ± 9.8 mg/dL, $P < 0.001$) from baseline to 3 months post–LVAD implantation were noted. Mechanical circulatory support was also associated with significant improvements in functional status (assessed with a 6-minute walk test and NYHA functional class) and quality of life (measured by the Minnesota Living with Heart Failure and Kansas City Cardiomyopathy questionnaires). Compared to historical rates of risk with the HeartMate XVE, patients receiving the HeartMate II had lower risks of bleeding

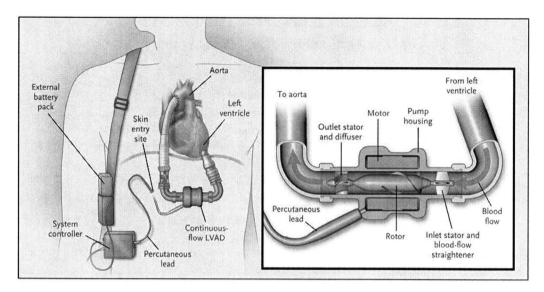

Figure 15.3. Implanted, continuous axial flow LVAD; inset shows the components and direction of blood flow in the LVAD. The continuous axial flow HeartMate II LVAD consists of an inflow conduit surgically attached to the LV apex and an outflow conduit anastomosed to the ascending aorta. Oxygenated blood from the lungs passes through the left ventricle, is continuously drawn from the ventricular apex into the internal axial flow blood pump, through the inflow conduit. It is then pumped into the ascending aorta, by the spinning of the rotor, via the outflow conduit, where it enters the systemic circulation. The pump is typically placed within the anterior abdominal wall. The percutaneous lead, via an electrical cable, connects the pump to an external systemic controller and battery packs, worn on a belt or waist pack. Miller LW, Pagani FD, Russell SD, et al. HeartMate II Clinical Investigators. Use of a continuous-flow device in patients awaiting heart transplantation. *N Engl J Med.* 2007;357:885–896. With permission from the Massachusetts Medical Society.

Figure 15.4. Outcomes over time for patients implanted with the continuous flow LVAD. Patient rate of survival at the time of pump support was 75% at 6 months and 68% at 12 months and the median duration of LVAD support was 126 days

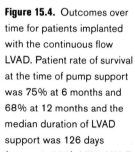
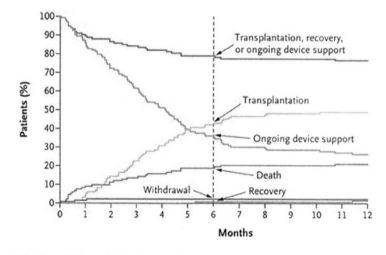

(range, 1–600). Miller LW, Pagani FD, Russell SD, et al. HeartMate II Clinical Investigators. Use of a continuous-flow device in patients awaiting heart transplantation. *N Engl J Med.* 2007;357:885–896. With permission from the Massachusetts Medical Society.

requiring reexploration (0.78 vs 1.47 events per patient year), RV failure requiring a RV assist device (0.08 vs 0.30), drive-line infection (0.37 vs 3.49), stroke (0.19 vs 0.44), and nonstroke neurologic events (0.26 vs 0.67).

The extension of continuous flow devices from bridge-to-transplant to destination therapy patients is appealing due to their estimated durability of ≥ 5 years.[10] An NIH-sponsored destination therapy trial with 2:1 randomization of the continuous follow HeartMate II to the pulsatile XVE was recently terminated due to an interim analysis finding superiority of the continuous flow device.[45] The longer duration of implants achieved with the continuous flow device, however, still has posed challenges. In particular, although the size of driveline penetration of the skin is smaller, there is a persistent potential for driveline or device pocket infections that may require recurrent intravenous or chronic oral suppression antibiotics.

Whereas the pulsatile HeartMate XVE has an internal textured surface that promotes formation of a pseudoneointima that may resist thrombosis,[44] this does not exist in the continuous axial flow HeartMate II pump. To offset a risk of device thrombosis formation and either *in situ* pump obstruction or embolic clinical events, at present, patients receiving the HeartMate II are recommended to receive both warfarin and aspirin orally, indefinitely. In practice, bleeding, especially from a gastrointestinal source, is a more common clinical problem than thrombosis in patients on and off anticoagulation. Similar to increased gastrointestinal bleeding from aortic valve malformations with high shear stress in native aortic valve stenosis,[45] this may be related to an acquired form of von Willebrand's disease due to a high pump-associated shear stress that can increase proteolysis of von Willebrand factor (vWF) multimers.[46] Thus, decreased activ-

ity of vWF may affect the ability to induce platelet aggregation and unmask subclinical sources of bleeding. When clinically significant bleeding is manifest, it is common to discontinue oral anticoagulation in Heart-Mate II patients; however, this is at an uncertain risk of subsequent thromboembolic events.

Patient Profiles and Suggested Clinical Criteria

Although augmentations in technical device design have contributed greatly to the success of mechanical circulatory support device therapy with substantial improvements in patient outcomes, the importance of patient selection and patient management, along with assessing the appropriate time frame for intervention, is a key factor in predicting prolonged patient survival and improvement in quality of life. Table 15.3 includes suggested criteria for LVAD placement in patients who are candidates for bridge-to-transplant or destination therapies.

On behalf of the INTERMACS registry, Kirklin and coworkers[47] proposed a classification of different patient subtypes who could potentially benefit from mechanical circulatory support device implantation, in general, and LVAD in many cases, in particular (Table 15.4). Seven profiles have been defined for patients "failing" conventional therapies.

Profile 1 includes patients with life-threatening hypotension, critical organ hypoperfusion, altering the normal functioning of the liver and kidney, despite rapidly escalating doses of inotropic therapy. Definitive intervention with a temporary circulatory support (IABP, Impella, Tandem Heart, CPS) may be required within hours. In the absence of a reversible etiology, this patient profile may be bridged to a long-term

Table 15.3: Suggested Criteria for LVAD Placement as Bridge-to-Transplant or Destination Therapies

Inclusion Criteria: LVAD (HeartMate II) Bridge-to-Transplant
- Eligible for transplant
- Body surface area $\geq$ 1.2 m^2
- NYHA class IV heart symptoms
- On inotropic support, if tolerated, with progressive end-organ dysfunction

Inclusion Criteria: LVAD Destination Therapy
- Ineligible for cardiac transplant
- Patients with advanced and unacceptable heart failure symptoms (class IIIB or class IV) despite maximum medical and pacemaker/defibrillation therapy
- LVEF < 25%
- Peak VO2 consumption < 14 mL/kg/min or < 50% of predicted VO2 max with attainment of anaerobic threshold, if not contraindicated due to intravenous inotropes, angina, or physical disability
- Body surface area > 1.2 m^2
- Progressive cardiorenal syndrome without correctable cause, including responsive to intravenous inotropes

Table 15.4: INTERMACS: Profiles for Patient Selection

Profile Descriptions	Time Frame for Intervention/LVAD*
1: Critical cardiogenic shock—*crash and burn*	Within hours
2: Progressive decline on inotropic support—*sliding on inotropes*	Within few days
3: Stable but inotrope dependent—*dependent stability*	Over a period of days to weeks
4: Resting symptoms—recurrent advanced HF	Over a period of weeks to few months
5: Exertion intolerant	Variable
6: Exertion limited—*walking wounded*	Variable
7: Advanced NYHA class III—patients, clinically stable and indulging in meaningful activity, limited to mild physical exertion with a history of decompensation	Not currently indicated

*May not require an LVAD if other interventions could lead to reversal of clinical profiles: for example, revascularization, temporary percutaneous support device; presence of life-threatening ventricular arrhythmias may accelerate the time frame for intervention.

Adapted from Kirklin JK, Naftel DC, Stevenson LW, et al. INTERMACS profiles of advanced heart failure: The current picture. *J Heart Lung Transplant.* 2009;28:535–541. With permission from Elsevier.

mechanical support with an LVAD or cardiac transplantation once hemodynamic stability and critical organ perfusion is achieved.

Profile 2 describes patients with progressive impairment in function (renal, nutritional, and circulatory) despite ongoing intravenous inotropic support as well as those intolerant to inotropic infusions. Diuretic resistance, consistently inadequate tissue perfusion resulting in refractory volume overload, or ischemia may contribute to ventricular arrhythmias. This profile may need definitive therapy within a few days of declining patient status. Worsening renal function as determined by a decline in creatinine clearance, and chronic volume overload may necessitate initiation of ultrafiltration or dialysis (Figure 15.5).

Profile 3 describes patient status to be "clinically stable" with IV inotropic infusions (at home) and/or a temporary circulatory

support device (in hospital) but with manifest repeated inability to wean from support due to critical noncardiac end-organ dysfunction or symptomatic hypotension.

Profile 4 patients have circulatory congestion at rest or during activities of daily living. Inotropic support at home may provide relief from resting symptoms but frequent rehospitalizations may require escalation of therapy. Profiles 1 through 4 are most likely to demonstrate features of cardiorenal syndrome—deteriorating renal function in the presence of HF.

Conclusion

Although the first LVAD in humans was placed over 40 years ago, mechanical circulatory support devices are still in a very active phase of clinical and technical devel-

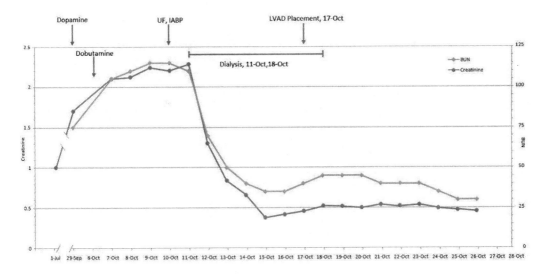

Figure 15.5. Renal function in individual before and following LVAD placement. Changes in creatinine and BUN are shown vs time in a 58-year-old female with nonischemic cardiomyopathy and progressive cardiorenal syndrome who had normal baseline renal function. Despite intravenous inotropes and percutaneous mechanical support, dialysis was required prior to and temporarily following LVAD placement.

IABP = intra-aortic balloon pump; LVAD = left ventricular assist device; UF = ultrafiltration

opment. In the case of LVADs, considerations of right HF, thrombosis versus bleeding, and infection persist. An optimal support device would be completely implanted without driveline or power line penetration of the skin barrier. Limited wearable battery life, although not life threatening, still affects patient quality of life. Of note, the current clinical evidence is almost entirely in patients with systolic dysfunction and not in those with HF and preserved systolic function.

In the future, advances in adjunct antithrombotic pharmacology, biocompatible pump surfaces, techniques for complete pump implantation, and battery life will all contribute to better patient outcomes. It is likely that application of mechanical support devices for bridge-to-recovery indications will increase as definitive stem cell, gene, and associated pharmacologic therapies permit regeneration of native myocardial function. Finally, it is anticipated that a spectrum of devices will evolve with increased durability, performance, and safety, as well as reduced size and cost.

References

1. Hillege HL, Nitsch D, Pfeffer MA, et al; Candesartan in Heart Failure: Assessment of Reduction in Mortality and Morbidity (CHARM) Investigators. Renal function as a predictor of outcome in a broad spectrum of patients with heart failure. *Circulation*. 2006;113: 671–678.

2. Heywood JT, Elatre W, Pai RG, Fabbri S, Huiskes B. Simple clinical criteria to determine the prognosis of heart failure. *J Cardiovasc Pharmacol Ther*. 2005;10:173–180.

3. Fonarow GC, Adams KF Jr, Abraham WT, Yancy CW, Boscardin WJ. Risk stratification for in-hospital mortality in acutely decompensated heart failure: classification and regression tree analysis. *JAMA*. 2005;293:572–580.

4. Heywood JT, Fonarow GC, Costanzo MR, Mathur VS, Wigneswaran JR, Wynne J. High prevalence of renal dysfunction and its impact on outcome in 118,465 patients hospitalized with acute decompensated heart failure: a report from the ADHERE database. *J Card Fail*. 2007;13:422–430.

5. Forman DE, Butler J, Wang Y, et al. Incidence, predictors at admission, and impact of worsening renal function among patients hospitalized with heart failure. *J Am Coll Cardiol*. 2004;43:61–67.

6. Cowie MR, Komajda M, Murray-Thomas T, Underwood J, Ticho B. Prevalence and impact of worsening renal function in patients hospitalized with decompensated heart failure: results of the prospective outcomes study in heart failure (POSH). *Eur Heart J*. 2006;27: 1216–1222.

7. Dembitsky WP, Moore CH, Holman WL, et al. Successful mechanical circulatory support for noncoronary shock. *J Heart Lung Transplant*. 1992;11:129–135.

8. Hochman JS, Sleeper LA, Webb JG, et al. Early revascularization in acute myocardial infarction complicated by cardiogenic shock. SHOCK investigators. Should we emergently revascularize occluded coronaries for cardiogenic shock? *N Engl J Med*. 1999;341:625–634.

9. Thiele H, Sick P, Boudriot E, et al. Randomized comparison of intra-aortic balloon support with a percutaneous left ventricular assist device in patients with revascularized acute myocardial infarction complicated by cardiogenic shock. *Eur Heart J*. 2005;26:1276–1283.

10. Baughman KL, Jarcho JA. Bridge to life: cardiac mechanical support. *N Engl J Med*. 2007;357:846–849.

11. Copeland JG, Smith RG, Arabia FA, et al; CardioWest Total Artificial Heart Investigators. Cardiac replacement with

a total artificial heart as a bridge to transplantation. *N Engl J Med.* 2004;351: 859-867.

12. Holman WL, Kormos RL, Naftel DC, et al. Predictors of death and transplant in patients with a mechanical circulatory support device: a multi-institutional study. *J Heart Lung Transplant.* 2009;28:44-50.

13. Hunt SA, Abraham WT, Chin MH, et al; American College of Cardiology; American Heart Association Task Force on Practice Guidelines; American College of Chest Physicians; International Society for Heart and Lung Transplantation; Heart Rhythm Society. ACC/AHA 2005 Guideline Update for the Diagnosis and Management of Chronic Heart Failure in the Adult: A report of the American College of Cardiology/American Heart Association Task Force on Practice Guidelines (Writing Committee to Update the 2001 Guidelines for the Evaluation and Management of Heart Failure): developed in collaboration with the American College of Chest Physicians and the International Society for Heart and Lung Transplantation: Endorsed by the Heart Rhythm Society. *Circulation.* 2005;112:e154-e235.

14. Rose EA, Gelijns AC, Moskowitz AJ, et al; Randomized Evaluation of Mechanical Assistance for the Treatment of Congestive Heart Failure (REMATCH) Study Group. Long-term mechanical left ventricular assistance for end-stage heart failure. *N Engl J Med.* 2001;345: 1435-1443.

15. Boucek MM, Aurora P, Edwards LB, et al. Registry of the International Society for Heart and Lung Transplantation: twenty-fourth official adult heart transplant report—2007. *J Heart Lung Transplant.* 2007;26:769-781.

16. Lietz K, Long JW, Kfoury AG, et al. Outcomes of left ventricular assist device implantation as destination therapy in the post-REMATCH era: implications for patient selection. *Circulation.* 2007;116:497-505.

17. Jaski BE, Lingle RJ, Kim J, et al. Comparison of functional capacity in patients with end-stage heart failure following implantation of a left ventricular assist device versus heart transplantation: results of the experience with left ventricular assist device with exercise trial. *J Heart Lung Transplant.* 1999;18:1031-1040.

18. Haft J, Armstrong W, Dyke DB, et al. Hemodynamic and exercise performance with pulsatile and continuous-flow left ventricular assist devices. *Circulation.* 2007;116(11 suppl):I8-15.

19. Mancini D, LeJemtel T, Aaronson K. Peak VO(2): a simple yet enduring standard. *Circulation.* 2000;101:1080-1082.

20. Dennis C, Hall DP, Moreno JR, Senning A. Reduction of the oxygen utilization of the heart by left heart bypass. *Circ Res.* 1962;10:298-305.

21. DeBakey ME. Left ventricular bypass pump for cardiac assistance. Clinical experience. *Am J Cardiol.* 1971;27:3-11.

22. Norman JC, Brook MI, Cooley DA, et al. Total support of the circulation of a patient with post-cardiotomy stone-heart syndrome by a partial artificial heart (ALVAD) for 5 days followed by heart and kidney transplantation. *Lancet.* 1978;1:1125-1127.

23. Helman DN, Rose EA. History of mechanical circulatory support. *Prog Cardiovasc Dis.* 2000;43:1-4.

24. Jaski BE, Kim J, Maly RS, et al. Effects of exercise during long-term support with a left ventricular assist device. Results of the experience with left ventricular

assist device with exercise (EVADE) pilot trial. *Circulation.* 1997;95:2401-2406.

25. Dew MA, Kormos RL, Roth LH, et al. Life quality in the era of bridging to cardiac transplantation. Bridge patients in an outpatient setting. *ASAIO J.* 1993;39: 145-152.

26. Levin HR, Oz MC, Chen JM, Packer M, Rose EA, Burkhoff D. Reversal of chronic ventricular dilation in patients with end-stage cardiomyopathy by prolonged mechanical unloading. *Circulation.* 1995;91:2717-2720.

27. Burnett CM, Duncan JM, Frazier OH, Sweeney MS, Vega JD, Radovancevic B. Improved multiorgan function after prolonged univentricular support. *Ann Thorac Surg.* 1993;55:65-71.

28. Altemose GT, Gritsus V, Jeevanandam V, Goldman B, Margulies KB. Altered myocardial phenotype after mechanical support in human beings with advanced cardiomyopathy. *J Heart Lung Transplant.* 1997;16:765-773.

29. Frazier OH, Benedict CR, Radovancevic B, et al. Improved left ventricular function after chronic left ventricular unloading. *Ann Thorac Surg.* 1996;62: 675-681.

30. Müller J, Wallukat G, Weng YG, et al. Weaning from mechanical cardiac support in patients with idiopathic dilated cardiomyopathy. *Circulation.* 1997;96:542-549.

31. Nakatani S, McCarthy PM, Kottke-Marchant K, et al. Left ventricular echocardiographic and histologic changes: impact of chronic unloading by an implantable ventricular assist device. *J Am Coll Cardiol.* 1996;27: 894-901.

32. Scheinin SA, Capek P, Radovancevic B, Duncan JM, McAllister HA Jr, Frazier OH. The effect of prolonged left ventricular support on myocardial histopathology in patients with end-stage cardiomyopathy. *ASAIO J.* 1992;38:M271-M274.

33. Zafeiridis A, Jeevanandam V, Houser SR, Margulies KB. Regression of cellular hypertrophy after left ventricular assist device support. *Circulation.* 1998;98: 656-662.

34. Loebe M, Hennig E, Muller J, Spiegelsberger S, Weng Y, Hetzer R. Long-term mechanical circulatory support as a bridge to transplantation, for recovery from cardiomyopathy, and for permanent replacement. *Eur J Cardiothorac Surg.* 1997;11 suppl:S18-S24.

35. Dipla K, Mattiello JA, Jeevanandam V, Houser SR, Margulies KB. Myocyte recovery after mechanical circulatory support in humans with end-stage heart failure. *Circulation.* 1998;97: 2316-2322.

36. Mancini DM, Beniaminovitz A, Levin H, et al. Low incidence of myocardial recovery after left ventricular assist device implantation in patients with chronic heart failure. *Circulation.* 1998;98:2383-2389.

37. Birks EJ, Tansley PD, Hardy J, et al. Left ventricular assist device and drug therapy for the reversal of heart failure. *N Engl J Med.* 2006;355:1873-1884.

38. Dembitsky WP, Tector AJ, Park S, et al. Left ventricular assist device performance with long-term circulatory support: lessons from the REMATCH trial. *Ann Thorac Surg.* 2004;78:2123-2129.

39. Miller LW, Pagani FD, Russell SD, et al; HeartMate II Clinical Investigators. Use of a continuous-flow device in patients awaiting heart transplantation. *N Engl J Med.* 2007;357:885-896.

40. John R, Kamdar F, Liao K, Colvin-Adams M, Boyle A, Joyce L. Improved survival and decreasing incidence of adverse events with the HeartMate II

left ventricular assist device as bridge-to-transplant therapy. *Ann Thorac Surg.* 2008;86:1227-1234.

41. Saito S, Westaby S, Piggot D, et al. End-organ function during chronic nonpulsatile circulation. *Ann Thorac Surg.* 2002;74:1080-1085.

42. Radovancevic B, Vrtovec B, de KE, Radovancevic R, Gregoric ID, Frazier OH. End-organ function in patients on long-term circulatory support with continuous- or pulsatile-flow assist devices. *J Heart Lung Transplant.* 2007;26:815-818.

43. Slaughter MS, Rogers JG, Milano CA, et al., HeartMate II Investigators. Advanced heart failure treated with continuous-flow left ventricular assist device. *N Engl J Med.* 2009;361:2241-2251.

44. Dowling RD, Park SJ, Pagani FD, et al. HeartMate VE LVAS design enhancements and its impact on device reliability. *Eur J Cardiothorac Surg.* 2004;25:958-963.

45. Vincentelli A, Susen S, Le Tourneau T, et al. Acquired von Willebrand syndrome in aortic stenosis. *N Engl J Med.* 2003;349:343-349.

46. Klovaite J, Gustafsson F, Mortensen SA, Sander K, Nielsen LB. Severely impaired von Willebrand factor-dependent platelet aggregation in patients with a continuous-flow left ventricular assist device (HeartMate II). *J Am Coll Cardiol.* 2009;53:2162-2167.

47. Kirklin JK, Naftel DC, Stevenson LW, et al. INTERMACS profiles of advanced heart failure: the current picture. *J Heart Lung Transplant.* 2009;28:535-541.

Practical Management of Cardiorenal Syndrome
A Patient-Centered Approach

16

TARIQ A. KHAN

J. THOMAS HEYWOOD

The Acute Decompensated Heart Failure National Registry (ADHERE) study cast a bright spotlight on the effect of renal dysfunction on patients admitted with heart failure (HF). Two of the 3 most important predictors of mortality were markers of renal function blood urea nitrogen (BUN) and creatinine. Coupled with a systolic blood pressure < 115 mm Hg, significant renal dysfunction was associated with a 10-fold increase in mortality compared with those with more normal renal function and blood pressure (2.3% vs 22.5%).[1] These disturbing data can be viewed another way, however; 80% of these high-risk patients survive to hospital discharge. So renal dysfunction in HF is not necessarily a death sentence. It can be managed successfully in most patients.

As can be seen from the preceding chapters there are multiple mechanisms for the development of cardiorenal syndrome (Table 16.1). Therefore, the therapy for cardiorenal syndrome cannot be standardized; it must be individualized to address the unique set of problems for the patient at hand.[2] That said, a systemic approach to discover the particular cardiovascular derangement is mandatory for 2 reasons:

1. In many instances cardiorenal syndrome is reversible if the immediate cause can be identified and addressed.
2. The appearance of cardiorenal syndrome can be a true medical emergency; a precious window of opportunity may be missed and appropriate therapy can become unsuitable if renal dysfunction progresses to multiorgan failure.

What follows is one approach for the patient with cardiorenal syndrome. Once

The Cardiorenal Syndrome: A Clinician's Guide to Pathophysiology and Management, 1st ed. © 2012 J. Thomas Heywood and John C. Burnett Jr., eds. Cardiotext Publishing, ISBN: 978-0-9790164-7-9.

Table 16.1: Potential Causes of Cardiorenal Syndrome

Impaired Renal Perfusion
- Hypovolemia (reduced filling pressures resulting in decreased CO)
- Cardiogenic shock (reduced CO with low systemic blood pressure; usually normal systemic vascular resistance)
- Vasodilatory shock (reduced systemic blood pressure with normal or near normal CO; significant reduction in systemic vascular resistance)
- Reduced CO due to neurohormonal activation and greatly increased afterload; significant increase in systemic vascular resistance
- Reduced renal perfusion due to high central venous pressures
- Renal artery stenosis

Intrinsic Renal Disease
- Longstanding renal dysfunction due to diabetes mellitus, hypertension, etc
- Diuretic resistance

---

the physiologic derangement is understood (when possible), then appropriate therapy can be instituted.

Causes of Cardiorenal Syndrome

Although cardiorenal syndrome is far from completely understood, several key features have been identified.[3] Significant reduction in renal perfusion will impair renal performance and severe HF provides a milieu in which this can occur. The kidney can function adequately across a wide range of car-

diac outputs but when cardiac index falls below 1.5 L/min/m[2] then renal function declines.[4] Several distinct mechanisms can impair cardiac output (CO) in HF including hypovolemia (reduced preload), reduced contractility, or a marked increase in afterload. Renal perfusion is also reduced when central venous pressure is markedly elevated. Firth and colleages[5] demonstrated this elegantly in an animal model in 1988. Central venous pressures > 20 mm Hg resulted in a marked decline in GFR, which was reversed when pressures were reduced. Mullens and colleages[6] also reported that an elevated right atrial pressure was strongly predictive of renal dysfunction in those with advanced HF. Systemic hypotension may also lead to reduced renal function. Again, this can be multifactorial including hypovolemic shock, cardiogenic shock due to a marked reduction in cardiac performance, or vasodilatory shock with relatively preserved CO but inappropriate peripheral vasodilation.[7]

Comorbidities are common in HF patients and may result in intrinsic renal disease independent of, but contributing to, the HF syndrome. In the ADHERE database both diabetes and hypertension were extremely common, 73% and 44%, respectively.[8] In addition over 60% had at least moderate kidney injury as defined by the Modification of Diet in Renal Disease equation.[9] Loss of renal function can result in salt and water retention, which can lead to acute HF decompensation. Therapies that improve CO such as inotropes in patients with primarily renal disease are counterproductive in that the CO is already normal and exposes them to the risks of inotropes such as arrhythmias and myocardial ischemia. Chronic use of diuretics can also result in hypertrophy of the distal tubule cells in the nephron, which may increase reabsorption of salt and water resulting in diuretic resistance, another manifestation of cardiorenal syndrome.[10]

Management of the Patient with Acute Cardiorenal Syndrome

Because of the many potential etiologies of cardiorenal syndrome and potential treatments, which may be diametrically opposed, a systematic approach to the HF patient presenting with worsening renal function (WRF) is critical. To focus this evaluation 5 key questions must be answered about the patient at hand.

1. What is the fluid status of the patient; is hypovolemia present?
2. Is there systemic hypotension (systolic blood pressure < 80 mm Hg)?
3. What is the cardiac output?
4. Is the central venous pressure markedly elevated?
5. Is there a history of, or evidence for, intrinsic renal disease?

Evaluation of volume status and the early recognition of hypovolemia is important because intercurrent gastrointestinal illness and iatrogenic volume depletion are common yet rapidly correctable. A focused history and physical examination that look for postural blood pressure changes, flat neck veins and absence of rales, and a third heart sound should be adequate to identify most cases of hypovolemia. When the fluid status is in doubt, then a limited echocardiogram can often resolve the issue. Vigorous collapse of the inferior vena cava during respiration, a transmitral E wave < the A wave, and an E wave deceleration time > 200 milliseconds strongly suggests low filling pressures in HF with WRF.[11] The recognition of hypovolemia is critical because rapid volume replacement of 500 to 1000 cc of normal saline can improve CO by restoring normal preload, and hence blood pressure and renal

perfusion. Hemodynamic monitoring to determine volume status may be necessary in some circumstances when uncertainty remains (Table 16.2).

Once hypovolemia has been ruled out or corrected, then systolic hypotension should be addressed. Clearly, the lower the systolic blood pressure the more urgently this should be corrected if renal perfusion is to be restored before irreversible damage occurs. In those with less severe hypotension, blood pressure may be restored with dobutamine if there is a history of severe left ventricular (LV) dysfunction. Profound hypotension may require pressor support with norepinephrine and/or epinephrine. The appearance of cardiorenal syndrome coupled with hypotension is a true medical emergency that requires rapid action but also hemodynamic data to address the underlying cardiovascular abnormality. Knowledge of the CO is very useful to tailor therapy to the individual patient. The ESCAPE trial did not show a benefit with hemodynamic monitoring of patients, however, very few patients in the trial had severe renal dysfunction (average creatinine 1.5 mg/dL, BUN 34 mg/dL).[12] Knowing the CO can be important for decision making for several reasons. When the cardiac index is < 1.5 L/min/m^2 then renal function is difficult to maintain. The use of dobutamine or milrinone in this instance can rapidly improve renal function and stabilize the patient. The resolution of renal dysfunction by improving CO with inotropes demonstrates adequate renal reserve and confirms a cardiac basis for cardiorenal syndrome.

The use of dopamine in cardiorenal syndrome has been the subject of much debate. For a long time low–dose dopamine was given to improve renal blood flow.[13] Randomized trials in acute renal dysfunction due to acute tubular necrosis, however, did not show benefit.[14] However, a study by

Table 16.2: Management of Cardiorenal Syndrome

Cause of Cardiorenal Syndrome	Volume Status	Cardiac Output	SVR	Treatments
Hypovolemia	⇊	↓	↓ or normal	Stop diuretic Volume replacement
Excess vasoconstriction	↑ or normal	⇊	⇈	↑ RAS blockade Nitroprusside Nesiritide Nitroglycerin
Cardiogenic shock	↑ or normal	⇊	↑ or normal	Dobutamine Dopamine Norepinephrine LVAD
Excessive vasodilation	↑ or normal	↓ or normal	⇊	Dopamine Norepinephrine Vasopressin LVAD
Diuretic resistance	⇈	↓ or normal	normal	Diuretic combination Ultrafiltration Nesiritide?
Intrinsic renal disease	⇈	normal	normal	Ultrafiltration Hemodialysis Renal transplantation

Elkayam et al[15] clearly demonstrated that dopamine improves renal blood flow markedly in patients with HF although these patients did not have significant renal dysfunction. Therefore, in clinical situations where CO is low and renal blood flow is impaired, dopamine may be a reasonable choice.

Because of the problematic long-term outcomes with inotropes and poor progno-sis associated with renal dysfunction, strong consideration should be given to more definitive therapy such as cardiac transplantation or left ventricular assist device (LVAD) placement. Use of LVADs can restore renal function and is associated with improved prognosis.[16,17]

Knowledge of the CO and calculation of systemic vascular resistance can give further insight into the pathophysiology of cardiorenal syndrome. A small minority may have hypotension without profound reduction of CO; hence, calculated systemic vascular resistance is very low due to peripheral vasodilation, mimicking septic shock. Chatterjee[7] has coined the phrase *pseudosepsis syndrome* to describe this phenomenon in HF patients, often with renal dysfunction. The etiology of the syndrome is unclear but appears to result in renal hypoperfusion from low blood pressure and shunting of blood to the periphery. This syndrome may be seen after bypass surgery in patients with marked LV dysfunction and is often resistant to norepinephrine infusion. Argenziano et al[18] described a beneficial response to vasopressin infusions in such patients with improved blood pressure and reduced requirements for norepinephrine. Because of hypotension and vasodilation, ACE inhibitors (ACEIs), angiotensin receptor blockers (ARBs), or other vasodilators should be discontinued in these patients until they stabilize.

On the other hand, patients may present with cardiorenal syndrome with low normal blood pressure coupled with a very elevated systemic vascular resistance. Although much less common in the era of ACEIs, it can be seen when ACEIs are not used out of concern for renal dysfunction or when an intercurrent gastrointestinal illness results in an abrupt withdrawal of ACE inhibition. Patients present with poor urine output, WRF, and cold extremities. Vasodilators are critical here because of the profound vasoconstriction producing increased afterload and reduced CO. Intravenous vasodilators such as nitroprusside or nesiritide may be employed until the patient can be placed on ACEIs. Some may require short-term inotropic support as vasodilators are added. Cardiac output can more than double in such patients with attendant improvement in renal perfusion and function. This syndrome can also

be seen in rare patients who acutely decompensate during the initiation of beta-blocker therapy.

The role of nesiritide in the management of decompensated HF is controversial. Although it lowers filling pressures and improves symptoms acutely, 2 meta-analyses raised concerns that the drug increased 30-day mortality and was associated with WRF.[19,20] Since the publication by Sachner-Bernstein et al,[20] new data about the drug has appeared. The NAPA trial evaluated nesiritide in 279 patients with LV dysfunction undergoing bypass and valve surgery. Compared to the placebo group those receiving nesiritide developed less renal dysfunction, had reduced length of stay, and had lower mortality.[21] Ritter et al[22] reported that low-dose nesiritide (0.0025–0.005 μg/kg/min) was associated with improved renal function in patients with elevated creatinine compared with the standard dose (0.01 μg/kg/min). The ASCEND trial, which enrolled over 7000 patients, demonstrated that nesiritide did not increase 30-day mortality. In addition, there was no significant change in serum creatinine compared to placebo. Unfortunately, improvement in dyspnea with the drug did not reach the prespecified level of significance, 0.0025.[23]

An important practical consideration is the method used to measure CO. The gold standard remains invasive monitoring with a pulmonary artery catheter. Recent concerns about complications and the publication of the ESCAPE trial have led to a dramatic reduction in its use.[24] This does not mean a pulmonary artery catheter should never be used, and the hemodynamic information it provides can be invaluable in managing critically ill HF patients. In the patient with cardiorenal syndrome a single measurement of CO may be sufficient to determine hemodynamics and guide initial therapy.[25] In this instance a bedside echocardiographic determination of CO can be quicker, less expensive, and noninvasive. The most accurate technique involves pulsed Doppler interrogation of the LV outflow tract (LVOT) and measuring the time velocity integral (TVI)—LVOT TVI cm/sec (Figure 16.1). This number is then multiplied by the outflow tract area just below the aortic valve (cm²) to determine the stroke volume, LVOT TVI x LVOT area = stroke volume (cm³/sec). The stroke volume is then multiplied by the heart rate

to determine CO. In general LVOT TVI < 10 cm/sec suggests severe reduction in CO.

When hypovolemia has been ruled out and adequate renal perfusion ensured with normal blood pressure and CO, then intrinsic renal disease should be considered as the cause of renal dysfunction. Indeed, given the advanced age and frequent comorbidities in the HF population it would be surprising if intrinsic renal disease was not common. A renal etiology of cardiorenal syndrome is

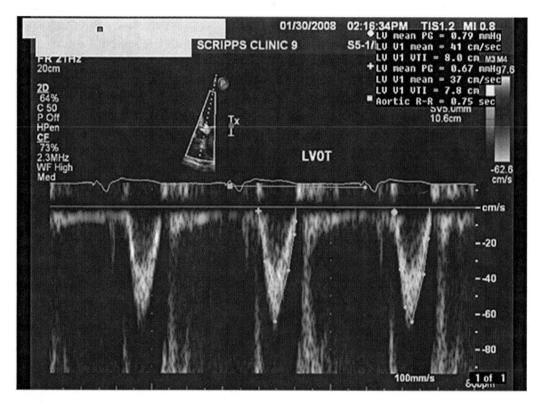

Stroke Volume = LV Time Velocity Integral x LV outflow track Area   = 8 cm/sec x 3.1 cm2 = 24.8 cm3
Cardiac Output = Stroke Volume x Heart Rate = 24.8 cm3 x 80 beat/min = 1984 cm3/min = 1.98 Liters/min

Figure 16.1. Cardiac output can be estimated noninvasively using Doppler echocardiography. In this technique the flow through the LVOT is measured using pulsed Doppler, termed the LV outflow track time velocity integral (LVOT TVI, cm/sec). The area of the LVOT is then measured in the parasternal long axis view (cm²) (not shown). The stroke volume then equals the LVOT TVI multiplied by the outflow track area. The CO is obtained in the standard fashion by multiplying the stroke volume by the heart rate.

more likely when there is evidence for long-standing renal dysfunction. Significant proteinuria (> 1 g/day) also strongly suggests an intrinsic renal disorder.

Once the kidney is identified as the cause of renal dysfunction, this diagnosis has important implications for therapy. Diuretics can and should be used as long as the patient remains volume overloaded, although meticulous care should be taken to avoid overdiuresis and hypotension. In a Cochrane review, continuous infusions of furosemide were shown to increase urine output to a greater extent than intermittent therapy.[26] In the recently completed Diuretic Optimization Strategies Evaluation in Acute Heart Failure (DOSE) trial a strategy of low versus high or continuous versus every 12-hour administration of furosemide was evaluated.[27] In this important study furosemide given at 2.5 times the daily outpatient dose showed a significant reduction in weight loss and more net volume reduction. This was coupled to an increased incidence of a rise of serum creatinine of $\geq$ 0.3 mg/dL at 72 hours (14% vs 23%, $P = 0.041$). However, there was no significant difference in serum creatinine between the high- and low-dose groups at 7 days. In some instances bumetanide or torsemide may be more effective than furosemide and may be tried if urine output is inadequate. Another technique to deal with renal resistance is the addition of a distal tubular diuretic to block sodium reuptake in this area of the nephron. Metolazone or hydrochlorothiazide can be used. However, the response to this therapy is unpredictable and can result in tremendous diuresis and electrolyte abnormalities. Therefore, it is best to use a single dose of these agents and then observe their effect rather than giving them daily. An intravenous-form thiazide (chlorothiazide) is available for those who cannot take oral agents.

When renal dysfunction is profound then the option of dialysis is available as either a temporary or permanent therapy for cardiorenal syndrome. Short of dialysis for patients who do not respond adequately to diuretics, ultrafiltration is an important option (see Chapter 11). The reduction of severely elevated right-sided filling pressures via ultrafiltration may actually improve renal function and should be considered early in the very fluid-overloaded, diuretic-resistant patient.[28] In selected patients renal transplantation should be considered as the ultimate therapy for kidney-centered cardiorenal syndrome (see Chapter 13). Although many HF patients are not appropriate for renal transplant, some do extremely well with transplantation and may even see an improvement in cardiac function following renal transplantation.[29] This is especially true for younger individuals with nonischemic, hypertensive HF with associated renal failure (see Chapter 13).

Preventing Cardiorenal Syndrome

Renal dysfunction upon admission and WRF while in the hospital portend a very poor prognosis with increased length of stay and mortality. Therefore, the prevention of cardiorenal syndrome is a very important goal for the hospitalized patient. While most hospitalized patients are admitted with volume overload, it is very easy to overdiuresis a patient to the point that preload and CO are impaired. Volume status and renal function should be carefully monitored (at least twice a day) so that diuretics, ultrafiltration, and other vasoactive agents can be discontinued once the patient becomes euvolemic. Continuing diuretics or other preload-reducing therapy while the patient is euvolemic is unnecessary for most patients in the hospital and only increases the risk of renal insufficiency. When diuresis is begun at admission the patient is typically quite fluid over-loaded, with a large extracellular volume. As the diuresis proceeds fluid removed by the kidneys comes from the plasma vascular space with its limited volume, which is refilled from the extravascular volume. As plasma refill rate is equal to or greater than the urine output then filling pressures are maintained[30] (Figure 16.2). However, as the extravascular volume is normalized and the patient approaches euvolemia, then the plasma refill rate declines. At this point if diuretics are continued, hypovolemia can develop with its potentially significant negative impact on renal function. Increased monitoring of the patient when edema has resolved and the neck veins are normal, as well as twice daily renal function checks, will allow the clinician to discontinue diuretics before filling pressures decline significantly.

Conclusion

In a sense all HF is a manifestation of cardiorenal syndrome. The cardiovascular system evolved over millions of years to maintain an exquisitely balanced aquatic milieu within land-dwelling creatures in a wide range of water and sodium conditions. Heart failure appears when the system fails, usually because of cardiovascular disease, to regulate this balance. Present therapies can restore this balance in many patients, but not in all, especially when the kidney, a much more complex organ than the heart, is responsible. If the progress made in the latter half of the twentieth century in HF is to be continued, the kidney should be a major focus of research. If renal function could be restored and GFR increased reliably in the future, then care of the sickest HF patients would be greatly improved. Drugs that restore renal function or implanted devices that could even partially replace the kidney's

maintenance of fluid and electrolyte balance would change HF management profoundly and save tens of thousands of lives.

References

1. Fonarow GC, Adams KF Jr, Abraham WT, Yancy CW, Boscardin WJ. Risk stratification for in-hospital mortality in acutely decompensated heart failure: classification and regression tree analysis. *JAMA*. 2005;293:572–580.

2. Heywood JT. The cardiorenal syndrome: lessons from the ADHERE database and treatment options. *Heart Fail Rev*. 2004;9:195–201.

3. Ronco C, Haapio M, House AA, Anavekar N, Bellomo R. Cardiorenal syndrome. *J Am Coll Cardiol*. 2008;52: 1527–1539.

4. Ljungman S, Kjekshus J, Swedberg K. Renal function in severe congestive heart failure during treatment with enalapril (the Cooperative North Scandinavian Enalapril Survival Study [CONSENSUS] trial). *Am J Cardiol*. 1992;70:479–487.

5. Firth JD, Raine AE, Ledingham JG. Raised venous pressure: a direct cause of renal sodium retention in oedema? *Lancet*. 1988;1:1033–1035.

6. Mullens W, Abrahams Z, Skouri HN, et al. Elevated intra-abdominal pressure in acute decompensated heart failure: a potential contributor to worsening renal function? *J Am Coll Cardiol*. 2008;51: 300–306.

7. Chatterjee K. The Swan–Ganz catheters: past, present, and future. A viewpoint. *Circulation*. 2009;119:147–152.

8. Adams KF Jr, Fonarow GC, Emerman CL, et al; ADHERE Scientific Advisory Committee and Investigators. Characteristics and outcomes of patients hospitalized for heart failure

A. Initial Therapy for Heart Failure with Excess Extracellular Fluid and Adequate Plasma Refill Rate

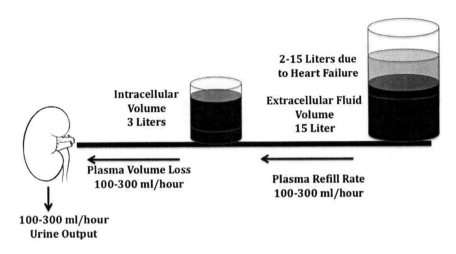

B. Hypovolemia with Continued Diuresis and Inadequate Plasma Refill Rate

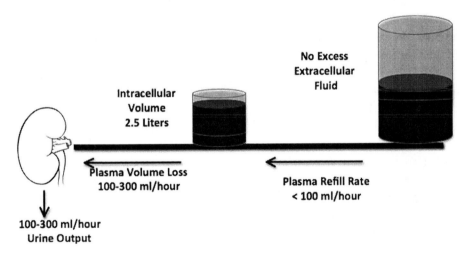

Figure 16.2. (a) In the fluid overloaded state of ADHF extracellular volume is increased, often by many liters. Volume removal either by diuretics or ultrafiltration removes fluid from the plasma compartment. This compartment is refilled from the extracellular fluid. The rate of fluid movement into the plasma compartment is called the plasma refill rate (PRR). As long as the PRR equals or exceeds the rate of fluid removal, preload is maintained and CO and blood pressure are preserved. (b) As fluid removal continues the excess volume in the extracellular space normalizes and the PRR declines. If fluid removal continues and exceeds the PRR then plasma volume is reduced, often precipitously with attendant reduction in blood pressure and CO. Cardiorenal syndrome can thus be precipitated by continued diuresis in the patient who has become euvolemic.

in the United States: rationale, design, and preliminary observations from the first 100,000 cases in the Acute Decompensated Heart Failure National Registry (ADHERE). *Am Heart J.* 2005;149:209-216.

9. Heywood JT, Fonarow GC, Costanzo MR, Mathur VS, Wigneswaran JR, Wynne J. High prevalence of renal dysfunction and its impact on outcome in 118,465 patients hospitalized with acute decompensated heart failure: a report from the ADHERE database. *J Card Fail.* 2007;13:422-430.

10. Kaissling B, Stanton BA. Adaptation of distal tubule and collecting duct to increased sodium delivery. I. Ultrastructure. *Am J Physiol.* 1988;255:F1256-F1268.

11. Nagdev AN, Merchant RC, Tirado-Gonzalez A, Sisson CA, Murphy MC. Emergency department bedside ultrasonographic measurement of the caval index for noninvasive determination of low central venous pressure. *Ann Emerg Med.* 2010;55: 290-295.

12. Shah MR, O'Connor CM, Sopko G, Hasselblad V, Califf RM, Stevenson LW. Evaluation Study of Congestive Heart Failure and Pulmonary Artery Catheterization Effectiveness (ESCAPE): design and rationale. *Am Heart J.* 2001;141:528-535.

13. Szerlip HM. Renal dose dopamine: fact and fiction. *Ann Intern Med.* 1991; 115:153-154.

14. Bellomo R, Chapman M, Finfer S, Hickling K, Myburgh J. Low-dose dopamine in patients with early renal dysfunction: a placebo-controlled randomised trial. Australian and New Zealand Intensive Care Society (ANZICS) clinical trials croup. *Lancet.* 2000;356:2139-2143.

15. Elkayam U, Ng TM, Hatamizadeh P, Janmohamed M, Mehra A. Renal vasodilatory action of dopamine in patients with heart failure: magnitude of effect and site of action. *Circulation.* 2008;117:200-205.

16. Khot UN, Mishra M, Yamani MH, et al. Severe renal dysfunction complicating cardiogenic shock is not a contraindication to mechanical support as a bridge to cardiac transplantation. *J Am Coll Cardiol.* 2003;41:381-385.

17. Stevenson LW, Miller LW, Desvigne-Nickens P, et al; REMATCH Investigators. Left ventricular assist device as destination for patients undergoing intravenous inotropic therapy: a subset analysis from REMATCH (Randomized Evaluation of Mechanical Assistance in Treatment of Chronic Heart Failure). *Circulation.* 2004;110:975-981.

18. Argenziano M, Choudhri AF, Oz MC, Rose EA, Smith CR, Landry DW. A prospective randomized trial of arginine vasopressin in the treatment of vasodilatory shock after left ventricular assist device placement. *Circulation.* 1997;96:II-286-290.

19. Sackner-Bernstein JD, Skopicki HA, Aaronson KD. Risk of worsening renal function with nesiritide in patients with acutely decompensated heart failure. *Circulation.* 2005;111:1487-1491.

20. Sackner-Bernstein JD, Kowalski M, Fox M, Aaronson K. Short-term risk of death after treatment with nesiritide for decompensated heart failure: a pooled analysis of randomized controlled trials. *JAMA.* 2005;293:1900-1905.

21. Mentzer RM Jr, Oz MC, Sladen RN, et al; NAPA Investigators. Effects of perioperative nesiritide in patients with left ventricular dysfunction undergoing cardiac surgery: the NAPA trial. *J Am Coll Cardiol.* 2007;49:716-726.

22. Ritter HG, Redfield MM, Burnett JC, Chen HH. Nonhypotensive low-dose nesiritide has differential renal effects compared with standard-dose nesiritide in patients with acute decompensated heart failure and renal dysfunction. *J Am Coll Cardiol.* 2006;47(11):2334–2335.

23. O'Connor CM, Starling RC, Hernandez AF, et al. Effect of nesiritide in patients with acute decompensated heart failure. *N Engl J Med.* 2011;365:32–43.

24. Binanay C, Califf RM, Hasselblad V, et al; ESCAPE Investigators and ESCAPE Study Coordinators. Evaluation study of congestive heart failure and pulmonary artery catheterization effectiveness: the ESCAPE trial. *JAMA.* 2004;294:1625–1633.

25. Northridge DB, Findlay IN, Wilson J, Henderson E, Dargie HJ. Non-invasive determination of cardiac output by Doppler echocardiography and electrical bioimpedance. *Br Heart J.* 1990;63:93–97.

26. Salvador DR, Rey NR, Ramos GC, Punzalan FE. Continuous infusion versus bolus injection of loop diuretics in congestive heart failure. *Cochrane Database Syst Rev.* 2004;(1):CD003178.

27. O'Connor C, Felker GM. Study explores furosemide dosing options in patients with acute heart failure. No clear winner, but high-dose furosemide may be better for fluid overload. American College of Cardiology, ACC.10, 59th Annual Scientific Session, March 16, 2010. http://www.acc.org/media/acc _scientific_session_2010/press/tuesday /ACC10_Felker-OConnor8am.pdf. Accessed on April 17, 2010.

28. Mullens W, Abrahams Z, Francis GS, Taylor DO, Starling RC, Tang WH. Prompt reduction in intra-abdominal pressure following large-volume mechanical fluid removal improves renal insufficiency in refractory decompensated heart failure. *J Card Fail.* 2008;14:508–514.

29. Wali RK, Wang GS, Gottlieb SS, et al. Effect of kidney transplantation on left ventricular systolic dysfunction and congestive heart failure in patients with end-stage renal disease. *J Am Coll Cardiol.* 2005;45:1051–1060.

30. Boyle A, Sobotka PA. Redefining the therapeutic objective in decompensated heart failure: hemoconcentration as a surrogate for plasma refill rate. *J Card Fail.* 2006;12:247–249.

Index

CPSIA information can be obtained at www.ICGtesting.com
Printed in the USA
BVOW051850260312

285982BV00003B/2/P